Handbook of
Surgery

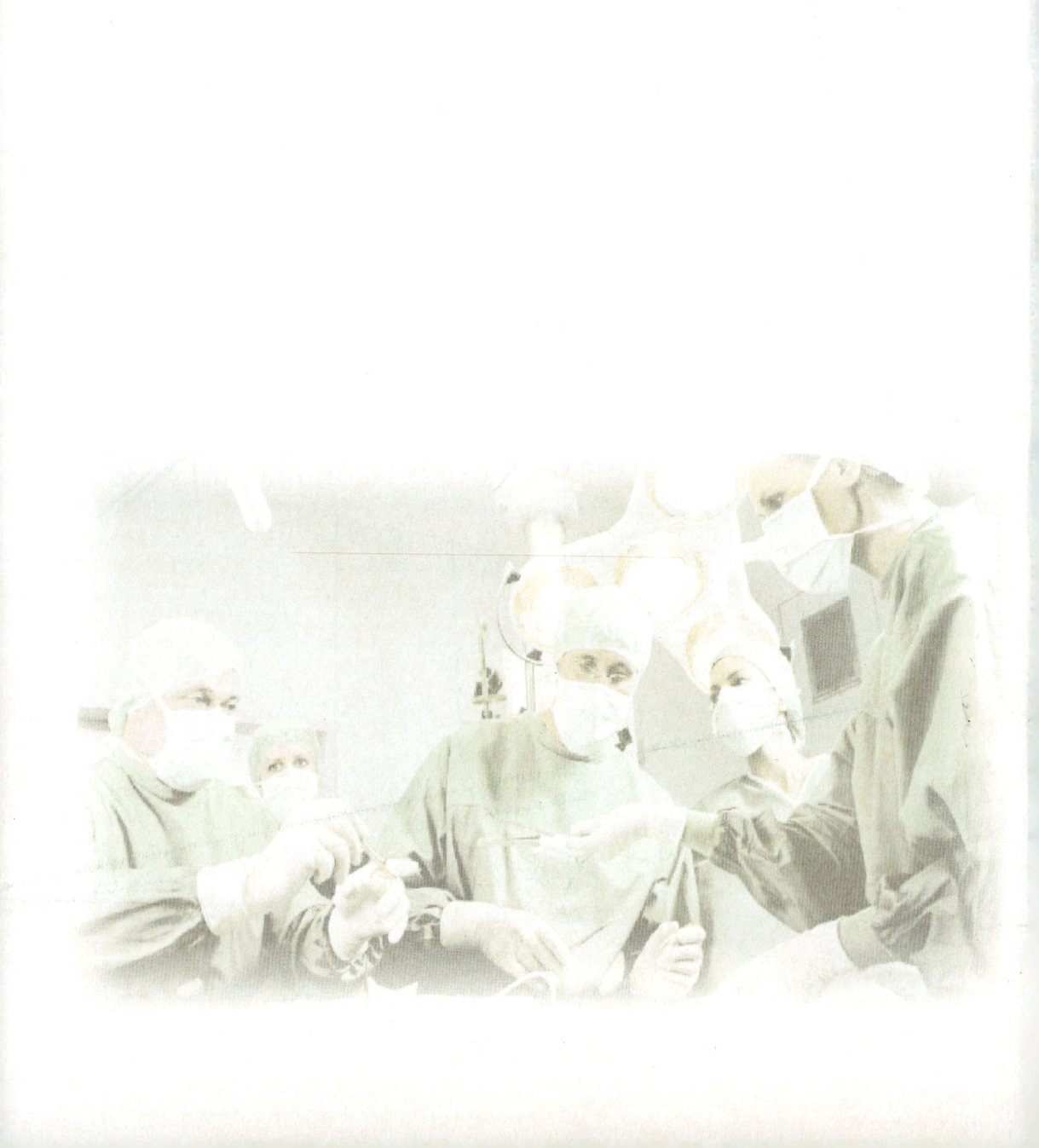

Handbook of
Surgery

Sudhir Kumar Jain MS FRCS FICS FACS

Professor of Surgery
Maulana Azad Medical College
New Delhi

Vivek Manchanda MS MCh

Assistant Professor of Pediatric Surgery
Chacha Nehru Bal Chikitsalaya
Delhi

Raman Tanwar MS FMAS

MCh Urology Registrar
Department of Urology
PGIMER and Dr RML Hospital
New Delhi

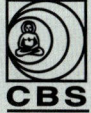

CBS Publishers & Distributors Pvt Ltd

New Delhi • Bengaluru • Chennai • Kochi • Kolkata • Mumbai
Hyderabad • Jharkhand • Nagpur • Patna • Pune • Uttarakhand

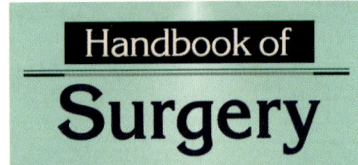

ISBN: 978-81-239-2422-9

Copyright © Authors and Publishers

First Edition: 2014
  Reprint: 2018

Published by Satish Kumar Jain and produced by Varun Jain for
CBS Publishers & Distributors Pvt Ltd
4819/XI Prahlad Street, 24 Ansari Road, Daryaganj, New Delhi 110 002, India.
Ph: 23289259, 23266861, 23266867 Website: www.cbspd.com
Fax: 011-23243014   e-mail: delhi@cbspd.com; cbspubs@airtelmail.in.
Corporate Office: 204 FIE, Industrial Area, Patparganj, Delhi 110 092
Ph: 4934 4934   Fax: 4934 4935   e-mail: publishing@cbspd.com; publicity@cbspd.com

Branches

- **Bengaluru:** Seema House 2975, 17th Cross, K.R. Road,
  Banasankari 2nd Stage, Bengaluru 560 070, Karnataka
  Ph: +91-80-26771678/79   Fax: +91-80-26771680   e-mail: bangalore@cbspd.com
- **Chennai:** 7, Subbaraya Street, Shenoy Nagar, Chennai 600 030, Tamil Nadu
  Ph: +91-44-26680620, 26681266   Fax: +91-44-42032115   e-mail: chennai@cbspd.com
- **Kochi:** Ashana House, No. 39/1904, AM Thomas Road, Valanjambalam,
  Ernakulam 682 018, Kochi, Kerala
  Ph: +91-484-4059061-65   Fax: +91-484-4059065   e-mail: kochi@cbspd.com
- **Kolkata:** 6/B, Ground Floor, Rameswar Shaw Road, Kolkata-700 014, West Bengal
  Ph: +91-33-22891126, 22891127, 22891128   e-mail: kolkata@cbspd.com
- **Mumbai:** 83-C, Dr E Moses Road, Worli, Mumbai-400018, Maharashtra
  Ph: +91-22-24902340/41   Fax: +91-22-24902342   e-mail: mumbai@cbspd.com

Representatives

- **Hyderabad** 0-9885175004 • **Jharkhand** 0-9811541605 • **Nagpur** 0-9021734563
- **Patna** 0-9334159340 • **Pune** 0-9623451994 • **Uttarakhand** 0-9000660880

Printed at HT Media, Noida, UP, India

to

---

the Almighty God for giving us an opportunity to share our knowledge
our teachers for their guidance
our parents for their blessings and the values they have instilled in us
our wives and children for their unconditional support
our patients who have been our source of learning   and
our students who inspire us daily

Foreword

Surgery is a very important subject for undergraduate students of medical sciences. Many textbooks in the subject are available by International and Indian authors. However, students find it difficult to remember and reproduce the knowledge due to long text. It has been a felt need for a book that would provide the appropriate information in a comprehensible and reproducible manner.

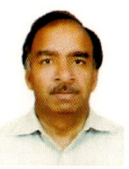

Handbook of Surgery by Prof Sudhir Kumar Jain, Dr Vivek Manchanda and Dr Raman Tanwar is an excellent effort to fill the void. Based on the vast knowledge and long experience in teaching, the authors have caught the pulse and provided the right prescription for the students of surgery.

The book covers all the important areas according to the prescribed curriculum and provides the information in point-wise manner that is easy to grasp and understand. The format of the book makes it very easy for the students to recollect the knowledge. The text is augmented by inclusion of well designed illustrations and tables which leave a long lasting impression on the reader.

I am sure the book will be an asset for not only the undergraduate students but act as a ready reference for postgraduates and clinicians. I recommend the book to all those interested in the subject of surgery.

Prof Anup Mohta
MS, MCh (pediatric surgery)
PGCHM, PGDMLS, FIMSA, MAMS
Director, Chacha Nehru Bal Chikitsalaya
Geeta Colony, Delhi 110031, India

Preface

General surgery is a rapidly growing science and it is a difficult task to summarize the subject in its entirety. There are numerous pathologies that require a surgical management but commoner conditions amongst them are limited and this book attempts to sensitize the naive mind to these more often encountered and relevant disease states. The *Handbook* tries to abridge the vast subject into easily readable and understandable notes which are based on the lectures taken by a teacher of eminence. These lectures are a result of extensive academic research and vast experience. The notes made from these lectures were compiled by two of his students who along with the author have revised updated and shortlisted topics relevant to a student of surgery.

The book contains information which focuses on topics of relatively greater relevance and helps the student focus on these topics. The point-wise yet detailed coverage of topics limited to areas of clinical and theoretical relevance is a beneficial adjunct to standard surgical text. Easy to grasp diagrams and flowcharts will make learning surgery easier and subsequent retention better. The *Handbook of Surgery* is an adjunct to the standard surgical text that will help the students revise, focus and cover additional useful points in an effective way.

Sudhir Kumar Jain
Vivek Manchanda
Raman Tanwar

Acknowledgements

Our deepest regards and thanks to our parents and families for being the pillars of our foundation and their blessings. Our heartfelt thanks to our wives Dr Deepti Jain, Dr Smita Manchanda, and Dr Kirti Vijay Rathore for their constant support during the course of this work. We would like to thank our teachers who have been a guiding light for us and our students who have helped us learn and grow on a daily basis. We express our gratitude towards our patients for vesting their faith in us and helping us to understand the subject beyond what books could express.

We are grateful for the support of Mr SK Jain, Managing Director; Mr YN Arjuna, Senior Director—Publishing, Editorial and Publicity, and his entire team at CBSPD comprising Mr PS Ghuman, Mrs Ritu Chawla, Mrs Baljeet Kaur, Mrs Preeti Khera, Ms Deepti, Ms Poonam and Mr Sunil Dutt. It is only due to the untiring team-work that the difficult task of bringing out this book has been achieved.

Sudhir Kumar Jain
Vivek Manchanda
Raman Tanwar

Contents

SECTION I

SECTION II

Contents

SECTION III

SECTION IV

SECTION V

SECTION VI

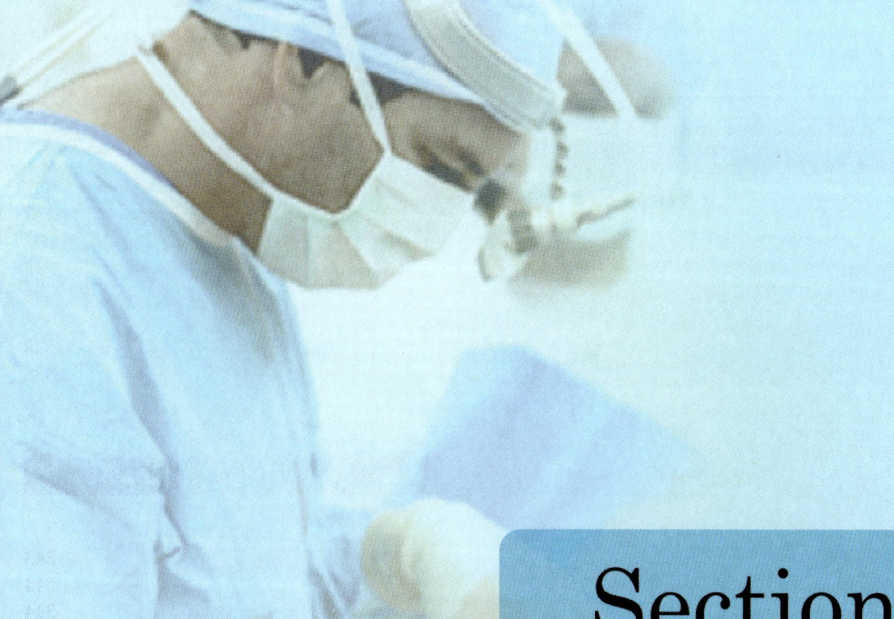

Section I

1

Fluids and Electrolytes in Surgical Patients

TOTAL BODY WATER (Fig. 1.1)

	Body weight %	Total body water %
Total	60	100
Intracellular	40	67
Extracellular	20	33
Intravascular	5	8
Interstitial	15	25

Composition of Fluids

	Plasma	Interstitial	Intracellular
Cations			
Na^+	140	146	12
K^+	4	4	150
Ca^{++}	5	3	10
Mg^{++}	2	1	7
Anions			
Cl^-	103	104	3
HCO_3^-	24	27	10
SO_4^-	1	1	–
HPO_4^-	2	2	116
Protein	16	5	40

Osmolality

- Plasma osmolality (P_{osm}) is a measure of body osmolality
- Usually P_{osm} (m Osm/l) = 2 × serum [Na] + glucose/18 + BUN/2.8
- Normal plasma osmolality is 289 m Osm/L

Control of Volume

- Effective circulating volume is defined as
  - Portion of ECF that perfuses organs
  - Usually equates to intravascular volume
- Third space loss occurs
  - Whenever there is abnormal shift of fluid from intravascular space to third space, e.g. bowel obstruction, pancreatitis

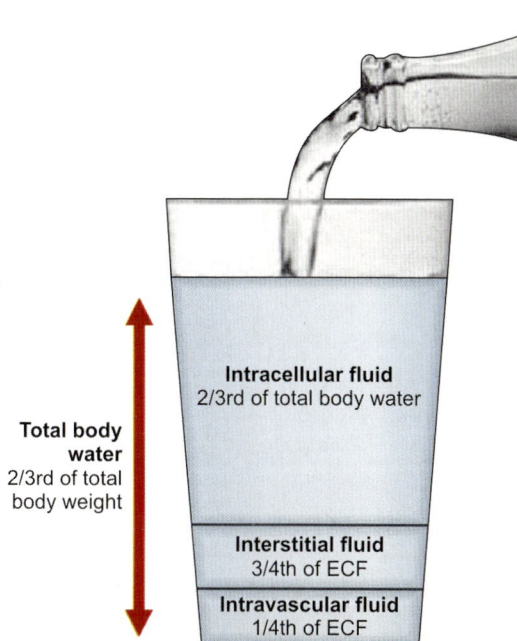

Total body water 2/3rd of total body weight

Intracellular fluid 2/3rd of total body water

Interstitial fluid 3/4th of ECF

Intravascular fluid 1/4th of ECF

Fig. 1.1: Distribution of total body water

- Volume control is mediated through
  - Osmoreceptors—day to day control
  - Baroreceptors—respond to pressure change
  - Neural input and output
  - Hormonal mediators

Osmoregulation

- Osmolality 289 mOsm/kg H_2O
- Osmoreceptor cells are situated in paraventricular/supraoptic nuclei
- Osmoreceptors control thirst and ADH secretion
- Small changes in P_{osm} leads to a large response
- Excess free water (P_{osm} 280) leads to
  - Thirst inhibition
  - ADH declines
  - Urine dilutes to U_{osm} 100
- Decreased free water (P_{osm} 295)
  - Thirst increases
  - ADH increases
  - Urine concentrates to U_{osm} 1200
- Change in U_{osm} = 95 × change in P_{osm}

Neural Mechanism

- Increased sympathetic tone leads to tachycardia and increased renal blood flow and decreased Na^+ reabsorption

Hormonal Mediators

Those hormones which participate in control of fluid and electrolyte are:
- Renin
- Aldosterone
- ANP
- Dopamine
- Hormonal effect leads to increased Na^+ and water reabsorption even when there is decrease in ECF.

Renin-Angiotensin System

- Renin is secreted when
  - Drop in blood pressure
  - Drop in Na^+ delivery to kidney (chloride mediated)
  - Increased sympathetic tone

Angiotensin II

- Increases vascular tone
  - Increases catecholamine release
  - Decreases renal blood flow
  - Increases Na^+ reabsorption
  - Stimulates aldosterone release

Aldosterone

- Release stimulated by
  - Angiotensin II
  - Increased K^+
  - ACTH
- Effect
  - Na^+ and water absorption in distal tubular segments

Normal Intake of Water

- 2000 ml
  - 1300 ml free water
  - 700 ml bound to food
- Additional water comes from catabolism

Water and Electrolyte Exchange

- Surgical patients prone to disruption:
  - Nil orally
  - Post anesthesia
  - Trauma
  - Sepsis
- Surgical patients have
  - Maintenance volume requirements
  - Ongoing losses
  - Volume excess/deficits
  - Maintenance electrolyte requirements
  - Electrolyte excess/deficits

Maintenance Requirements

- This includes:
  - Insensible losses
  - Urinary losses
  - Stool losses

Body weight	Fluid required
0–10 kg	100 ml/kg/d
Next 10–20 kg	50 ml/kg/d
Subsequent 20 kg	20 ml/kg/d
	15 ml/kg/d for elderly

- 70 kg man needs
  - 10 × 100 = 1000
  - 10 × 50   = 500
  - 50 × 20   = 1000
  - 2500 ml/day

Ongoing losses

- Nasogastric tube
- Drains
- Fistulae

- Third space losses
  - Concentration of electrolytes is similar to plasma in above losses
  - Replacement with isotonic fluids, e.g. ringer lactate

Volume Deficit—Acute

- Vital signs change
  - Blood pressure decreases
  - Heart rate increases
  - CVP become low
- Tissue changes not obvious
- Urine output low

Volume Deficit—Clinical Features in Chronic Losses

- Decreased skin turgor
- Sunken eyes
- Oliguria
- Orthostatic hypotension
- High BUN/creatinine ratio
- Hematocrit increases 6–8 points per litre deficit
- Plasma Na^+ may be normal

Volume Excess

- Over hydration
- Mobilization of third space losses back to the body compartments
- Signs
  - Weight gain
  - Pulmonary edema
  - Peripheral edema
  - S3 gallop

Fluid and Electrolyte Therapy

- Goal
  - Normal hemodynamic parameters should be restored
  - Normal electrolyte concentration achieved
  - Method–Replacement
    ◊ Replenish normal maintenance requirements
  - Ongoing losses
    ◊ Measure all losses in I/O chart
    ◊ Estimate third space losses
  - Deficits
    ◊ Estimate using vital signs
    ◊ Estimate using hematocrit
- The best estimate of the volume required is the patients response

- After therapy is started; observe
  - Vital signs
  - Urine output (0.5–1 ml/kg/hr)
  - Central venous pressure
- Time frame for replacement
  - Usually correct over 24 hours
  - For ill patients calculate over shorter period and reassess, e.g. 12 hours or 3 hours for emergency operative cases
  - Deficits — correct half the amount over a smaller period and reassess

Maintenance Electrolyte Requirements

- Na^+ 1–2 mEq/kg/d
- K^+ 0.5–1 mEq/kg/d
- Usually no K^+ is given until the urine output is adequate.
- Always give K^+ with care, in an infusion slowly—never bolus
- Ca^{++}, PO_4^-, Mg^{++} are not required for short term

Postoperative Fluid Therapy

- Check intravenous fluid regime ordered in operation form
- Assess for deficits by checking I/O chart and vital signs
- Maintenance requirements should be calculated
- Usually K^+ not started on first two days
- Monitor vital signs and urine output carefully
- Urine output is one of the best parameter
- CVP measurement is useful in difficult situations (5–15 cm H_2O)
- Body weight is measured in special situations, e.g. burns

Concentration Changes

- Changes in plasma Na^+ are indicative of abnormal total body water (TBW)
- Losses in surgery are usually isotonic
- Hypo-osmolar condition is usually caused by replacement with free water

HYPONATREMIA

- Usually excess free water is the cause
- Caused by free water replacement of isotonic losses
- Increased ADH secretion can lead to water retention
- Low intravascular volume states like cirrhosis/low albumin can also be the cause
- Infusion of excess solute, e.g. glucose can lead to intracellular water shifts to ECF

Clinical Features

- Depends on rapidity of sodium loss. If there is acute drop below 120 mEq/L.
  - Weakness
  - Fatigue
  - Confusion
  - Cramps
  - Nausea/vomiting
  - Headache/delirium/seizures/coma
  - Permanent CNS damage

Diagnosis of Hyponatremia

- Assess circulating volume
- Exclude hyperosmolar states
- Check for losses
- Check for excess free water replacement
- In difficult situations measure urine Na^+ (< 20 mEq/L)

Treatment of Hyponatremia

- Replace volume deficits in dehydration
- Restrict free water in overload
- Na^+ required = [Desired Na^+] – [Actual Na^+] × (TBW); TBW = $0.6 \times$ BodyWt
- Correct half the deficit over 12 hours and reassess

2 Nutritional Support

Nutritional support may supplement normal feeding, or completely replace normal feeding into the gastrointestinal tract.

Body composition varies in normal and catabolic state.
- Normal individual have:
  - 30% adipose tissue
  - 30% lean body mass
  - 30% extracellular water
- In catabolic states, body has:
  - 50–60% extracellular fluid
  - 20% lean body mass
  - 20% adipose tissue

Benefits of Nutritional Support
- It preserves nutritional status during catabolic state
- Prevention of complications of protein malnutrition
- There is decreased incidence of post-operative complications in well-nourished patients

Indications of Nutritional Support
- To prevent malnutrition in patients who have normal or near normal nutrition, but are likely to result in malnutrition, e.g.
  - Trauma patients
  - After major surgery
  - After severe burns
  - Ventilated patients
- To treat malnutrition

Assessment of Malnutrition
Clinical Examination
History
- Loss of appetite
- Changes in diet
- Loss of body weight
  - >10% loss of body weight which is unintensional during the last 6 months.
  - Beware of patients with ascites/edema, as they can have increased weight inspite of malnutrition.

Examination
- Evidence of muscle wasting
- Depletion of subcutaneous fat
- Peripheral edema, ascites
- Features of vitamin deficiency, e.g. nail and mucosal changes
- Ecchymosis and easy bruising
- Features of micronutrient deficiency

Anthropometric Measurements
- Weight and height
- Body mass index (BMI):
  19–25 kg/m^2 = Normal
  <19 kg/m^2 = Malnourished
  >25 kg/m^2 = Overweight
  >30 kg/m^2 = Obese
- Mid-arm muscle circumference (MAMC) = mid arm circumference
  - Triceps skin-fold thickness × 0.314
  - MAMC below 10th percentile is significant

- Fasting causes mobilization of fat stores
- Stressed patients — Proteolysis causes muscle wasting

Measurement of Organ Function

- Malnutrition can lead to impaired muscle strength which in turn leads to increased fatigability of small muscles especially of the hand.
- Impaired muscle function is measured by *Hand Grip Dynamometry*
  - Measured in non-dominant hand
  - Highest value of three readings is taken
  - Force-frequency characteristics of muscles and rate of recovery from fatigue after electrical stimulation of the ulnar nerve is measured
- Bioelectric impedance analysis measures adipose reserve, intracellular and extracellular water and third space fluid in a stable surgical patients
- **Indirect calorimetric tests:** Measures oxygen consumption, respiratory quotient

Anergy

- It is the loss of cutaneous responses to antigens, e.g. PPD, Candida
- Total leukocyte count ($<1800/mm^3$) is seen in malnutrition
- Decreased level of
  - S. Albumin ($t_{1/2}$ of 14–18 days) < 3 g/dL. As serum albumin has long half-life its level falls late in malnutrition
  - S. Transferrin ($t_{1/2}$ of 7 days) < 150 m-mol/L. It can be elevated in iron deficiency irrespective of nutritional status
  - S. Pre-albumin ($t_{1/2}$ of 3–5 days) <12 mg/dl. *It is the first to fall even in early stage of malnutrition. It is useful in ICU patients and should only be used if creatinine clearance is more than 50 ml per minute as levels of pre-albumin may be raised in renal failure inspite of poor nutritional status.*
  - S. Retinol binding protein ($t_{1/2}$ of 12 hours). Retinol binding proteins are bound to pre-albumin in circulation
  - Insulin like Growth Factor-1 (IGF-1)
  - Iron, calcium, magnesium, folic acid, vitamin B_{12}, 25-OH vitamin D
- Specific functional defects like increased prothrombin time

Urinary Creatinine Height Index

- It is measured by following formula:

$$\frac{\text{Actual 24 hours urinary creatinine excretion}}{\text{Ideal urinary creatinine excretion as per height}}$$

- Creatinine excretion is an indicator of muscle mass and total body nitrogen
- Value of urinary creatinine height index less than 80 suggests malnutrition

Requirements for Nutritional Support

- Adequate energy
- Protein nitrogen
- Water and electrolytes
- Trace elements
- Vitamins

Energy requirements

- 25–35 kcal per kg of body weight/day
- Should not exceed more than 40 kcal/kg/day

Energy Sources

- Hypertonic sugar
  - Glucose 10–50%
  - Fructose 15%
  - Insulin may be required when high concentration of glucose is used
- Fat emulsion
  - 1–2 grams/kg body weight/day
  - Given as intra-lipid 10% or 20%
  - Soyabean oil emulsion is commonly used which also contains egg lecithin
  - Glycerol is added to make it isotonic
  - 50% of the fatty acid content is linoleic acid
  - 500 units of heparin is used to facilitate fat utilization.

Nitrogen Source

- To meet substrate requirements for protein synthesis, the non-protein: nitrogen ratio of 150:1 should be maintained. This is required to prevent proteins from being used up to meet the caloric requirements
- Approximately 0.25 to 0.35 g of nitrogen per kilogram of body weight should be provided daily (to be adjusted depending on renal and hepatic function)

- 1 gm of nitrogen for every 150 kcal per day or 0.2 grams/kg/day is ideal
- 6.25 grams of protein gives 1gm of nitrogen
- Synthetic crystalline amino acids, e.g. L-amino acids are commonly used
- All amino acids are given but the ratio of essential amino acids and total amino acids should be 3:4
- Cationic amino acids should be avoided
- Optimum pH should be between 5–6.

Water

- 30–35 ml/kg/day

Electrolytes

- Sodium
- Potassium
- Chloride
- Calcium
- Magnesium

Routes of Nutritional Support

- Enteral route
- Parenteral route

INDICATIONS OF ENTERAL NUTRITION

1. When a patient cannot meet more than 70 per cent of nutritional requirement by oral route
2. Major head injury patients with glasgow coma scale less than or equal to 8
3. Major trauma involving torso, long bones, pelvis or chest

- *Advantages of enteral nutrition are:*
  - Economical and easy to administer
  - Safer with less complications
  - More physiological as gut is used for absorption of nutrients, thus maintaining the gut mucosal barrier function and gut immune function (secretion of IgA)
- *Indications:*
  - Low intestinal or colonic fistulae
  - Short bowel syndrome after massive resection of gut or post irradiation enteritis
  - Inflammatory bowel disease when elemental diet is indicated
  - Patient with profound anorexia
  - Patient who are unable to eat or swallow
  - Critically ill patients with normal gut

- *Intestinal access:*
  - Natural route:
    - ◊ Nasogastric tube
    - ◊ Oro-gastric tube
    - ◊ Naso-duodenal tube
    - ◊ Naso-jejunal tube

Post pyloric feeding is better than gastric feeding in cases of major surgery or trauma as there is delayed gastric emptying for several days in these patients. Post pyloric feeding can deliver much more calories with lower rates of infectious complications in comparison to gastric feeding.

Advantages of Nasogastric Tube

- It is less expensive.
- It can be used only in those patients with intact mentation and preserved laryngeal reflexes as gastric-oesophageal reflux is promoted by the presence of wide bore tube which makes gastro-oesophageal sphincter incompetent.
- Risk of aspiration is reduced by 25% if tube is placed in jejunum, but duodenal or jejunal placement requires image guidance (endoscopic/fluoroscopic).
- Tubes are susceptible to blockage by food residue or as a result of kinking or displacement.
- Not recommended for longer than 30 days.
- *Complications:* Oesophageal and gastric erosions, tube displacement, pulmonary aspiration, sinusitis, oesophageal stricture/perforation, pneumothorax, arrhythmias.

Invasive (percutaneous) procedure:
- Percutaneous gastrostomy/percutaneous jejunostomy.
- Indications
  - Impaired swallowing mechanisms
  - Oro-pharyngeal/oesophageal obstruction
  - Major facial trauma
  - Debilitated patients requiring nutritional support/hydration
- Contraindications:
  - Ascites
  - Coagulopathy
  - Gastric varices
  - Gastric neoplasm
  - Unsuitable location
- Size of tube to be placed: 18–28 Fr. Tubes made up of silicon or silicon coated tubes are preferred

- Complications:
  - Wound infection
  - Necrotizing fasciitis
  - Peritonitis
  - Leaks
  - Dislodgement
  - Bowel perforation
  - Enteric fistulas
  - Bleeding

Surgical gastrostomy and jejunostomy
- Contraindications to jejunostomy:
  - **Absolute:** Distal intestinal obstruction
  - **Relative:** Bowel wall edema, radiation enteritis, inflammatory bowel disease, severe immunodeficiency, bowel ischemia
- Complications:
  - Pneumatosis intestinalis
  - Small bowel necrosis

Types of Enteral Nutrition
- Oral dietary supplements
- Low-residue isotonic formulae:
  - First choice for stable patients with intact GI tract
  - Calories provided 1.0 kcal/ml
  - Daily requirement 1500–1800 ml
  - Low osmolarity
  - Carbohydrates, protein, electrolytes, water, fat and fat soluble vitamins (+/– Vit K) can be given
  - Non protein calories:nitrogen= 150:1
- Isotonic formulae with fibre:
  - Soy-based soluble/insoluble fibre
  - Advantages:
    ◊ Reduce incidence of diarrhoea
    ◊ Stimulate pancreatic lipases
    ◊ Degraded into short-chain fatty acids (SCFAs) by intestinal bacteria. SCFAs are trophic for the mucosa
- Immune-enhancing formulae:
  - Glutamine, arginine, branched chain amino acids, nucleotides and beta-carotene added
- Calorie-dense formulae:
  - Implies a greater caloric value for the same volume, but a higher osmolality
  - Approx. 1.5–2 kcal/ml is provided
  - Useful when fluid restriction is required
  - Provided as intra-gastric feeds

- High-protein formulae:
  - Isotonic/non-isotonic mixtures
  - Non protein calories(NPC):nitrogen ratio should be 80:1 to 120:1
  - Used for critically ill/trauma patients
- Elemental formulae:
  - Pre-digested nutrients, small peptides and paucity of fat
  - High osmolarity
  - Used in malabsorption, gut impairment, pancreatitis
  - Long term use not recommended
  - Expensive
- Renal-failure formulae:
  - Lower fluid volume
  - Decreased amounts of potassium, phosphorus, magnesium are given
  - Essential amino acids: Branched chain amino acid enriched and aromatic amino acid deficient solution are used
  - High non protein calories: nitrogen ratio (> 150:1)
  - No trace elements or vitamins are added.
- Pulmonary-failure formulae:
  - Fat accounts for 50% of total calories
  - Advantage: Reduced carbon dioxide production
- Hepatic failure formulae:
  - 50% of amino acids are branched chain amino acids, i.e. leucine, isoleucine, valine
  - To alleviate the risk of hepatic encephalopathy
- Polymeric feeds—whole protein, hydrolysate of starch, long-chain triglycerides are used
- Pre-digested chemical defined diets (monomeric/elemental feeds)—peptides, medium chain fatty triglycerides; required in patients with severe intestinal disease

Methods of Feeding
- **Infusion feeding:** By infusion pumps. Started initially at 50 ml/hr, increased gradually to 100 ml/hr.
- **Bolus feeding:** Has more side effects, e.g. bloating, diarrhoea.

Complications of Enteral Nutrition
- 12% overall complication rate.

- *Gastrointestinal* (10%)
  - Bloating/abdominal distension/cramps due to rapid administration of feeds.
  - Nausea and vomiting due to slow gastric emptying.
  - Diarrhoea
  - Constipation
  - Regurgitation
- *Infectious*
  - Aspiration pneumonia
  - Bacterial contamination
- *Mechanical*
  - Malposition of feeding tube
  - Sinusitis
  - Ulcerations/erosions
  - Blockage of tubes
  - Unwanted removal of tubes
- *Others*
  - Drug interactions, e.g. theophylline, warfarin, methyldopa.
  - Vitamin, mineral, trace elements deficiency.

Parenteral Nutrition

- Allows greater caloric intake, but is more expensive, has more complications and needs more technical expertise.
- Can be supplemental or total.
- Indicated for patients with non-functional or non-accessible GI tract.
- Healthy well-nourished patients can be maintained on intravenous fluids only for up to 10 days before significant protein catabolism starts.
- *Indications:*
  - Prolonged paralytic ileus after
    ◊ Major surgery (>7–10 days)
    ◊ Multiple injuries/abdominal trauma
    ◊ Ileus accompanying medical disorders
  - Intestinal fistulas (both internal or external)
    ◊ Enteroenteric
    ◊ Enterocolic
    ◊ Enterovesical
    ◊ High output enterocutaneous (>500 ml/day)
  - Short bowel syndrome which occurs after massive resection
    ◊ <100 cm short bowel without colon/ileocaecal valve
    ◊ <50 cm short bowel with intact ileocaecal valve and colon
  - Malabsorption
  - Functional GI disorders
    ◊ After cerebrovascular accident
    ◊ Idiopathic diarrhoea
    ◊ Psychogenic vomiting
    ◊ Anorexia nervosa
  - Malignancy
  - Critically ill patients requiring nutritional support for >5 days or in whom enteral nutrition is contraindicated
  - Failed attempt at enteral nutrition
- *Contraindications:*
  - Hemodynamic instability
  - Severe metabolic derangement
  - Good nutritional status
  - Enteral nutrition is feasible
  - End of life, irreversibly decerebrate or dehumanized patients
  - Cardiac failure
  - Hepatic failure
  - Blood dyscrasias
  - Grossly impaired fat metabolism
  - Uncontrolled diabetes

Differences in metabolism of nutrients delivered by the parenteral route:

- Nutrients bypass the liver as they are supplied directly to the systemic route and the intricate steps of processing and storage cannot take place in the usual manner
- The induction of enteric hormones is not possible and overall nutrient disposal is less efficient

Routes of Parenteral Nutrition

- Via peripheral vein
- Via central vein: The central line is to be placed so that the tip of the catheter lies in superior vena cava. This can be achieved by inserting the catheter through
  - Subclavian vein
  - Internal jugular vein
  - Brachiocephalic vein

The two routes differ in:

- Composition of feed

- Primary caloric source
- Potential complications
- Method of administration

Peripheral Route

- *Indications:*
  - If nutritional support is needed for < 2 weeks
  - Mildly stressed patients
  - Low caloric requirements
  - Needs large amounts of fluid
  - Central line is contraindicated or impossible to insert
- *Advantages:*
  - Avoids risks of central venous catheters
- *Disadvantages:*
  - Higher incidence of thrombophlebitis
- Nutrients that can be used
  - 3% amino acid solution
  - 5% dextrose solution
  - Isotonic fat emulsion
- Limitation
  - 1500 kcal/day
  - 100 grams proteins/day
- Thrombophlebitis can be reduced by:
  - Use of isotonic solution
  - Use of heparin
  - In line filtration
  - Use of cortisol
  - Use of fine bore cannula
  - Reduction of osmolality
  - Proper buffering of solution
  - Use of locally applied *glycerol trinitrate* patches

Central Parenteral Route

- Central parenteral nutrition is indicated
  - If nutrition is needed for > 2 weeks
  - If hyperosmolar solution is needed
  - In absence of peripheral veins
  - For unusual nutritional requirement with volume restriction
- Silastic catheters are used because
  - They are non-irritant
  - They do not encourage fibrin formation
- Nutrients that can be provided:
  - Safe delivery of hypertonic solution is possible
  - 3–15% amino acid solution

- 5–50% dextrose solution
- 10–20% fat emulsion
- Electrolytes—sodium, potassium, calcium, magnesium
- Vitamins
- Trace metals
- Nutrients provided through parenteral nutrition can be divided into
  - Macronutrients
    ◊ Combination of lipids and carbohydrates in ratio 50:50
    ◊ Nitrogen sources are L-amino acids
  - Micronutrients
    ◊ Electrolytes
    ◊ Trace elements
    ◊ Vitamins

What to do before Starting TPN

- Nutritional assessment
- Venous access evaluation
- Baseline weight
- Baseline lab investigations
  - Full blood count
  - Coagulation screen
  - Blood sugar
  - Kidney and liver function tests
  - Ca^{++}, Mg^{++}, PO_4^{2-}
  - Lipid profile
  - Other tests when indicated

Steps to Ordering TPN

See Fig. 2.1.

Determine total fluid volume

- Cater for maintenance and ongoing losses. It should take care of normal maintenance requirements
  - By body weight
  - Alternatively, 30 to 50 ml/kg/day
- Add ongoing losses based on I/O chart
- Consider insensible fluid losses also, e.g. add 10% for every degree Celsius rise in temperature.

Determine caloric needs

- "Too much of a good thing causes problems"
  - Not more than 4 mg/kg/min dextrose (less than 6 g/kg/day)
  - Not more than 0.7 mg/kg/min lipid (less than 1 g/kg/day)

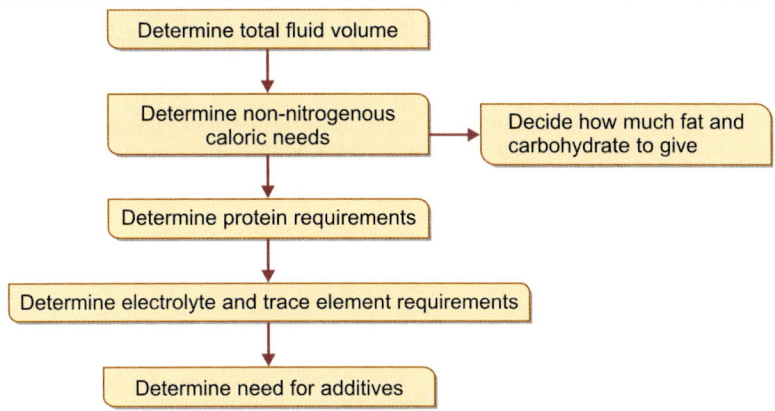

Fig. 2.1: Steps of ordering TPN

- Fats usually form 25 to 30% of calories
  - Not more than 40 to 50%
  - Increase usually in severe stress
  - Aim for serum TG levels < 350 mg/dl or 3.95 mmol/l
- Carbohydrates usually form 70–75% of calories

Determine protein requirements

- Based on calorie: nitrogen ratio
  - Normal ratio is 150 cal: 1g nitrogen
  - Critically ill patients 85 to 100 cal:1g nitrogen
- Based on degree of stress and body weight
  - Non-stress patients   0.8 g/kg/day
  - Mild stress   1.0 to 1.2 g/kg/day
  - Moderate stress   1.3 to 1.75 g/kg/day
  - Severe stress   2 to 2.5 g/kg/day
- Based on nitrogen balance
  - Aim for positive balance of 1.5 to 2 g/kg/day

Determine electrolyte requirements

- Cater for maintenance + replacement needs
  - Na^+ 1 to 2 mmol/kg/d (or 60–120 meq/d)
  - K^+ 0.5 to 1 mmol/kg/d (or 30–60 meq/d)
  - Mg^{++} 0.35 to 0.45 meq/kg/d (or 10 to 20 meq/d)
  - Ca^{++} 0.2 to 0.3 meq/kg/d (or 10 to 15 meq/d)
  - PO_4^{2-} 20 to 30 mmol/d

Determine trace elements requirements

- Total requirements not well established
- Commercial preparations exist to provide
  - Zn   2–4 mg/day
  - Cr   10–15 µg/day
  - Cu   0.3–0.5 mg/day
  - Mn   0.4–0.8 mg/day

Determine need for additives

- Vitamins
  - Give 2–3 times that recommended for oral intake
  - Or give 1 ampoule multi vitamin per 1l bag of TPN
  - Multi vitamin does not include vitamin K
    ◊ Can give 1 mg/day or 5–10 mg/wk
- Insulin
  - Can give initial soluble insulin based on sliding scale according to blood or plasma glucose estimation q6h (keep <11 mmol/l)
  - Once stable, give 2/3 total requirements in TPN and review daily
  - Alternate regimes
    ◊ 0.1 U per g dextrose in TPN
    ◊ 10 U per liter TPN initial dose
- Other medications

Overfeeding

- Overestimation of caloric requirements
- Can lead to clinical deterioration due to:
  - Increased oxygen consumption
  - Increased CO_2 production and thus, prolonged ventilator support
  - Fatty liver
  - Suppression of leukocyte production
  - Hyperglycemia
  - Increased risk of infection.

Monitoring

- **Clinical review**
  - Clinical examination
  - Vital signs
  - Fluid balance
  - Catheter care

- – Sepsis review
- – Blood sugar profile
- – Body weight
- **Laboratory tests**

– Full blood count	Weekly, unless indicated
– Kidney function tests	Daily until stable, then twice a week
– Ca^{++}, Mg^{++}, PO_4^{2-}	Daily until stable, then twice a week
– Liver function test	Weekly
– Iron profile	Weekly
– Lipid profile	Once or twice a week
– Nitrogen balance	Weekly

  Nitrogen Balance = $N_{input} - N_{output}$

where

N_{input} = (protein in g/6.25)

N_{output} = 24h urinary urea nitrogen + non urinary N losses

(Estimated normal non-urinary nitrogen losses about 3–4 g/d)

Complications

- Catheter related
- Nutritional/metabolic
- Effects on other organs

Catheter related complications

- At the time of insertion:
  - – Pneumothorax if pleura is punctured
  - – Air embolism
  - – Injury to subclavian artery leading to haematoma formation or haemothorax
  - – Neurological injury leading to brachial plexus injury
  - – Cardiac arrhythmia if tip of catheter touches SA node
  - – Catheter misplacement
  - – Catheter embolism
  - – Thoracic duct injury
- Late complications:
  - – Catheter infections
    - ◊ Insertion site contamination may be due to

- Catheter contamination
- Improper insertion technique
- Use of catheter for non-feeding purposes
- Contaminated TPN solution
- Contaminated tubing
  - – Catheter displacement
  - – Catheter occlusion
  - – Central venous thrombosis

Metabolic complications

- Hyperglycemia
- Hypoglycaemia
- Hypophosphatemia
- Hypercalcemia
- Hyperkalemia
- Hypernatremia or hyponatremia
- Acidosis
  - – If excessive cationic amino acids (arginine, lysine, histidine) are used
  - – Excess of lipids may lead to rise in ketone levels
  - – Fructose or sorbitol metabolism
- Deficiencies of folate, zinc, magnesium, trace elements, vitamins

Effects on Other Organs

- If hyperosmolar solution is used, may lead to cerebral dehydration
- Hepatobiliary disease
  - – Hepatic steatosis
  - – Cholestasis
  - – Acalculous cholecystitis
- Endocarditis (secondary to catheter sepsis)
- Osteomyelitis (secondary to catheter sepsis)
- Pulmonary embolism following central venous thrombosis
- Septicemia

Stopping TPN

- Stop TPN when enteral feeding can restart
- Wean slowly to avoid hypoglycaemia
- Monitor blood sugars during weaning
  - – Give IV Dextrose 10% solution at previous infusion rate for at least 4 to 6 hrs.
  - – Alternatively, wean TPN while introducing enteral feeding and stop when enteral intake meets total nutritional requirement.

3 Shock

DEFINITION

It is an acute clinical state characterized by inadequate cellular perfusion leading to cellular damage and failure of major organ systems. It can also be defined as decreased tissue respiration with inadequate consumption of oxygen and excretion of carbon dioxide at cellular level.

Basic pathology in shock is inadequate (not always low) cardiac output for the metabolic needs of the tissue.

Causes of Shock

- Central or cardiogenic shock (pump failure)
- Hypovolemic shock. Treatment of this type of shock needs volume replacement
- Peripheral failure of venous return. This type of shock needs drug therapy to increase the peripheral vascular tone.

Cardiogenic Shock (Pump Failure)

This is associated with low cardiac output, e.g. myocardial infarction, cardiac contusion, tension pneumothorax, cardiac tamponade, pulmonary embolus. This type of shock needs cardiac stimulation either by pharmacological or mechanical means.

Peripheral Failure

- True hypovolemia
  - Loss of blood, e.g. external or internal haemorrhage
  - Loss of plasma, e.g. in burns
  - Loss of extracellular volume
- Peripheral pooling of blood (apparent hypovolemia)
  - Neurogenic shock, e.g. spinal injury, vasovagal attack
  - Anaphylactic shock, e.g. antigen-antibody reaction like drug allergy
  - Septic shock, e.g. endotoxic shock

Signs and Symptoms

The patient is
- Restless, anxious, confused
- Thirsty
- Pale
- Cold sweating
- Cyanosed with a rapid feeble pulse
- Hypotensive
- Low urine output
- Hyperventilating
- Central venous pressure is reduced, except in cardiogenic shock when it can be increased.
- Tachycardia, except in cardiogenic shock when heart rate can be normal or decreased.
- Pulmonary artery wedge pressure is decreased in hypovolemic shock, but increased in cardiogenic shock.
- Cardiac output is reduced, but in early stages it can be increased due to hyper-dynamic circulation.

Management
- General
- Specific

General Measures
Maintain **ABCDE**
- **A** – Airway
- **B** – Breathing
- **C** – Circulation
- **D** – Disability assessment
- **E** – Expose the patient for complete examination

Airway maintenance
- Remove any debris and foreign body from the oral cavity and throat
- Gentle throat suction to remove mucus or vomitus
- Prevent tongue from falling backward by chin lift/jaw thrust
- If the patient is unable to maintain airway, consider intubation/tracheostomy

Maintain breathing
- Give 100% oxygen
- If the breathing effort is inadequate, artificial respiration is to be given by
  - Mouth-to-mouth breathing
  - Respiratory bag after intubation
  - Mechanical ventilator

Maintain circulation
- Control obvious haemorrhage
- Insert two large bore IV cannulas
- Take blood sample for grouping and cross matching
- Start IV infusion
  - Normal saline or ringer lactate
  - Plasma expanders or colloids like dextran 70, haemaccel, hydroxyethyl starch can be used if there is any delay in getting blood in cases of major blood loss
  - Whole blood in moderate to severe blood loss to maintain haemoglobin above 10 gm/dl or hematocrit more than 30%

Hemorrhage
Classification
Depending on nature of blood vessels
- Arterial
  - Bright red colour
  - Blood gushes out and is pulsatile

  - Pulsation of artery can be seen
  - Can be easily controlled as artery is easily seen
- Venous
  - Dark red colour
  - Neither pulsatile nor jets out, rather blood oozes out of the wound
  - Difficult to control as the vein gets retracted
- Capillary
  - Red colour
  - Slow ooze

Depending on time of hemorrhage
- Primary
  - At the time of surgery
  - Reactionary bleeding is 6–12 hours after surgery
  - Causes of reactionary hemorrhage
    - ◊ Hypertension in post-op period
    - ◊ Sneezing
    - ◊ Coughing
    - ◊ Retching
- Secondary
  - 5–7 days after surgery
  - Due to infection leading to sloughing of vessel wall.

Depending on duration of haemorrhage
- Acute haemorrhage
  - Occurs suddenly, e.g. oesophageal variceal bleed
  - Chronic haemorrhage
- Slow bleeding over long period, e.g. piles, chronic duodenal ulcer.

Depending on the nature of bleeding
- External or revealed hemorrhage, e.g. epistaxis, hematemesis
- Internal or concealed haemorrhage, e.g. splenic rupture, ruptured ectopic pregnancy

Stages of Hemorrhage
1. Mild hemorrhage (Class I)
   a. <15% of blood loss (<750 ml in 75 kg man)
   b. Signs and symptoms
      i. Slight tachycardia (<100/min)
      ii. Slight confusion
2. Moderate hemorrhage (Class II)
   a. 15–30% of blood loss
   b. Signs and symptoms
      i. Tachycardia (>100/min)

ii. Blood pressure—normal or slightly low
iii. Anxious
iv. Respiratory rate increased (20–30/min)
v. Urine output decreased (20–30 ml/hr)
3. Severe hemorrhage (Class III)
   a. 30–40% of blood loss
   b. Signs and symptoms
      i. Greater tachycardia (>120/min)
      ii. Hypotension
      iii. Tachypnea (respiratory rate > 30–40/min)
      iv. Oliguria (urine output 5–15ml/hr)
      v. Anxious
      vi. Confused
4. Exsanguinating hemorrhage (Class IV)
   a. >40% of blood loss
   b. Signs and symptoms
      i. Confused and lethargic
      ii. Weak low volume pulse
      iii. Respiratory rate > 35/min
      iv. No urine output
   c. At >50% of loss of blood volume
      i. Patient is unconscious
      ii. Blood pressure is not recordable
      iii. Peripheral pulses are not palpable

Treatment

Up to 1L or < 20% of blood volume loss

- Use of blood as replacement is not required
- Crystalloids alone or crystalloids in combination with colloids (in ratio 2:1) are transfused
- If crystalloids alone are used, 3–4 times the volume of blood lost needs to be transfused

because crystalloids go into the extracellular fluid compartment.

Up to 1–2 L or 20–40% of blood volume loss

The fluids are transfused in the following order till the patient is adequately resuscitated:

- 1L crystalloid (0.9% NaCl) over 30–60 minutes
- 1L colloid solution (dextran 70 or Hemaccel®) over 30–60 minutes
- Two red cell concentrate to restore oxygen carrying capacity

> 40% of blood volume loss

- Whole blood transfusion is required
- 4.5% albumin infusion will help retain the crystalloids in intravascular compartment for a longer time because albumin has longer half-life than other colloids

Local Methods to Control Hemorrhage

- Pressure and packing
- Position and rest, e.g. limb elevation
- Tourniquets
  - Pneumatic
  - Rubber bandage
  - Contraindicated in venous hemorrhage or in patient with peripheral vascular disease

Surgical Methods to Control Hemorrhage

- Artery forceps
- Suture ligature
- Cautery coagulation
- Clips
- Surgical glues and coagulation activators

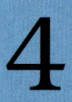

4   Wound Healing

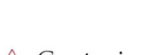

Disruption of the continuity of tissues due to loss or destruction of tissue.

Three basic types of wound healing are:

1. *Primary:* Wound margins are opposed. Healing is without complications and minimal new tissue formation.
2. *Delayed primary:* Wound is left open initially and edges approximated 4–6 days later.
3. *Secondary:* Wound margins are not approximated. Defect in the wound is filled with granulation which gets covered with epithelium.

Etiology

- Accidental trauma
- Surgical trauma
- Physical agents
- Chemical agents

Wound Healing

- Restoration of the continuity of disrupted tissue
- Destroyed tissue replaced by living tissue

Types of Wound

- **Rank and Wakefield classification:**
  - Tidy wounds
  - Untidy wounds
- **Other classifications used to categorise wounds:**
  - Closed
    - ◊ Contusion
    - ◊ Abrasion
    - ◊ Hematoma
  - Open
    - ◊ Incised
    - ◊ Lacerated
    - ◊ Penetrating wound
    - ◊ Crushing wound

Wound Management

- Primary suturing
- Wound excision with primary suturing
- Wound excision with delayed primary suturing
- Secondary suturing

Factors Affecting Wound Healing

General Factors

- *Age:* Healing is delayed in old age.
- *Nutrition:* Delayed healing in malnutrition.
- *Vitamin deficiency:* Wound healing delayed in vitamin C deficiency
- Micronutrient deficiency
- Diabetic
- Uremia
- Immunocompromised patient
- Drugs—corticosteroids

Local Factors

- Poor blood supply leads to delayed wound healing
- Local infection

- Recurrent trauma
- Hematoma
- Faulty technique
- Tension

Classification of Wounds

- Clean
- Clean contaminated
- Contaminated
- Dirty

Wound Management

- Admission/observation
- Care of ABC—airway, breathing, circulation
- Antibiotics
- Tetanus prophylaxis
- Local treatment of wound

Wound Healing

- Primary intention
- Secondary intention

Three phases of wound healing are:

1. *Inflammatory phase:* This phase lasts for 4–6 days. There is haemostasis and inflammation. Exposed collagen fibres activate clotting cascades and inflammatory phase. There is scaffolding of fibrin clot. Cytokines and growth factors are attracted in it. Monocytes and macrophages attracted in to wound by complement. These activated macrophages mediate angiogenesis, fibroplasia and secrete collagenases.

2. *Proliferative phase:* Lasts from day 4 to 14. Production of collagen is the hallmark. There is epithelialization of the wound from basal epithelial cells at the wound margin. There is laying down of fibroblast in the wound.

   Fibroblast secrete type III collagen, elastin fibers. Later on tissue fibroblast becomes myofibroblast. These myofibroblast induces tissue contraction.

3. *Remodeling phase:* Type III collagen is replaced by type I collagen. Strength of wound increases by collagen organisation and cross linking of collagen.

Stages of Wound Healing

- Epithelialization (24–72 hours)
- Wound contraction (4–14 days) by myofibroblasts
- Connective tissue formation starts after the 5th day
  - Proliferation of fibroblasts
  - Laying down of collagen
  - Capillary budding
  - Secretion of mucoploysaccharides bind collagen fibres
- Scar formation

$$\text{Protocollagen} \xrightarrow[\text{+ Fe + Vitamin C}]{\text{Protocollagen hydroxylase}} \text{Collagen}$$

Surgeon's Role in Wound Management

- Minimise adverse effects of wound
- Remove or repair damaged tissue
- Harness the process of wound healing to restore function

Tidy Wounds

- By sharp instruments
  - Surgical incision
  - Cut from glass/knives
- No devitalized tissue
- Wound single/clean cut
- Primary healing
- Fractures not common
- Underlying arteries/nerves may be cut

Untidy Wounds

- Caused by crushing, tearing, avulsion, burns
- Devitalized tissue present in the wound
- Skin margins irregular
- Tendons/arteries/nerves exposed (damaged but not cut)
- Associated fractures common
- Managed by wound excision
  - Aim is to convert an untidy wound into a tidy wound.

5   Management of Burns

- Epidermis
  - Protection from desiccation
  - Protection from bacterial entry
  - Protection from toxins
  - Fluid balance: avoiding excess evaporative loss
  - Neurosensory
  - Social-interactive
- Dermis
  - Protection from trauma due to elasticity and durability
  - Fluid balance through regulation of skin blood flow
  - Thermoregulation through control of skin blood flow
  - Growth factors for epidermal replication and dermal repair

Management of Burns

- Stop the burning process
- Treat carbon monoxide toxicity
- Manage airway injury
- Manage pulmonary problems from smoke
- Correct chest wall restriction
- Recognize the burn induced plasma shift
- Begin fluid resuscitation for major burns
- Correct blood flow restriction from burn tissue compression

Stop the Burning Process

Flame Burns

- Eliminating any ongoing burning (i.e. from burning clothes)
- Synthetics in clothes can retain heat which needs to be neutralized
- Cover with dry clean sheets

Chemical Burn

- Chemicals continue to burn if in contact with skin
- Remove chemically contaminated clothing
- Continuous flushing with water

Management of Airway and Pulmonary Problems

Smoke Inhalation

- Major cause of morbidity and mortality
- Often life threatening
- Effects of smoke inhalation must be recognized and aggressively managed

Smoke Exposure

- Carbon monoxide toxicity—immediate peak symptoms
- Upper airway injury with potential obstruction—peak symptoms can be delayed for an hour or more
- Lower airway injury with impaired gas exchange—peak symptoms can be delayed for hours

Carbon Monoxide Toxicity

Pathophysiology

- Carbon monoxide binds to the hemoglobin molecule
- Displaces oxygen from hemoglobin
- Decreased oxygen delivered to tissue.

Risk Factors

- Any exposure to smoke
- Any exposure to fumes

Diagnosis

- A high index of suspicion
- A carboxyhemoglobin level exceeding 10% of total
- Unexplained metabolic acidosis

Treatment of Carbon Monoxide Exposure

- Awake patient
  - High flow oxygen by mask (FiO_2 100%) until carboxyhemoglobin < 5%
- Treatment of carbon monoxide exposure in unconscious patient
  - Intubate
  - Provide 100% oxygen via ventilator
  - Hyperbaric oxygen therapy is used if patient is not responding to 100% oxygen

Cyanide Toxicity

- Cyanide is found in smoke of burning polyurethane
- Diagnosis requires high index of suspicion
- Unexplained severe metabolic acidosis
- Treatment
  - Cardiopulmonary support
  - Sodium nitrite i.v. (300 mg)
  - Thiosulfate is also given which binds to cyanide to form thiocynate

Upper Airway Injury

Risk Factors

- **Oral burn:** Rapid swelling of tongue and mucosa impeding airway patency
- **Supraglottic edema:** Progression to obstruction
- **Cord and infra-glottic edema:** Progression to obstruction

Diagnosis

- History of smoke exposure or exposure to high temperature, e.g. explosion
- Direct laryngoscopic evidence of injury
  - Edema and erythema with decreasing airway lumen is noted on initial assessment
  - Symptoms of stridor, dyspnea (often delayed in onset)

Treatment

- 100% oxygen
- Airway support
- Early intubation may be required
- Transfer to burn center if smoke inhalation injury suspected

Impaired Breathing from Deep Chest Wall Burn

- Chest wall escharotomy may be required to relieve the restriction

Restoring and Maintaining Hemodynamic Stability

- Loss of plasma volume is rapid after a burn injury as fluid collects in the burn tissue
- Early fluid resuscitation is required for burns exceeding 20% of body surface.

Assessment

- Estimate percent (%) of body surface burned "Rule of Nine" (Fig. 5.1).

Aim of resuscitation

- Maintain:
  - Blood Pressure > 90 systolic
  - Urine output 0.5–1.0 ml/kg/hr
  - Pulse < 130
  - Temperature > 37°C

Fluid resuscitation protocol

- Establish and maintain adequate circulation
- Burns > 20% TBS require initial fluid resuscitation
- Use at least one large bore intravenous catheter
- Foley catheter
- Nasogastric tube
- Begin Ringer's Lactate

Amount of fluids (Parkland formula)

- 4 cc/kg/%TBS burn in 24 hours
- Giving half of the estimate in first 8 hours

Modify protocol

- Fluid requirements are greater to prevent burn shock
  - Massive burns

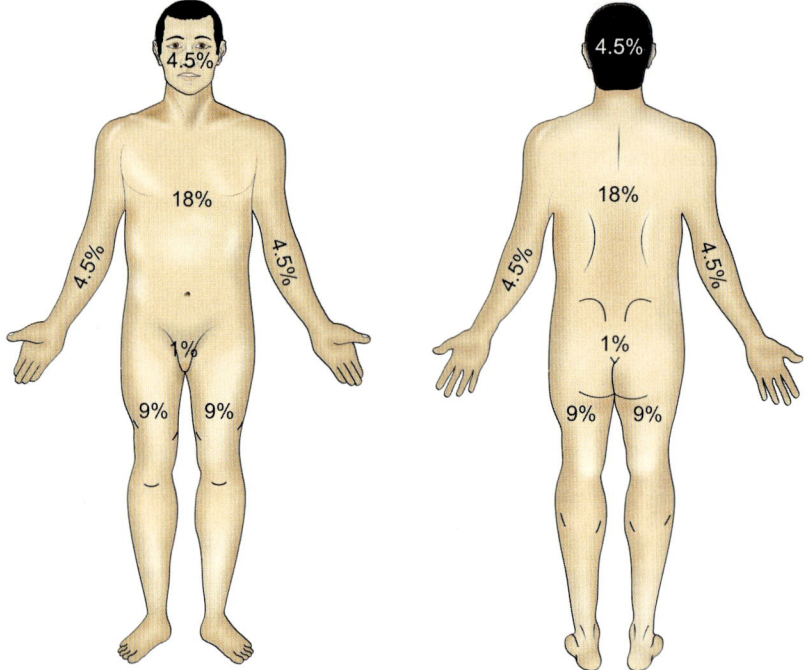

Fig. 5.1: Area of burn

- – Inhalation injury
- – Shock, and in elderly patients
- Colloids

Degree of Burn

Burn wounds can be divided into four degrees depending upon thickness of skin involvement.

1. *First degree:* Only superficial layer of epidermis is involved
2. *Second degree:* Deep layer of epidermis involved, however, skin appendage may remain intact.
3. *Third degree:* Whole of epidermis and dermis involved.
4. *Fourth degree:* Structures below dermis involved.

Transfer Criteria to a Burn Center

- Partial thickness burns greater than 10% total body surface area (TBSA)
- Burns that involve the face, hands, feet, genitalia, perineum
- Third degree burns in any age group
- Electrical burns, including lightening injury
- Chemical burns
- Patients with pre-existing medical disorders that could complicate management

- Any patient with traumatic injury (such as fractures)
- Any burned children if the hospital initially receiving the patient does not have qualified personnel or equipment for children.

Superficial partial thickness burn (Fig. 5.2)

- Clean, remove small blisters; apply grease gauze and soft gauze dressing (occlusion, absorbent dressing, changed daily).
- On face, perineum, apply bacitracin or neomycin ointment
- Use of a synthetic adhesive dressing which seals the wound and decreases pain
- Water-soluble topical antibiotic if the wound is grossly contaminated or if one is unsure if the wound is superficial or deep
- Prophylactic systemic antibiotics are not needed.

Deep partial thickness (deep second degree) burn

- Admit to burn centre due to size, i.e. > 15% TBS
- Too big for cold dressings (avoid hypothermia)
- Gently clean, debride loose tissue
- Use grease gauze or use silver sulfadiazine
- Dry gauze dressing changed at least daily

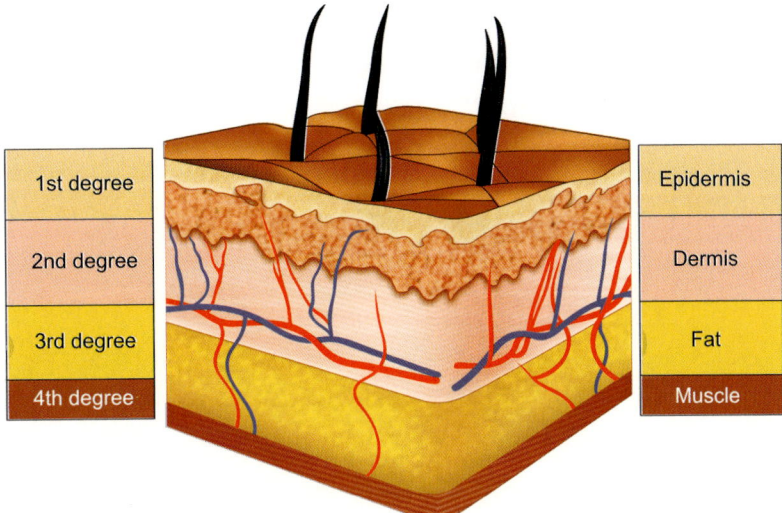

Fig. 5.2: Degree of burns

Full thickness burn
- High risk for infection due to the presence of dead tissues and lack of blood flow

- Surgical excision and grafting will be needed
- Initial use of a silver sulphadiazine dressing or cream is required

6 Metabolic Response to Surgery

- In order to mount a metabolic response to injury, the body uses glucose, fat and protein as a fuel.
- Even though protein is used as a fuel in stress, its depletion is detrimental
  - Use of protein as a fuel should be minimised.

Protein and Amino Acid Metabolism

Protein

- 15% body weight—1/2 of which is intracellular
- Present in the form of enzymes, transport, hormones, immune function, muscle
- It is not usually used as a source of energy
- When needed it is converted to glucose to be used as a fuel
- Total protein turnover — 300 g/day
- Obligatory N loss in urine — 12 g/day or 80 g protein/day
- Nitrogen balance
  - N balance = N intake – N output
  - Negative in starvation, injury, severe infection
- If protein is depleted via proteolysis, then ability to adapt in stress is compromised
- Protein depletion results in
  - Decreased wound healing
  - Decreased immune response
  - Defective gut-mucosal barrier
  - Decreased mobility/respiratory effort

Homeostatic Responses to Stress

- Designed to maintain homeostasis
- Same response in controlled or uncontrolled stress
- Trigger mechanisms:
  - Volume loss
  - Tissue damage
  - Pain
  - Fear
- Volume loss and tissue underperfusion
  - Pressure and stretch receptors activated
  - Heart rate and stroke volume increased
  - ADH/Aldosterone secreted—Renal and hypothalamic mechanism
  - Need for adequate resuscitation
- Tissue damage
  - Most important trigger
  - Neural pathways from wound reach hypothalamus
  - Efferents go to pancreas → Increased glucagon and decreased insulin secretion
  - Efferents to adrenal leads to increased cortisol and catecholamine
  - Release of cytokines
- Pain and fear
  - Increased levels of catecholmines
  - Fight or flight response
- Elective operation
  - Minimal tissue damage
  - Pain/fear managed
  - Less hypotension

- Infection rare
- Stress response is controlled
- Trauma
  - Major tissue damage
  - Excessive Pain/fear
  - Hypotension common
  - Infection common
  - Stress response uncontrolled

Table 6.1: Response to starvation vs injury

Parameter	Starvation	Trauma
Major fuel	Fat	Mixed
Ketone production	+++	+/−
Hepatic urea production	+	+++
Negative N balance	+	+++
Gluconeogenesis	+	+++
Muscle proteolysis	+	+++
Hepatic protein synthesis	+	+++

Triggers	Response
Volume loss	— Neurohormonal response
Tissue damage	— Inflammatory response
Pain and fear	— Neurohormonal response

Mediators of Stress Response

- Neurohormonal arm
  - Catecholamines, glucocorticoids, glucagon, ADH, aldosterone
    Inflammatory arm
  - Cytokines, complement, eicosanoids, PAF

Neurohormonal Arm

- Counterregulatory hormones
  - Catecholamines
    ◊ Maintain circulation
    ◊ Hepatic glycolysis, lipolysis, gluco-neogenesis
  - Glucagon
    ◊ Glycogenolytic, gluconeogenic
  - Glucocorticoids/ACTH
    ◊ Mobilise muscle protein, gluconeo-genesis
  - ADH and aldosterone
    ◊ Retain water and Na$^+$

Inflammatory Arm–Cytokines

- TNF-alpha, IL-1, IL-2, IL-6, IFN-gamma
- Local effects — para or autocrine
- Response to tissue injury
- Cytokines

- In elective surgery — confined to wound
- Trauma/sepsis-spill over/endocrine effect
- Cytokines—local effect
  - Promote wound healing
  - Stimulate angiogenesis
  - White cell migration
  - Ingrowth of fibroblasts
  - Localize the wound
- Cytokines — spill over
  - Mobilization of amino acids, stimulation of acute phase protein synthesis
  - Increase WBC counts/hypoferremia
  - Fever, subjective discomfort, sleep
  - Cytokines — severe trauma/sepsis
  - Increased organ vascular permeability
  - Multiple organ dysfunction
  - Hypotension

Stress Response

- The stress response may be classified as a adrenergic corticoid phase
- When the patient recovers the adrenergic corticoid phase changes to an anabolic phase

Adrenergic-Corticoid Phase

- ACTH and cortisol is increased which in turn mobilizes protein and leads to gluconeogenesis
- Catecholamines
  - Circulatory adjustment
  - Metabolic response if prolonged
- Aldosterone and ADH
  - Salt and water retention
- ↓ Insulin and ↑ glucagon (via epinephrine)
  - Gluconeogenesis
  - Cytokines confined to wound
- Remains until the surgical insult is corrected
- Hypermetabolism: BMR increases
  - 10–15% in elective operation
  - 25% in long bone fracture
  - 200% in 50% burn
- Altered glucose metabolism
  - Normal/low insulin and insulin resistance
  - Persisting hyperglycemia
  - Injured tissue uses glucose
- Altered protein metabolism
  - Extensive muscle protein release

- – Extensive urine N loss
- – Reduced by feeding
- Altered fat metabolism
  - – Accelerated lipolysis via hormone sensitive lipase
  - – Ketosis blunted

Anabolic Phase

- ↓ Gluconeogenesis
- ↓ Catecholamines
- ↓ Aldosterone and ADH
- Salt and water loss
- ↑ Insulin and ↓ glucagon
- Protein anabolism
- Cytokine reduction

Elective Operations

- Adrenergic corticoid phase
  - – Period of catabolism lasts 1–3 days
- Anabolic phase starts from the 3rd day onwards and continues upto the 6th day
  - – Positive N balance
  - – Protein synthesis
  - – Recovery of lean mass

Nutritional support for elective operations

- Because the adrenergic-corticoid phase is short in elective, uncomplicated surgery- nutrition with 5% dextrose is enough for up to 5–7 days

Nutritional support for severe stress

- The adrenergic-corticoid phase is prolonged in
  - – Severe injury
  - – Malnourished patients
  - – Infected patients
- Nutritional therapy is needed

Stress Responses

- The response is affected by
  - – Malnutrition
  - – Age
  - – Gender
  - – Infection

Consequences of Malnutrition

- Metabolic response needs increased energy expenditure
- If intake < expenditure — increased protein/fat mass lost

- Loss of 15% body weight interacts with disease process to
  - – Compromise immune response — sepsis, multi-organ failure
  - – Poor wound healing
  - – Edema due to ↓ albumin
  - – Reduced mobility, ↓ respiratory muscle strength and vital capacity → pneumonia
  - – Altered GI function/breached mucosal barrier

Normal Postoperative Infusion

- Energy provided as dextrose
- 1 L of D5W – 50g or 170 kcal
- Typical postoperative patient gets 500 kcal/d
- Enough to stimulate pancreatic insulin
- Not enough to support a severe stress reaction
- Need for nutritional support to match energy
- Expenditure if stress is prolonged

Metabolic Response to Trauma/Severe Surgical Stress

- Unfed trauma patients rapidly use their protein and fat stores resulting in increased susceptibility to effects of hemorrhage, operations and infection resulting in organ system failure, sepsis and death
- Malnourished patients are at greater risk

Determinants of Host Responses to Surgical Stress

Age

- Fat mass increases with age
- Loss of muscle mass
- Loss of strength with immobility
- Decreased sensitivity to perturbations
- Decreased effectiveness to maintain homeostasis

Gender

- Lean body mass less in females
- N loss more pronounced in muscular males

Invasive Infection

- May complicate any operation/injury
- Results in increased metabolic rate, fever, hyperventilation, etc.
- Nutritional depletion synergistic

Metabolic Response to Trauma/Severe Surgical Stress

It can be divided into four phases:

1. *Injury phase:* There is retention of NaCl and water and increased urinary loss of nitrogen and potassium. There is increased metabolic rate, breakdown of body fat stores and lean body mass. There is increased oxygen consumption and energy requirement varying from 10–100% depending upon severity of trauma. Injury phase lasts for 5–7 days. There is increased secretion of ACTH, growth hormone, prolactin, ADH, cortisol and aldosterone. Tumor necrosis factor (TNF), Interleukin 1, 3, 6 are released from monocytes, macrophages and lymphocytes.

2. *Turning point:* Occurs between 5–10th day. Nitrogen and potassium balance go from negative to positive. Sodium and water balance goes from positive to negative as hormonal changes are reversed.

3. *Nitrogen anabolic phase:* Corticosteroid levels have returned to normal. Under the effect of insulin, body and liver proteins are laid down. This phase may last for 4–5 weeks.

4. *Fat anabolic phase:* In this phase fat is replaced and its composition in the body returns to normal.

7 Acute Respiratory Distress Syndrome (ARDS)

- First described by Ashabaugh in 1967

Definition

ARDS is manifested as "Non-cardiogenic pulmonary edema" characterized by
- Acute onset
- Bilateral pulmonary infiltrates on Chest X-ray
- Pulmonary artery wedge pressure less than 19 mmHg
- Impaired oxygenation characterized by ratio of PaO_2 to FiO_2 less than 200
- ARDS is basically transudation of capillary fluid in to lung interstitial tissue which is diffuse and multilobar

Key Features of ARDS

- Diffuse pulmonary infiltrates
- Reduced lung compliance
- Hypoxemia refractory to increased inspired oxygen concentration
- Ventilation/perfusion mismatch which is significant
- Pulmonary capillary wedge pressure is less than 18 mm of Hg.

Pathophysiology

- Can result from
  - Direct pulmonary injury, e.g. pulmonary infection, aspiration
  - Indirect pulmonary injury e.g. sepsis, pancreatitis, multiple trauma
- Mediated by
  - Free oxygen radicals and proteolysis enzymes released by neutrophils
  - Cytokines, complement system and endo-toxins

Goals of Treatment of ARDS

- Diuretics to reduce lung edema
- Inspired oxygen concentration should be less than 60% to avoid oxygen toxicity
- Peak inspiratory pressure should be limited to 40 cm of water to avoid lung barotrauma
- Ventilation perfusion mismatch should be reduced by positive end-expiratory pressure
- Systemic oxygen delivery should be main-tained.

8 Postoperative Pulmonary Complications

Following changes occur during general anesthesia which predisposes patients to increase incidence pulmonary complications:

- Increase in right to left shunting of pulmonary blood flow
- Depression of ciliary activity of the bronchial mucosa
- Diaphragmatic elevation leading to reduced functional residual capacity and under-ventilation of lung bases
- Elevation of the diaphragm occurs due to following factors:
  - Increase in intra-abdominal pressure from GI distension
  - Pain causes reflex contraction of abdominal musculature

- Increase in bronchial secretions in habitual smokers (Table 8.1)

Postoperative pulmonary complications which are commonly seen are
- Pulmonary collapse and consolidation
- Aspiration pneumonitis
- Pneumothorax
- Pleural effusion
- Pulmonary embolism
- Respiratory insufficiency

Pulmonary Collapse

- Occurs due to impaired ventilation of lung bases and accumulation of bronchial secretions
- It can be
  - Patchy
  - Basal

Table 8.1: Patients at risk of pulmonary complications

Risk factor	Mechanism
Obesity	↓ Functional residual capacity
Chronic obstructive airway disease	↑ Bronchial secretion
	↓ Ciliary activity
Chronic smokers	↑ Bronchial secretion
	↓ Ciliary activity
Restrictive airway disease	↓ Vital capacity
Elderly patients	Aspiration
Cystic Fibrosis	Bronchial obstruction by secretions
Operative damage to recurrent laryngeal nerve ineffective cough	Aspiration

- Segmental
- Total
- Infection leading to consolidation commonly supervenes in the collapsed segment
- Infective organisms which are commonly seen are:
  - *H. influenza*
  - *Streptococcus pneumoniae*
  - *Staphylococcus aureus*
  - Coliforms or *Pseudomonas* occasionally
- Clinical features
  - Mild cases
    ◊ Asymptomatic
    ◊ Mild pyrexia
    ◊ Productive cough
  - Severe cases
    ◊ Tachypnea
    ◊ Cyanosis
    ◊ Dullness due to percussion over affected region and bronchial breathing
- Management
  - Prevention
    ◊ Chest physiotherapy to every post-operative patient
    ◊ Steam inhalation
    ◊ Deep breathing exercises (by use of incentive spirometer)
  - Treatment
    ◊ Antibiotics — start empirically with amoxycillin, till culture report is available
    ◊ Oxygen administration by mask
    ◊ Humidification of secretions by steam inhalation
    ◊ Chest physiotherapy
    ◊ In severe cases bronchoscopy and clearing of secretions by suction may help
    ◊ If secretions in airway persist, then mini-tracheotomy through crico-thyroid membrane may be needed. This will help by frequent tracheal toilet to clear secretions
    ◊ If hypoxemia persists, assisted ventilation may be required

Pulmonary Aspiration

- Minor aspiration may lead to pneumonia or pulmonary abscess
- Massive aspiration of gastric contents into broncho-pulmonary tree may be serious, often accompanied by cardio-respiratory arrest and high mortality
- Massive aspiration occurs during
  - Induction of anaesthesia
  - Endotracheal intubation
  - Recovery from general anaesthesia
- Risk factors
  - Patient undergoing anaesthesia with full stomach
  - Acute gastric dilatation
  - Paralytic ileus
- Clinical features
  - Patient markedly cyanosed
  - Increased respiratory rate with laboured breathing
  - Crepitations and decreased air entry over lung bases
- Treatment
  - Vigorous toilet suction of tracheobronchial tree
  - 100 percent oxygen through intermittent positive pressure ventilation
  - Bronchodilators like salbutamol through nebuliser
  - Methylprednisolone
  - Appropriate broad spectrum antibiotics as per culture report

Post-operative Pneumothorax

- It can occur
  - During insertion of central venous catheter
  - In patient on positive pressure ventilation
  - As a complication of laparoscopic hiatal hernia surgery like fundoplication
  - After thoracic sympathectomy and pulmonary surgery
  - After kidney surgery via intercostal or flank approach if pleura is breached
- Treatment
  - Insertion of intercostal underwater-seal drain with negative suction

9 | Infectious Diseases

- Caused by *Mycobacterium tuberculosis* which was discovered by Robert Koch in 1882 in Germany.

Primary Routes of Spread

- Direct spread to lungs by droplet infection
- From tonsils to lymph nodes in the neck
- From small gut to mesenteric lymph nodes
- Trans-placental spread
- Inoculation in the skin via BCG vaccination.

Mycobacteria

- Grows well at 37°C in LJ (Lowenstein Johnson) medium
- On direct smear they can be seen after staining by ZN (Ziehl Neelson) stain
- Growth in culture media takes 6–8 weeks
- Polymerase chain reaction (PCR) can give more rapid diagnosis.

Pathology

- The primary lesion of disease is a tubercular follicle which is a collection of chronic inflammatory cells and giant cells around the area of caseation necrosis.
- Surgeons usually see tuberculosis as local manifestation of:
  - Tubercular lymphadenitis
  - Urogenital tuberculosis
  - Intestinal tuberculosis
  - Bone and joint tuberculosis

Clinical Features

- General
  - Generalised lethargy and weakness
  - Patient feels sick
  - Lassitude
  - Poor appetite
  - Loss of weight
  - Evening rise in temperature which is low grade with night sweats
- Local features–Depend on the site involved
  - *Lymph node*
    - ◊ Cervical region commonly involved
    - ◊ Lymph nodes are enlarged, non-tender and initially discrete, but become matted to each other due to peri-adenitis later in the course of the disease
    - ◊ Caseating necrosis may progress to cold abscess. Further progression of the disease leads to rupture of the abscess so that it forms a *Collar Stud Abscess* with distinct superficial and deep components
    - ◊ The abscess when burst, opens over the skin (either spontaneously or iatrogenic) and may lead to "sinus" formation
  - *Intestinal*
    Types of intestinal tuberculosis:
    - **a. Ulcerative type:** There are multiple ulcers in the intestine placed trans-

versely. The clinical presentation is intermittent episodes of diarrhoea.

b. **Stricture type:** There are single or multiple strictures in the ileum.

c. **Ulcero-stricturing type:** There are ulcers and strictures in the small gut.

d. **Hyperplastic type:** Usually occurs in ileocaecal junction when infection occurs due to low virulent organisms and patient has high immunity.

Intestinal tuberculosis occurs either by Mycobacterium tuberculosis due to ingestion of infected sputum from open pulmonary case or by Mycobacterium bovis due to ingestion of unpasteurised milk.

◊ May present as acute or sub-acute intestinal obstruction

◊ May present as perforation peritonitis due to perforation of ulcers

◊ On examination, ileocecal mass may be palpable in right iliac fossa in hyperplastic type

- Investigations
  - Blood
    ◊ Leucocytosis with increase of lymphocytes
    ◊ Increased ESR
  - *Tuberculin test* using PPD — Area of induration:
    ◊ < 5 mm – Anergy
    ◊ 5–10 mm – Indeterminate
    ◊ >10 mm – Positive
    ◊ >15 mm – Strongly positive
  - *Diagnosis can be confirmed only by demonstrating AFB in*
    ◊ Biopsy
    ◊ Direct smear
    ◊ Culture
    ◊ PCR assay in tissue
- Treatment
  - Antitubercular drugs (ATT) as per DOTS policy for 6 months
    ◊ First 2 months — Intensive phase using 4 drugs (rifampicin, isoniazid, ethambutol and pyrazinamide).
    ◊ Next 4 months — Maintenance phase using 2 drugs (rifampicin and isoniazid).

Pathology

- Common in children and young adults
- Source of infection—tonsil
- Human bacillus responsible in more than 70% cases
- In 90% cases tuberculous process is only limited to one side

Stages of Infection

- In early disease there are discrete lymph nodes, later they get matted together
- Enlarged lymph nodes with matting
  - Multiple
    ◊ One or more groups
    ◊ Same region/different triangles
- Later stages— caseous changes
  - Matted lymph nodes with cystic areas
- Cold abscess/collar stud abscess
- Collar stud abscess with secondary infection
- Sinus or fistula formation

Clinical Presentations

- Lump in the neck
  - Painless
  - Painful: In case of complications
- Constitutional symptoms
- Fever
  - Low grade
  - Evening rise
  - Night sweats
- Anorexia
- Signs of general malaise
- Pulmonary symptoms

Approach in Management

- Examine other lymph nodes
- Catchment area
- Systemic review
- Abdominal examination: Liver/spleen

Differential Diagnosis

- Lymph node enlargement in the neck
  - Tuberculosis
    ◊ Early stage — firm, discrete lymph nodes
  - Hodgkins
  - Non hodgkins
  - Metastatic disease
- Cystic lump in the neck
  - Tuberculosis
    ◊ Caseous necrosis

- Branchial cyst
- Thyroglossal cyst
- Abnormal openings in the neck
  - Tuberculosis
    ◊ Sinuses/fistula
  - Branchial fistula
  - Thyroglossal fistula

Investigations
Laboratory Investigations
- Blood for C/P
- ESR

Tissue Diagnosis
- Most important step is FNAC/biopsy of lymph node
- Histological features
  - *Granulomatous lesions:* Central area of giant cells containing tubercle bacilli surrounded by a zone of epitheloid cells
  - *Tubercle:* A granuloma surrounded by fibrous tissue undergoing central caseous necrosis
  - Healing occurs by fibrosis and calcification.

Others
- Tuberculin test
- Culture and sensitivity of tuberculous aspirate
- Chest X-Ray

Treatment
- General management
  - Attention to nutrition and general health
- Specific measures
  - Anti-tuberculous drugs

Anti-Tuberculous Drugs
- First line drugs
  - Rifampicin 10–20 mg/kg
  - Isoniazid 15 mg/kg
  - Ethambutol 15 mg/kg
  - Pyrizinamide 20–30 mg/kg
- Second line drugs
  - Streptomycin
  - Quinolones
  - Cephalosporins
  - Only warranted if there is resistance to any of the first line drugs or in case of MDR-TB

- Baseline investigations
  - ESR
  - LFT
  - CXR
  - Fundoscopy
- Duration
  - 04 drug combination for 02 months
    ◊ Rifampicin + Isoniazid + Ethambutol + Pyrazinamide
    - 02 drug combination for 04 months (at least)
    ◊ Rifampicin + Isoniazid

Indications for Surgery
- Abscess
- Sinuses and fistulae

TUBERCULAR EPIDIDYMO-ORCHITIS

Clinical Features
- 2/3rd of the cases have a past history of tuberculosis or active tuberculosis
- Dull aching pain in the scrotum
- Enlarged irregularly nodular (craggy) firm and non-tender epididymis
- Scrotal skin may be:
  - Free
  - Adherent to epididymis
  - May have a cold abscess
  - Sinus or ulcer on the posterior aspect of the scrotum
- Vas may be beaded due to submucous tubercles
- Lax hydrocele may be present in 30% of cases
- On per rectal examination irregular indurated seminal vesicle may be palpable

Investigations
- Complete hemogram with ESR
- X-ray chest
- Urine examination
- USG guided FNAC from the epididymis
- CT urography to rule out renal involvement

Treatment
- Administration of ATT and application of scrotal support

Surgery
May be indicated in the presence of:
- Residual disease
- Scrotal sinus
- If testicular involvement is present

ANATOMICAL BASIS OF PRESENTATION OF COLD ABSCESSES AT VARIOUS SITES

From Cervical Vertebrae

Retropharyngeal

- Bulge over the pharynx
- Lies behind the pre-vertebral fascia and is central in position in contrast with the acute retropharyngeal abscess which lies to one side of midline and is anterior to the pre-vertebral fascia

At the Posterior Border of the Sternocleidomastoid (SCM)

- Abscess tracks laterally behind pre-vertebral fascia
- Appears in posterior triangle of neck near the posterior border of SCM (Bezold's abscess)
- **In the mediastinum:** Abscess tracks down to posterior mediastinum
- **Back of the neck:** Tracks along posterior division of spinal nerve and appears on one side of the neck and back
- **Axilla:** Tracks under the pre-vertebral fascia, enters open mouth of axillary sheath and then tracks along branches of nerves and arteries.

From Thoracic Vertebrae

- May remain pre-vertebral in posterior medias-tinum
- Tracks down in posterior mediastinum to enter one of the three openings:

a. Behind lateral lumbocostal arch
↓
Tracks down between anterior layer of thoracolumbar fascia and quadratus lumborum
↓
May remain here behind kidney
↓
May extend forward and anteriorly along the 12th thoracic, ilioinguinal and iliohypogastric nerve
↓
Extend into lower and anterior abdominal wall

b. Behind medial lumbocostal arch
↓
Enters open end of psoas sheath

↓
After entering this sheath, goes down unimpeded up to insertion of psoas into lesser trochanter and appears in thigh as a swelling (pushing the femoral vessels laterally)

c. Behind median arcuate ligament

Cold abscess extends down into the abdomen along the aorta and can extend along its branches besides the thoracic nerves:

a. Upto anterior end of intercostal space in thorax or rectus sheath
b. Extends along lateral cutaneous branch of intercostal nerve and appears at mid-axillary line where lateral cutaneous nerve becomes subcutaneous
c. Extends along posterior division of thoracic nerve and appears over the back at one inch (along medial branch) or three inches (along lateral branch) from the midline.

From Lumbar Vertebrae

- Extends along aorta and its branches:
  - Along Internal pudendal artery into the ischiorectal fossa
  - Along superior gluteal artery and appears in the buttock
- Follows course of the lumbar nerve and appears in the thigh along the femoral or obturator nerve or in the back
- Extends between flat muscles of abdominal wall and presents in the triangle of Petit
- Extends along sheath of psoas or quadratus lumborum

TETANUS

- Caused by *Clostridium tetani* which is a gram positive anaerobic rod with terminal spores giving it a *drumstick* appearance.

Routes of Infection

- Division of umbilical cord in neonates by infected or rusted instruments
- Deeply contused wound contaminated with foreign body, soil or dirt and dead or necrotic tissue which reduces oxygen tension
- Road traffic accidents
- Agricultural injuries contaminated with soil
- Endogenous infection after septic abortion

Pathology

Tetano-spasmin

- It has high affinity for nerves.
- It reaches CNS by axons of motor nerve trunks.
- Toxin causes extreme hyper excitability of the motor neurons in anterior horn cells. This results in widespread and explosive reflex spasm in response to sensory stimuli.
- Toxin fixed to CNS cannot be neutralized. Only circulating toxin can be neutralized by the anti-toxin antibodies so anti-tetanus should be administered early in the course of disease.

Favourable Conditions for Growth of Organisms

- Low immunity
- Foreign body
- Injury
- Improper sterilization
- Devitalized tissue
- Anaerobic conditions in the wound

Special Types of Tetanus with Poor Prognosis

- Tetanus neonatorum
- Cephalic tetanus
  - Through wounds of face and head
  - Cranial nerves are involved
- Bulbar tetanus
  - Muscles of deglutition and respiration are involved
- Post-operative tetanus

Signs and Symptoms

- *Trismus* / Lock jaw – Most common condition due to contraction of masseter muscle
- Dysphagia due to spasm of pharyngeal muscles
- Neck rigidity
- *Opisthotonus* (arched back) due to rigidity of back muscles
- *Risus sardonicus* – Spasm of facial and jaw muscles
- Generalized convulsions – Muscles do not relax between convulsive attacks (differential of strychnine poisoning)
- Mild fever
- Tachycardia

Causes of Death

- Aspiration pneumonia
- Laryngeal spasm
- Respiratory arrest

Treatment

Prophylaxis

- Active immunization by tetanus toxoid
- Three injections
  - First – at the time of injury
  - Second – 6 weeks later
  - Third – 6–12 months after the second dose
- Booster – 10 years interval and at the time of wound. No booster is required if injury occurs within 5 years of completion of an active immunization course or booster dose
- If no immunization or booster dose taken for >10 years, then
  - Tetanus Immunoglobulin (TIG) 250 µg intramuscular (i.m.) indicated
  - Active immunization started at the same time using a different limb

Active Treatment

- Objective
  - To reduce the risk of mortality from spasm or pneumonia
- General
  - Isolation in dark room
  - Injection tetanus toxoid 0.5 ml i.m.
  - TIG 500 U i.m. to limit the effects of free toxin
  - Antibiotics, e.g. penicillin and metronidazole
- Specific
  - Mild cases (tonic rigidity alone)
    ◊ Sedation by barbiturates (e.g. diazepam)
    ◊ Muscle relaxation (e.g. Promazine)
  - Seriously ill patient (dysphagia and reflex muscle spasm)
    ◊ Treatment as for mild cases
    ◊ Nasogastric tube for nutrition
    ◊ Tracheostomy if the patient has difficulty in breathing
  - Dangerously ill patient (major cyanotic convulsions)
    ◊ Intubation and intermittent positive pressure ventilation (IPPV) after giving muscle relaxant (e.g. Pancuronium)

- Mortality can be reduced to 15% by
  - Proper nursing care
  - Prophylactic antibiotics
  - Active/passive immunization
  - Tracheostomy, if indicated
  - Assisted ventilation

GAS GANGRENE

- Causative organisms — mixed clostridia infection caused by both saccharolytic and proteolytic organisms
- True pathogens are
  - *Clostridium perfringens*
  - *Clostridium novyi*
  - *Clostridium septicum*

Pathology

- Various toxins produced are
  - α-toxin (Lecithinase) – Breaks down phospholipid component of RBC causing haemolysis
  - Collagenase
  - Hyaluronidase
  - Deoxyribonuclease
- Exotoxins cause cellulitis and myonecrosis. The necrosis of muscles leads to fermentation of muscle carbohydrates releasing lactic acid, hydrogen and CO_2. The discharge is initially odourless, which later becomes fishy. Initially all dead muscles are odourless and brick red in colour, but later become greenish black due to putrefaction.
- Spread of gangrene occurs due to
  - Exotoxin release
  - Ischemia from pressure from gas and exudate within a tight muscle compartment

Incidence

- Occurs only in wounds having reduced oxygen tension which is required for spore germination
- Low oxygen tension is found in
  - Severely contused and lacerated wounds with necrotic tissue
  - Devitalized wounds with impaired blood supply
  - Foreign bodies implanted in the depth of a wound
  - Wounds contaminated with soil
  - Coexisting infections with pyogenic organisms
- Majority of gas gangrene infections are exogenous and occur in
  - Large wounds as in agricultural injuries
  - Road traffic accidents
  - In compound fractures
  - War injuries
- Endogenous infection occurs due to contamination by bowel organisms as in
  - Following amputation for peripheral vascular disease when associated with incontinence
  - Criminal abortion
  - Following intestinal or biliary surgery

Clinical Features

- Acute onset
- Incubation period – 3 days (1 day to 4 weeks)
- Pain in the region of wound
- Fever, tachycardia, toxaemia, drowsiness
- Affected area is swollen, tense and tender
- There is fishy, foul smelling, serous or blood stained discharge
- Gas in underneath tissue is detected by crepitus or by X-ray examination
- Overlying skin may be
  - White
  - Red with bullae formation
  - Greenish black due to gangrene
- Terminal events
  - Jaundice
  - Haemolysis
  - Renal failure
- Mortality – 40%

Treatment

- General measures for treatment of shock
- Specific therapy
  - Antibiotics
  - Antitoxin
  - Surgical treatment
  - Hyperbaric oxygen

Antibiotics

- Benzyl penicillin is the drug of choice – 1–2 Mega units q4–6 hourly
- Metronidazole – Loading dose 15mg/kg i.v., not to exceed 4g/day; Maintenance dose –

7.5mg/kg PO/IV (over 1 hour) q 6 hourly for 2–3 weeks

- Clindamycin – 150–450 mg PO q6–8 hourly, not to exceed 1.8g/day; 1.2–2.7 g/day i.v./i.m. divided q6–12hrs; not to exceed 4.8g/day
- Vancomycin – 2 g/day divided q6–12hrs; may increase based on body weight or to achieve higher trough values; maintain trough values 15–20 mg

Antitoxin
- Anti-gas gangrene serum

Surgical treatment
- Evacuation of pus
- Excision of all necrotic tissue – aggressive excision is vital part of therapy
- In lower limbs, it usually amounts to amputation.

10   Madura Foot

- Chronic infective granulomatous condition of subcutaneous tissue of the feet
- It is more prevalent in tropical countries. In India, it is endemic in Madura district of South India

Causative Organisms

- Bacterial Mycetoma—filamentous organisms
  - *Nocardia madurae*
  - *Streptomyces madurae*
- Fungal mycetoma
- Madura mycosis

These organisms grow in soil and road dust

Portal of Entry

These organisms gain entry into human host through a trivial injury, e.g. prick into the skin and subcutaneous tissue in bare footed subjects

Effects of Infection

- Destruction of deeper tissues
- Appearance of multiple sinuses
- Escape of colored granules through sinuses

Clinical Features

- Firm painless pale subcutaneous nodules on the sole of the feet
- Vesicles appear on the nodule and nodules burst
- Formation of discharging sinuses with surrounding skin having bluish discoloration
- Discharge may be yellow (due to *Streptomyces*), red (due to *Nocardia*) or black (due to *Madura mycosis*)
- No lymphadenitis because filaments are too big to travel through lymphatics
- Grossly swollen foot with flattening of instep

X-Ray

- Multiple cystic cavitations in the bone without new bone formation (Honey comb appearance)

Treatment

- Dapsone 100 mg twice a day for two years
- Iodine helps in resolution of fibrosis
- Antibiotics, e.g. penicillin or tetracycline
- Surgery
  - Multiple incisions and drainage of sinuses

11 | Diabetic Foot

- Spectrum of foot disorders ranging from ulceration to gangrene occurring in diabetics as a result of peripheral neuropathy or ischemia or both

Incidence

- It is seen in 15–20% of diabetic patients
- It is more common in between 45–65 years of age

Pathophysiology

Three distinct processes lead to the problem of diabetic foot

- Ischemia due to macroangiopathy or microangiopathy
- Neuropathy — sensory, motor and autonomic
- Sepsis — glucose saturated tissue provides a good culture media for bacterial growth.

Ischemia

Macroangiopathy

- It is similar to atherosclerotic occlusive disease, except that:
  - It occurs at an early age
  - It involves men and women equally
  - Tibial and peroneal vessels are more commonly involved than aorta or iliac vessels

Microangiopathy

- It is characterized by
  - Thickening of arteriolar and capillary basement membrane leading to inability of capillaries to vasodilate in response to injury leading to functional ischemia of the skin
  - Basement membrane thickening leads to less migration of WBCs at the site of injury leading to infection and ulceration.

Autonomic Neuropathy

Inability to dilate small vessels in response to injury.

Clinical Features

Neuropathic Features

- Sensory disturbances
- Trophic changes
- Plantar ulceration
- Degenerative arthropathy known as "Charcot's Joints"
- Neuropathic ulcers are deep and painless. They are present over pressure points, e.g. plantar aspect of foot or big toe.
- Feet are warm
- All pedal pulses are present
- No intermittent claudication

Ischemic Features

- Rest pain and history of intermittent claudication
- Feet may be cold
- Reduced or absent pulses
- Ischemic ulcers are painful, present over toes or medial aspect of first or fifth metatarsal.

Sepsis can occur in both neuropathic and ischemic ulcers and can lead to

- Cellulitis
- Deep tissue abscess
- Osteomyelitis
- Gangrene

Usual organisms are *Staphylococci, Streptococci, E. coli* and anerobic bacteria.

Investigations

- Plain X-ray of the foot to rule out
  - Osteomyelitis – lytic lesions
  - Invasive soft tissue infection suggested by the presence of gas in subcutaneous tissue
- Ankle brachial index (ABI)
  - Ratio of ankle systolic blood pressure and arm systolic pressure (better of the two arms chosen).
  - ≥ 1.0 Normal
    - 0.5   Claudication
    - < 0.3 Severe ischemia
- Due to medial calcification, arteries are relatively incompressible and ABI may be falsely normal
- Digital blood pressure — 30–40 mmHg suggests adequate perfusion
- Transcutaneous oxygen tension of skin of foot if > 30 mm Hg, is consistent with wound healing
- Angiography to identify the site of block
  - MR angiography
  - Digital subtraction angiography

Management

Advice for Foot Care

Do's
- Carefully wash and dry feet daily
- Inspect feet daily for injury
- Meticulous care of toenails
- Use antifungal powder on feet daily.

Dont's
- Walk bare footed
- Wear ill fitted shoes
- Use a hot water bottle
- Ignore any foot injury.

Treatment

Aim is control of infection and removal of necrotic tissue.

- Broad spectrum antibiotics intravenously in the form of metronidazole, ampicillin and gentamicin. If renal function is impaired, a third generation cephalosporin can be used.
- Wound debridement
  - Local removal of callus or slough
  - Drainage of abscesses and removal of dead or necrotic tissue
- Control of blood sugar
- Dressings — initially with povidone iodine, later on with normal saline, calcium alginate or petroleum gauze dressings.
- If ischemic disease, arterial bypass using an autogenous saphenous vein grafting may be needed.

12 | Amputations

When the Limb is
- Dead
- Deadly
- Deformed

Dead
- Limb destroyed by severe trauma in blunt or crush injuries and reconstruction not possible
- Severe vascular injury of major vessels where reconstruction has failed or is not possible
- Gangren of limb due to severe peripheral vascular disease
- Severe rest pain or critically ischemic limb where limb cannot be salvaged.

Deadly
- Soft tissue sarcoma or bone sarcoma where limb preserving resection is not possible
- Subungual melanoma
- Infected spreading gangrene
- Gas gangrene
- End stage diabetic foot
- Actinomycosis of foot when medical treatment has failed
- Chronic osteomyelitis of foot not responding to treatment.

Deformed
- Deformed, shortened or unstable lower limb hampers the day to day life of the patient and patient wants the surgery.

Stump Length
- Should be of adequate length for fitting the prosthesis
- Hand should be preserved as much as possible
- Upper arm/forearm – 20 cm stump
- Below knee – 15 cm tibial stump
- Above knee – 25–30 cm stump
- Amputation through joint is more appropriately called disarticulation and should be avoided.

Site of Division
- Above knee – 11" from the tip of greater trochanter
- Below knee – 5–6" from the knee joint
- Above elbow – 8" from the tip of acromion
- Below elbow – 7" from tip of olecranon

Features of Ideal Stump
- Should be conical in shape
- No projecting bony spurs should be present
- No redundant muscle mass over stump
- Terminal scar should be transverse

- Skin should not be adherent to underlying structures
- Skin should not be loose or thin over the stump
- Free from tenderness
- Joint above stump should be fully mobile

Methods of Amputation

- **Guillotine method:** This method is used in case of infective pathology, wet gangrene or if line of demarcation is not clearly demarcated. Stump is left open till infection is fully controlled.
- **Flap method:** Stump is closed either by long posterior flap or by skew flap method

Complications of Amputation

- Bleeding
- Infection
  - In soft tissue
  - In bony stump
- Necrosis of skin flap
- Adherent scar
  - Infection
  - Suturing of skin
  - Necrosis of skin flaps
- Painful stump neuroma
- Phantom limb
- Causalgia — pain, tenderness and redness at the end of stump
- Jactitation — intermittent distressing spasms in the stump
- Stiffnes of proximal joint

13 | Examination of an Ulcer

An ulcer is defined as break in the continuity of surface epithelium due to some pathological process leading to necrosis or death of cell. It has a floor, a base, edges and margins.

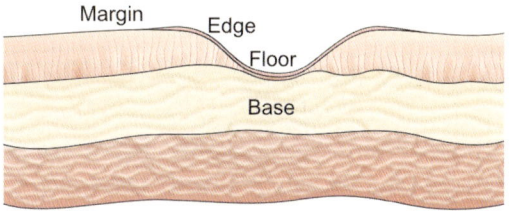

Fig. 13.1: Parts of an ulcer

CLASSIFICATION OF ULCER

Based on Stage of Healing

- **Spreading or active ulcer:** This type of ulcer has sero-purulent discharge with surrounding inflammation without any granulation tissue.
- **Healing ulcer:** This type of ulcer has slopping edge with red granulation tissue without any discharge.
- **Non healing ulcer:** Ulcer with no tendency to heal with pale granulation tissue.

On Duration

Ulcer can be acute or chronic. Any ulcer present for less than 12 weeks of duration is known as acute and if it is more than 12 weeks of duration it is known as chronic.

Ulcer can become chronic in following conditions:
- Poor general condition of patient like anemia and malnutrition
- Patient having immunosuppression like HIV, patient on long term corticosteroid therapy, patient on immunosuppressive therapy like post transplant, patient suffering from diabetes or uremia.
- If there is source of chronic irritation of the ulcer, e.g. carious tooth or with foreign body, e.g. mesh
- Ulcer occurring in an irradiated area
- Ulcer associated with arterial or venous disorders
- Ulcer associated with neuropathy
- If malignant change has occurred in an ulcer, e.g. marjolins ulcer or ulcer associated with malignancy
- Ulcer associated with specific chronic infection like tuberculosis until unless chronic infection is taken care of.

Inspection

Size
- Measure in 2 dimensions with a measuring tape

Shape
- Oval, round, irregular

Number
- Single or multiple similar ulcers, e.g. bed sores.

Site

- **Varicose ulcer:** Gaiter's area above the medial malleolus
- **Rodent ulcers:** Above a line joining the angle of the mouth to the lobule of the ear
- **Trophic or naturopathic ulcers:** Weight bearing areas
- Bed sores over pressure points
- Ischemic (arterial ulcers)
- **T.B. ulcers:** In the neck over the site of tubercular lymphadenitis

Margin

- It is the *border* or *transition zone* of the skin around the ulcer.
- It is the *line demarcating* the ulcer from intact surrounding skin.
- There are 3 types of margins:
  - Healing margin
  - Inflamed margin
  - Fibrosed margin

Healing margin

- Shows 3 zones
  - Outer **white:** Zone of cornified epithelium
  - Middle **bluish:** Line of growing squamous epithelium without cornification
  - Inner **red:** Covered by a single layer of squamous epithelium

Inflamed margin

- It is characterized by spreading irregular red margin with inflamed surrounding skin.

Fibrosed margin

- There is marked fibrosis with thickened white skin margins without the blue line of healing epithelium.

Edge

- It is the junction between the floor and the margin of the ulcer.
- It has thickness and can be palpated.
- There are 5 types:
  - **Sloping edge:** Healing ulcer
  - **Punched edge:** Trophic ulcer
  - **Undermined edge:** Tuberculous ulcer
  - **Everted edge:** Malignant ulcer
  - **Raised (heaped) edge:** Rodent ulcer

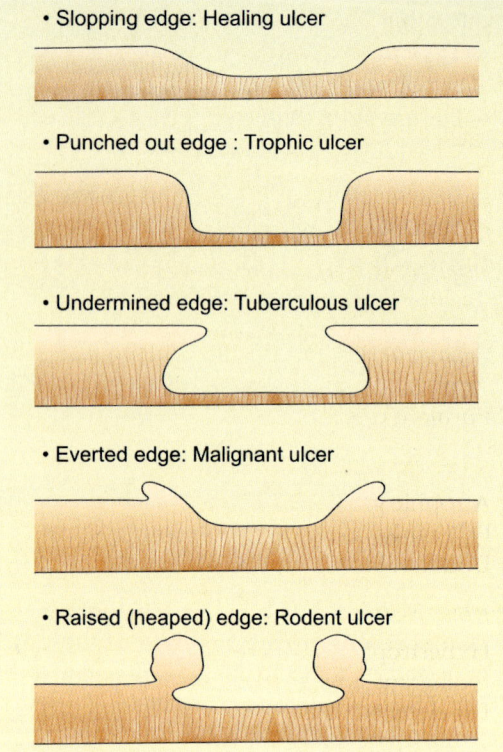

- Slopping edge: Healing ulcer
- Punched out edge : Trophic ulcer
- Undermined edge: Tuberculous ulcer
- Everted edge: Malignant ulcer
- Raised (heaped) edge: Rodent ulcer

Fig. 13.2: Types of edges in an ulcer

Sloping Edge

- It is seen in a healing ulcer.
- Granulation tissue is slightly below the skin surface and the skin gradually thins out.

Punched Edge

- In a trophic ulcer, tissue destruction is equal in all planes from skin to bone so the edge is vertical. It is seen in decubitus ulcer/gummatous ulcer.

Undermined Edge

- Tissue destruction is deeper to the skin so that the skin overhangs the ulcer. It is classically seen in a tubercular ulcer.

Raised Everted Edge

- Malignant tissue grows very fast and overhangs the skin; the ulcer itself is raised above the skin level. It is seen in squamous cell carcinoma.

Raised not Everted Edge (Rolled in)

- In a rodent ulcer due to tissue destruction

Floor

- It is the exposed visible surface of the ulcer.

- One should note:
  - Type of granulation tissue
  - Amount of slough (necrotic tissue)
  - Nature of discharge

Healthy Ulcer Floor

- Healthy granulation tissue
- No slough
- Small amount of serous discharge

Spreading or Infected Ulcer Floor

- Unhealthy granulation tissue
- Areas of slough
- Purulent discharge

Chronic Non-healing Ulcer Floor

- Atrophic granulation tissue
- Pale white
- Does not bleed on touch

Chronic Non-healing Ulcer Floor can also Show

- Hypertrophic granulation tissue or proud flesh
- Exuberant growth above the skin surface
- Excessive serosanguinous or purulent discharge

Surrounding Skin

- **Infected ulcers:** Red, shiny and edematous
- **Varicose ulcer:** Dark pigmented skin (lipo-dermatosclerosis)
- **Tuberculous ulcers:** Multiple scars and puckering
- **Ulcer within a large scar:** Marjolin's ulcer

Marjolin's Ulcer

- Aggressive ulcerating squamous cell carcinoma presenting in an area of previously traumatized, chronically inflamed, or scarred skin.
- They are commonly present in chronic wounds including burn injuries, venous ulcers, ulcers from osteomyelitis, and post radiotherapy scars. In these ulcers although malignant there is no involvement of regional lymph nodes as lymphatics in the area of ulcer have been destroyed by chronic inflammation.
- The term was named after French surgeon, Jean Nicolas Marjolin, who first described the condition in 1828. The term was later coined by J C De Costa.

Palpation

Surrounding Skin should be Palpated

- For raised temperature by back of the hand
- For tenderness by gentle finger palpation

Edge

- **Soft:** Healing ulcer
- **Firm:** Non-healing ulcer
- **Hard:** Malignant ulcer

Floor

- Bleeding on touch
  - Pin point spots (healthy granulation tissue)
  - Profuse (malignant ulcer)
- Note whether slough is loose or fixed

Base

- It is the tissue on which the ulcer rests or lies
- It cannot be seen
- Palpate the consistency of the base
- Palpate the underlying structures
- **Small ulcers:** Pinch between fingers
- **Large ulcers:** Feel through the floor
- **Firm base:** Chronic fibrosis
- **Hard base:** Suspect malignancy

Fixity to Underlying Structures

- Move the ulcer in 2 different directions
- If over a muscle, contract the muscle or make it taut and retest the mobility at right angles to the muscle fibres

Regional Examination

Regional Lymph Nodes

- **Hard, discrete/matted, non-tender, fixed:** Malignant
- **Soft, tender:** Infective
- **Non- tender, matted:** Tuberculosis

Related Arteries, Veins and Nerves

- Test for varicose veins and peripheral vascular disease

Nearby Joint Movement

- Active and passive
- **Restricted movement:** Muscle or tendon involvement or tenderness from inflammation

Systemic Examination

- **Cardiovascular system:** For evidence of CHF, murmurs
- **Respiratory system:** Crepitations , rales
- **Abdomen:** For splenomegaly, abdominal aortic aneurysm.

14 | Ingrowing Toe Nail

Toe nail is said to be ingrowing when edge of the nail digs into the toe substance at the lateral nail fold.

Predisposing Factors

- Tight fitting shoes causing pressure on the lateral nail fold
- Cutting the nail too short and convexly rather than transversely
- Excessive sweating of feet
- Poor hygiene.

Pathology

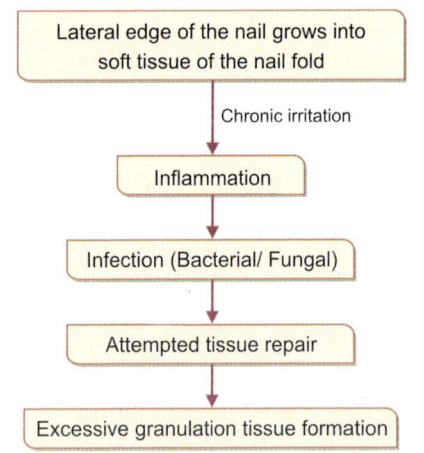

Fig. 14.1: Etiopathogenesis of ingrowing toe nail

Presentation

- Nail fold riding up on to the nail
- Grossly infected, painful nail fold with cellulitis and discharging granulation tissue
- Toe is swollen and wide due to edematous skin at the nail fold
- Skin of the lateral nail fold may be reddish blue

Management

Conservative

- In early cases
- Remove all source of pressure
- Daily packing of lateral groove with gauze soaked in antiseptic solution, to help the nail grow out from the nail fold
- Nail edge may be lifted out of its groove by elevation with a sharp instrument

Surgery

- Avulsion of whole nail
- Avulsion of the side of the nail that is ingrowing
- Wedge resection of the 25% of the width of the nail and the nail bed of the affected side
- Zadek's operation – done in recurrent cases.
  - Entire nail bed is removed surgically so that the nail does not regrow.

15 Sterilization and Disinfection

- It can be defined as complete destruction of all microorganisms including spores, viruses and mycobacterium.
- After effective sterilization the probability of a viable microorganism surviving is 1 in a million times.
- The term is applied only to equipments.

Methods of Sterilization

- Steam
- Hot air
- Ethylene oxide
- Low temperature steam and formaldehyde (LTSF)
- Gamma rays irradiation.

Steam

- *Principle:* Steam under pressure attains higher temperature than boiling water. This is so because temperature attained is directly related to pressure (Charles' Law)
- Used only for metallic instruments
- Autoclave machines are used to generate high pressure steam
- Instruments should be cleaned thoroughly before autoclaving
- Instruments are autoclaved at either
  - 121°C for 15 minutes at pressure of 15 lbs/sq. inch (psi) or
  - 134°C for 3 minutes at pressure of 30 lbs/sq. inch (psi)
- Total cycle of 30 minutes is involved which includes
  - Heating and time required to attain the desired pressure
  - Hold-up time (15 minutes)
  - Cooling
- Steam under pressure can kill all organisms except viruses responsible for *Spongiform Encephalopathy*. Non-disposable instruments exposed to a patient of Spongiform Encephalopathy should be autoclaved at 134°C for 18 minutes
- *Advantages:*
  - Short time
  - Low cost
  - Does not affect environment
  - No toxic residues
- *Drawbacks:*
  - Steam is corrosive to sharp instruments
  - Cannot be used for endoscopes and for other delicate instruments
- *Disadvantages:*
  - High initial cost of installation
  - Operator at risk of getting burnt
  - Regular maintenance of machine needed
- Instruments, gowns and towels are sterilized by steam.

Sterilization by Hot Air

- Dry heat kills all microorganisms at 160°C when allowed for a holding time of 2 hours or more.
- *It is used for:*
  - Ointments
  - Powders
  - Sharp instruments
  - Non-aqueous liquids
  - Air tight containers
  - Ophthalmic instruments with fine cutting edges
- *Hot air sterilization is contraindicated for:*
  - Aqueous fluids
  - Rubber and plastics
- *Advantages of hot air sterilization are:*
  - Less corrosive than steam
  - Non-toxic
  - Dry heat cabinet is simple to install
  - Low in operating cost
- *Disadvantages of hot air sterilization are:*
  - Long time required
  - High temperature not suitable for many materials.

Sterilization by Ethylene Oxide (EO)

- Highly penetrative
- Does not cause corrosion of instruments
- It can destroy all bacteria, spores and viruses
- Used in industries/hospitals as a low temperature sterilization method
- *Drawbacks:*
  - Toxic
  - Irritant
  - Mutagenic
  - Carcinogenic
  - Flammable
  - Expensive
- *ETO is used for:*
  - Wrapped/unwrapped heat sensitive equipment.
  - Ideal for electrical equipment.
  - Flexible — fibre-optic endoscopes.
  - Photographic equipment.
  - Medical devices made up of plastic and rubber, e.g. syringes catheters.
  - Laparoscopic hand instruments
- *Not advised for:*
  - Ventilator equipment
  - Items soiled with organic material

Sterilization by Low Temperature Steam and Formaldehyde (LTSF)

- It uses combination of dry saturated steam and formaldehyde
- Low temperature of 73°C is used
- *Can be used for* heat sensitive equipment and for plastic items
- *Not used for:*
  - Items contaminated with body fluids, since hardened fixed protein deposits will result
  - Endoscopes and narrow bore tubings

Sterilization by Irradiation

- Gamma rays or accelerated electrons are used
- Industrial process
- Useful for large batches of similar single use items like catheters and syringes

Disinfection and Cleaning

- Disinfection is a process by which numbers of viable microorganisms are reduced to an acceptable level
- Some viruses and spores may not be inactivated
- Cleaning is a process of removing all visible foreign materials from objects and is an essential prerequisite for sterilization and disinfection
- Cleaning can be done by:
  - Water
  - Mechanical action
  - Detergents
  - Ultrasonic energy.

Efficiency of disinfection depends upon

- Prior cleaning
- Quantum of organic load and contamination
- Concentration and contact time of disinfectant
- Temperature
- pH.

Common Methods of Disinfection

2% Glutaraldehyde Solution

- Most convenient and effective solution
- Effective at a pH of 7.5 to 8.5
- Shelf life after preparation is 14 days
- In 10 minutes contact time, it disinfects by killing gram positive and gram negative bacteria and viruses
- Sterilizes in 4 hours
- Ideal for endoscopes and respiratory equipment
- Gloves should be used while handling the solution to prevent allergic reactions.

Boiling Water

- Kills vegetative bacteria, some viruses and some spores
- Soft water at 100°C for 5 minutes at normal pressure is satisfactory
- Suitable for proctoscopes, speculums and sigmoidoscopes.

Formaldehyde

- Broad spectrum antimicrobial agent
- Under optimal conditions of concentration, exposure time, and relative humidity, it can be used as a disinfecting agent
- Has limited sporicidal action
- *Used for* ventilators, suction pumps and incubators
- *Drawbacks:*
  - Hazardous substance
  - Explosive
  - Irritant to eyes, skin and the respiratory tract.

16 | Scrubbing, Gowning and Gloving Technique

- Effectively reduce the number of micro-organisms on the skin by mechanical washing.

Microorganisms on Skin

- **Transient:** Introduced by soil, dirt, contamination
- **Resident:** Under finger nails, deeper layers of skin, i.e. sweat gland, hair follicles and sweat glands
- Scrubbing removes
  - Most of transient bacteria
  - Resident bacteria from surface and just beneath skin.

Theatre Etiquettes

Preparation for Scrubbing

- Personal hygiene should be maintained
- Shower taken before entering theatre
- Healthy skin on hands, fingers, nails and arms
- No boil, abrasion or wound on hands
- Free from cold or URTI.

Finger Nails

- Short and not over tips of fingers
- Short nails are easy to clean
- Will not puncture gloves
- Free from nail polish as chipped nail polish can harbour bacteria
- No artificial nails should be worn as fungal growth can occur beneath them.

Jewellery

- Remove all jewellery, i.e. rings, watches, bracelets from hands and arms
- Keep them at a safe place or in pocket
- Dead skin accumulate beneath rings and watches.

Theatre Attire

- Scrub suit
- Surgical cap and face mask
- Eye wear/Wiser
- Shoes
- Protective wearing
- Plastic apron
- Lead apron.

Scrub Suit

- Street clothes not allowed
- Short sleeved cotton scrub suit
- Sleeves 4 inches above elbow
- Shirt tucked in trouser to avoid shirt tail flapping on sterile field
- Trouser legs not touching floor to avoid transport of bacteria.

Shoes

- Street shoes not allowed
- Close ended shoes
- Flip flops or open ended shoes not allowed
- Shoe cover for single use only.

Surgical Cap and Face Mask

- Surgical cap cover hair completely
- Including pierced ear rings
- Face mask cover nose and mouth completely.

Protective Clothing

- Lead apron if radiation exposure
- Plastic apron in every case.

Areas of the Operative Suite (Traffic Patterns)

- Unrestricted — street clothes permitted
- Semi-restricted — must have scrub attire and cap
- Restricted — masks required.

Food/Drink

- No food or drinks in patient care areas
- Food/drinks must be consumed in staff lounges.

Scrubbing

Agents

- Soap 5 minutes
- **Povidone iodine solution:** 2minutes (8 ml required)
- **Chlorhexidine solution:** 2 minutes (8 ml needed).

Desirable Properties of Scrubbing Agent

- Non irritating to skin
- Leaves minimum bacteria on skin
- Prolonged antibacterial effect on skin
- Should lather in hot, cold or hard water.

Scrub Technique

- Scrubbing do not include rinsing time
- Set water temperature
- Wet hands and forearms
- Hold soap in hands till scrubbing is complete

- Keep hands elevated above elbow throughout
- Turn off taps with elbows
- Keep hands elevated.
- Skin should be blotted dry
- Use 2 towels
- Towel should be folded
- Discard towel immediately.

Gowning Procedure

- Pick up gown from opened pack
- Gown is folded with the inside uppermost.
- Slide both arms into gown
- Not to touch outside the gown.
- All gowns must be in a good state.

Parameters of a Sterile Gown

- Gowns are considered sterile from waist level to chest level including sleeves to 2" above elbow
- Stockinette cuffs must be covered by sterile gloves
- Sterile persons must have hands in sight at all times.

Gloving Procedure

- **The open method:** Never touch outer portion of glove with naked skin.
- **Closed method:** At no stage, gloves is held with bare skin during gloving.

Once Gowned and Gloved

- Stand with hand palms together
- Above the waist
- Away from the gown.

At the End of the Sterile Procedure

- First remove the gown over the gloved hands
- Then the gloves
- Hands should then be washed and dried
- Gloves disposed off according to policy.

17 Fundamental Principles of Laparoscopy

- Procedures performed
  - Hepatobiliary, e.g. lap chole
  - Small bowel and colon resections
  - Solid organ removal
    - ◊ Splenectomy, Adrenalectomy, Donor Nephrectomy
  - Foregut surgery
    - ◊ Fundoplication, Esophageal resection
  - Inguinal hernia
  - Diagnostic laparoscopy and staging
  - Bariatric surgery
  - Thoracoscopy (VATS)
- Benefits
  - Shorter hospital stay
  - Decreased recovery time
  - Decreased recurrence rate (ventral hernia repair)
  - Decreased inflammatory response
  - Decreased adhesion formation
  - Less wound-related morbidity
  - Less incidence and size of hernias
- New complications
  - Trocar injury
  - Longer operative times
  - Cancer recurrence in port sites
- Technology and surgical skill
  - Advanced simultaneously to permit more advanced cases
  - 1993 Lap cholecystectomy
  - 2005 Lap total colectomy and j-pouch
- Technology
  - Video scope and image production
  - Camera
  - Monitors
  - Light source
- Surgical skills
  - Knowledge of anatomy from laparoscopic perspective
  - Generation of surgeon weaned in MIS

Technology Used

- Three chip camera
  - One chip used for each of the three colors
  - Image regenerated on a high-resolution RGB monitor
- CCD (Charge coupled device)
  - Optimizes field view with limited lens size
- Rod lens (Scope)
  - Hopkins rod lens system
  - Laparoscope
  - Flexible or rigid
  - Angled scopes
    - ◊ Straight and oblique viewing scopes
  - Size of scope
    - ◊ 10 mm
    - ◊ 5 mm
    - ◊ 3 mm
    - ◊ Smaller (1.9 mm)

- Fiber optic light source
  - High-intensity light source (xenon) transmitted in a zigzag pattern along a fiber optic cable to the laparoscope

Access Techniques

- Open, Hassan's technique
  - Small incision through skin and fascia and direct view of peritoneum
- Closed, Veress needle technique
  - Needle with safety shield placed through a small skin incision
- "Opti-view" technique
  - Direct visualization of abdominal wall layers while inserting

Veress Technique

- Closed, Veress needle technique
- Needle with safety shield placed through a small skin incision
- Insufflate abdomen with CO_2
- Exchange needle for trocar

Pneumoperitoneum

- Carbon dioxide
  - Rapidly absorbed, non-flammable, inert
  - Easily eliminated
  - Suppresses combustion
- Carbon dioxide
  - Decreased venous return
  - Decreased cardiac output, direct myocardial depressant
  - Increased afterload

Orientation

- Positioning
- Trocars, camera and surgeon
  - Triangulation of instruments
  - Camera behind and in center of work
  - Camera-target-monitor axis
  - Align field of view and direction of view with target and monitor
- Visual cues from known anatomy
  - Orientation changes with camera position
  - Know where you are in the box

Limitations of Instruments

- Only 4 degrees of freedom
  - Up and down (pitch)
  - Right and left (yaw)
  - Back and forth, in a circle (roll)

Section | II

18 | Aneurysm

It can be defined as a localized dilated sac filled with blood which directly communicates with the lumen of the artery and is usually caused by weakness of the wall of the artery.

Etiology

a. **Congenital:** It is caused by the deficiency of elastic lamina. They usually occur in cerebral arteries leading to their rupture and subarachnoid hemorrhage.

b. **Acquired:** Causes of acquired aneurysm are:

1. **Traumatic:** The trauma is usually penetrating in nature, but can also be blunt. Trauma to artery can also occur due to displaced fracture fragment.
2. Degenerative etiology can be due to atherosclerosis or cystic medial necrosis
3. Hypertension
4. **Infective etiology:** Infective etiology can be due to bacterial infection leading to mycotic aneurysm. It can be a complication of subacute bacterial endocarditis in which arterial wall becomes weak either due to abscess formation or due to infected embolus resting upon arterial wall. It can also occur in cases where an artery traverses tubercular cavity in a lung. Rarely it can be seen in an artery located near the base of a peptic ulcer.
5. The syphilitic infections which are rarely seen these days can also lead to aneurysm.

Types of Aneurysm

1. **True aneurysm:** In this variety there is actual dilatation of artery which can be symmetrical or eccentric
2. **False aneurysm:** The sac is formed by condensed periarterial fibrous tissue which communicate with the lumen of artery.

Types of True Aneurysm

a. **Fusiform:** There is uniform expansion of entire circumference of arterial wall along the long axis of artery.
b. **Saccular:** There is expansion of part of the circumference of the arterial wall.
c. **Dissecting aneurysm:** Blood dissects its way along a tunnel between layers of artery.

Clinical Features

a. There is a swelling situated along the course of an artery.
b. The swelling shows an expansile pulsation.
c. If the artery is compressed proximal to swelling, the pulsation ceases and the swelling reduces in size.
d. A thrill may be palpable over the swelling.
e. A systolic bruit may be audible over the swelling.

Effects of Aneurysm

a. Pressure on adjacent structures e.g. distal edema due to pressure on veins or altered sensation due to pressure on nerves. The under lying bone, e.g. vertebrae may get eroded or underlying tubular structures may get compressed. The overlying skin may get stretched or undergoes necrosis leading to ulceration.

b. Thrombosis
c. Rupture
d. Ischemia

Investigation

CT or MR angiography is the investigation of choice.

Treatment

a. **Arterial ligation:** Simple ligation of an artery immediately above and below the aneurysm prevents embolization and rupture. The procedure, however, carries the risk of distal ischemia if sufficient collaterals are not present.

b. **Anel's method of ligation:** The ligature is applied just above the sac.

c. **Hunter's method of ligation:** The ligature is applied just proximal to the sac, but above the branch of artery.

d. **Bradors ligature:** The ligature is applied below the sac.

e. **Antylus' method:** Two ligatures are applied one proximal and one distal to the sac.

f. **Aneurysmorrhaphy (Matas):** This is suitable for saccular aneurysms which are small mouthed. The diseased sac is excised and the defect in the artery is closed by lateral suture of healthy arterial wall.

g. **Reinforcement:** The aneurysm is wrapped with fascia or with some synthetic material to strengthen it. This method is used in intracranial aneurysms.

h. **Excision of aneurysm** and arterial grafting is the treatment of choice in aortic aneurysm.

Abdominal Aortic Aneurysm

a. Commonest type of large vessel aneurysm
b. Seen in 2% of population at autopsy
c. 95 % are seen below renal artery
d. 95% are due to atherosclerosis

Presentation

a. It may be asymptomatic.
b. It may cause various symptoms.
c. It can present as ruptured aneurysm as life threatening emergency.

Asymptomatic

1. Mostly it is an incidental diagnosis.
2. Repair is only done if the diameter is more than 55 mm.
3. The incidence of rupture is less than 1% if diameter is less than 55 mm.
4. If diameter is more than 70 mm chances of rupture increase to more than 20%.

Symptomatic

1. It can present as back or abdominal discomfort.
2. It can present as pain in the thigh or groin due to nerve compression.
3. Pressure effects.
4. Symptoms due to distal embolization.
5. Inflammation of aneurysm wall.

Rupture

The anterior rupture occurs in 20% of cases. Anterior rupture results in free bleeding into the peritoneal cavity and only few patients survive to reach the hospital.

Posterolateral rupture occurs in 80% of cases. It produces retroperitoneal hematoma. The combination of resistance offered by retroperitoneum and moderate hypotension stops bleeding for sometime. Patient is in great pain but conscious. If urgent surgery is not performed the patient will die. Timely surgery can save 50% of patients.

Investigation

CT or MR angiography

Treatment

1. Open surgical repair
2. Endoluminal procedure

19 Thromboangitis Obliterans (Buerger's Disease)

Felix Von Winiwarter first described Thrombo-angitis Obliterans (TAO) in 1879. However, Leo Buerger in 1908 published the series of several cases and the disease is known as Buerger's disease.

Definition

It is an inflammatory non atherosclerotic occlusive disease involving small and medium sized arteries and veins. It mainly involves distal vessels of extremity.

Epidemiology

a. Young adult males of less than 45 years are mainly affected.
b. All patients are smokers.
c. Females are affected in less than 10 percent of cases.
d. Tobacco use has been incriminated as a factor in the development of the disease.
e. If the patient continues to smoke there is progression of the disease with 40 percent amputation rate.
f. If the patient stops smoking a good no. of patients go in to remission.
g. Genetic factors has been incriminated but not yet proven as increased expression of HLA-A9, HLA-B8, HLA-B40 is seen.

Histopathological Features

Tunica Albugenia

1. There is increased no. of fibroblasts.
2. There is proliferation of endothelial lining of vasa vasorum.

Tunica Media

1. There is lymphocyte infiltration.
2. Internal elastic lamina remains intact.

Tunica Intima

1. Proliferation of intima
2. Proliferation of intima leads to intimal cushioning
3. Intimal cushioning leads to narrowing of lumen

Lumen of Vessel

1. There is occlusion of lumen by highly cellular thrombus.
2. There is micro abscess formation and multi-nucleated giant cells in thrombus.

Clinical Features

1. Patient presents with progressive chronic ischemia of the lower limb
   Patient can present with
   - Intermittent claudicating pain of different grades
     Grade I → Pain appears on walking but disappears as patient continue to walk.

Grade II → Pain appears on walking but patient can manage to walk with pain.

Grade III → Pain appears on walking certain distance and is forced to take rest

Grade IV → Rest pain

- Non healing ulcers of foot
- Gangrene of toe/foot
- Nutritional changes in lower limb in the form of atropy of muscles

Involvement of all four limbs is seen in 43 percent of cases.

2. Patient can give history of Reynaud's phenomenon affecting the upper limb.
3. There might be history suggestive of migratory superficial thrombophlebitis.

Olin's Criteria for Diagnosis of TAO

1. Age less than 45 years
2. Current or recent history of smoking
3. Features of distal extremity ischemia, e.g. claudication, rest pain, or ischemic ulcers
4. Exclusion of autoimmune disease, hypercoagulable stage, diabetes mellitus
5. Exclusion of proximal source of embolization by echocardiography, or angiography
6. Consistent arteriographic findings in the form of:
   - Multiple segmental arterial involvement (skip lesions)
   - Smooth vessel wall in non-affected arteries
   - Abrupt or smoothly tapered arterial occlusions
   - Tortuous corkscrew collaterals
   - Normal proximal vessels

Investigations

1. Rule out autoimmune disorders, e.g. ESR, antinuclear antibodies, rheumatoid factor, complement level estimation.
2. Rule out hypercoagulable state by estimating antithrombin III, antiphospholipids antibodies, protein C and protein S estimation
3. Doppler study to estimate Ankle Brachial Index(ABI). ABI is measured by the ratio of ankle systolic pressure divided by higher of the two readings of brachial systolic pressure. Normal ABI is more than 1.

Treatment Outline

1. Patient is advised to stop smoking.
2. Patient should continue regular graded exercises just short of pain.
3. Heel of the shoe can be raised to relax tendo-achillis and calf muscles.
4. **Drug treatment:**
   - Pentoxyphylline 400 mg twice daily to improve microcirculation and to reduce blood viscosity.
   - Cilostazole 100 mg twice daily, is a vasodilator and its mode of action is to inhibit phospho-diestrase resulting in increase in microcirculation.
   - Low dose aspirin is started to reduce incidence of intravascular thrombosis.
   - Intravenous Iloprost (Prostacyclin analogue) and prostaglandin E1 are useful in critically ischemic limb and can help avoid amputation.
5. Lumbar sympathectomies have a role in patient with severe rest pain or non healing ulcers. It can be performed by open or laparoscopic method. It involves removal of L1 to L4 ganglion. It helps by increasing circulation of the skin. It has little role in patients with intermittent claudication.
6. Therapeutic angiogenesis by vascular endothelial growth factor (VEGF) and basic fibroblast growth factor (bFGF). Intramuscular injection of VEGF165 is given.
7. **Omentopexy:** Pedicle omentum is brought down up to ankle through subcutaneous tunnel. Omentum helps in the neo-vascularization of muscles.
8. Care of ischemic foot by
   - Protection from thermal or mechanical trauma
   - Use of properly fitted shoes, i.e. neither too tight or too loose
   - Local infection even trivial should be properly treated

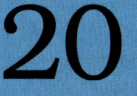

20 Peripheral Vascular Disease (PVD)

Incidence: Peripheral vascular disease (PVD) is a common disease.

- Occurs in approximately 1/3rd of the patients over 70 years of age
- Strong association with coronary artery disease, smoking and diabetes mellitus
- Progressive disease in 25% with progressive intermittent claudication/limb threatening ischemia
- Outcomes can be
  - Impaired quality of life
  - Limb loss
  - Premature mortality
- Buerger's disease is unheard in less than 45 years of age.
- Raynaud's patients will usually remember symptoms starting before 30 years of age.

Risk Factors for PVD: Framingham Heart Study

- Data from the Framingham heart study of 381 men and women who were followed for 38 years revealed that the odds ratio for developing intermittent claudication was:
  - 2.6 for diabetes mellitus
  - 1.2 for each 40 mg/dL (1 mmol/L) elevation in the serum cholesterol concentration
  - 1.4 for each 10 cigarettes smoked per day
  - 1.5 for mild and 2.2 for moderate hypertension
  - In addition, diabetic patients had worse arterial disease and a poorer outcome than nondiabetics

Outcomes in PVD Patients

See Fig. 20.1.

Diagnostic Modalities

- History
- Physical
- Ankle Brachial Index (ABI)
- Non-invasive vascular laboratory
- **Angiography:** MRA, CT, DSA

Initial Assessment

- Identifying risk factors and symptoms
- Pulse palpability (Palpate all pulses)
- Further assessment relies on functional non-invasive testing and radiological imaging
  - Determine not only the anatomic, but also the physiological aberration of peripheral vascular flow.

Intermittent Claudication

- Derived from the latin word for limp
- A reproducible discomfort of a defined group of muscles that is induced by exercise and relieved with rest
- Occurs due to mismatch in supply and demand
- Site of pain depends upon the location of the disease
  - Buttock, thigh, calf or foot claudication, either singly or in combination.

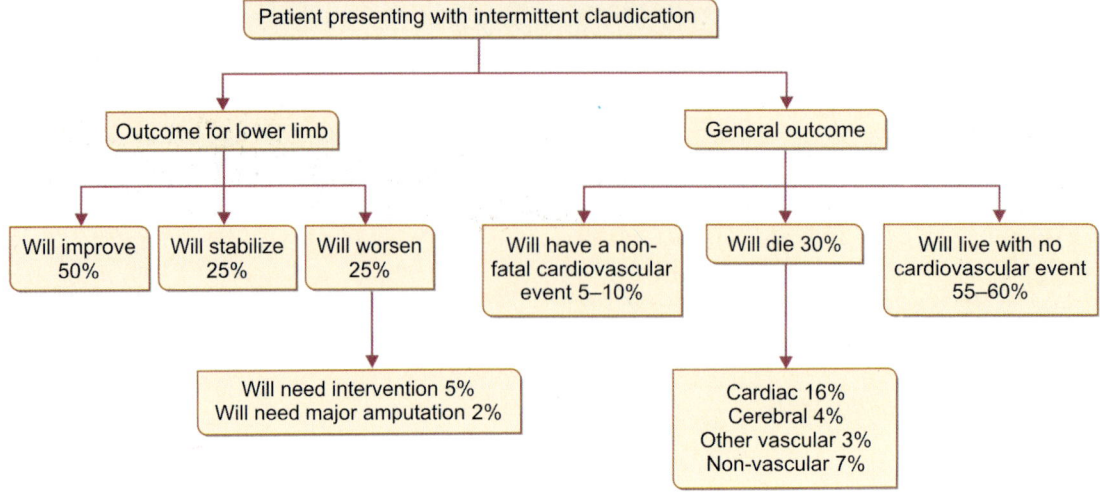

Fig. 20.1: Flowchart showing outcome of claudication of lower limb

PVD Etiology

- Large arteries
  - Atherosclerosis
  - Thromboembolism
  - Trauma
  - Arteritis of various types including
    - ◊ Fibromuscular dysplasia
    - ◊ Takayasu's disease
- Medium and small vessel occlusions
  - Diabetes
  - Buerger's disease
  - Chronic recurrent trauma
  - Multiple small emboli
  - Collagen vascular diseases
  - Pseudoxanthoma elasticum
  - Drug Reaction
  - Vasospasm
- Specific to certain anatomical sites
  - Cystic adventitial disease of the popliteal artery
  - Popliteal artery entrapment
  - Iliac endofibrosis (seen in cyclists)
- Various neurovascular compression syndromes affecting the upper limb
  - Cervical rib
  - Costoclavicular syndrome
  - Hyperabduction syndrome

Features of Lower Limb Ischemia

- Intermittent claudication
- Rest pain
- Coldness, numbness, paresthesia, color changes
- Ulceration/gangrene
- Temperature changes
- Decreased sensation
- Decreased function or loss of function
- Pulsation decreased or loss of pulsations
- Bruit
- Venous refilling prolonged

PVD Differential Diagnosis

- Deep venous thrombosis
- Musculoskeletal disorders
  - Osteoarthritis
  - Restless leg syndrome
- Peripheral neuropathy
- Spinal stenosis (pseudo-claudication)
  - Worse with erect posture (lordosis), better sitting or lying down
  - Can find relief by leaning forward and straightening the spine (pushing a shopping cart or leaning against a wall)

Differential Diagnosis of Intermittent Claudication

See Table 20.1.

Location

Buttock/Hip

- Usually indicates aorto-iliac occlusive disease (Leriche's syndrome)
- Some cases have thigh claudication also

Table 20.1: Differential diagnosis of intermittent claudication

Claudication	Intermittent claudication	Venous claudication	Neurogenic
Quality of pain	Cramping	"Bursting"	Electric shock like
Onset	Gradual, consistent	Gradual, can be immediate	Can be immediate, occurs even after first step, inconsistent in nature
Relieved by	Standing still	Elevation of leg	Sitting down, bending forward
Location	Muscle groups (Buttocks, thigh, calf)	Whole leg	Poorly localized, can affect whole leg
Legs affected	Usually one	Usually one	Often both

- Question diagnosis of bilateral disease if erectile dysfunction is not present

Thigh

- Occlusion of the common femoral artery leads to claudication in the thigh, calf, or both.

Calf

- Symptoms in upper 2/3 is usually due to Superficial Femoral Artery
- Lower 1/3 is due to Popliteal disease.

Physical Examination

- Trophic signs
  - Skin atrophy, brittle nails, hair loss, dependent rubor
  - Ulceration, gangrene
- Pulse examination to look for any absent or dimnished pulses.
- Elevation and dependency test (Buerger's test).

Table 20.2: Various values of venous filling and color return

	Color return(s)	Venous filling(s)
Normal	10	10–15
Adequate collaterals	15–25	15–30
Severe ischemia	>35	>40

Critical Limb Ischemia

- Persistent rest pain > 2weeks
- Ulceration/gangrene of toes and ankle systolic pressure < 50mm of Hg
- Toe systolic pressure < 30 mm Hg
- Trans-cutaneous O_2 pressure <10 mm of Hg
- Absence of arterial pulsation in big toe
- Structural or functional changes in skin capillaries of affected area

Non-Invasive Investigations

Ankle Brachial Index

- Cornerstone of lower extremity vascular evaluation
  - Blood pressure cuffs or Doppler is used
  - Ankle (Dorsalis pedis or posterior tibial) to brachial artery pressure is measured

Table 20.3: ABI in various stages of PVD

Normal	>0.96
Claudication	0.50 – 0.95
Rest pain	0.21– 0.49
Tissue loss	0.20
Significant change	0.15 or more

Limitations

- Non-compressible vessels
  - Diabetes
  - Renal Failure
  - ABI >1.5
  - Use toe-brachial index
    ◊ Normal >0.7
    ◊ Rest pain <0.2

Segmental Pressures

- Pneumatic cuffs at multiple levels
  - Doppler pressure at pedal artery
  - Drop >30 mmHg between levels
  - Drop >20 mmHg between limbs
- Reflects status of artery above drop in pressure
- Inaccurate with calcified vessels

Noninvasive Functional Assessment

- Targeted towards evaluating the arterial flow dynamics in the affected area, and are invariably supplemented with radiological depiction of anatomic abnormality

- Pressure measurements (ABI)
- Plethysmography
- Continuous wave Doppler

Duplex Doppler

- Non-invasive method of evaluating the blood vessels using sound waves, similar to ultrasonography and echocardiography
- Can obtain both anatomic and hemodynamic information
- Anatomical detail
  - Vessel wall
  - Intra-luminal obstructive lesions
  - Perivascular compressive structures
- **Doppler waveform analysis:** Hemodynamic information
  - Sensitivity of 92.6% and specificity of 97% (angiography gold standard)
  - Inaccurate at adductor canal and the aorto-iliac regions
  - 95% accuracy in the detection of bypass graft stenosis, but can overestimate stenosis
- Qualitative assessment of waveform analysis
  - Simple equipment
  - Not affected by medial calcinosis
  - Supplements segmental pressures

Pulse Volume Recordings

- Pneumatic cuffs at multiple levels
- Inflated to 65 mm Hg
- Extremity volume increases in systole
- Changes pressure in cuff
- Waveform analysis
- Not impacted by calcification
- Advantages
  - Widely available
  - Cheap
  - Reproducible
- Disadvantages
  - Technician dependent
  - Time consuming
  - Detection of collaterals is low
  - Presence of gas and calcification degrades images

Radiologic Imaging: MR Angiography (MRA) and CT Angiography (CTA)

- Digital subtraction angiography (DSA) (conventional angiography) remains the gold standard for evaluation of PVD

- Newer modalities that match its accuracy are rapidly evolving
- It is a matter of time before newer imaging replaces DSA, with the invasive angiographic techniques reserved for interventional procedures

Indications for Angiography

- When decision to intervene is taken on clinical grounds
- Angiography is a road map for surgery in
  - Limb threatened
  - Livelihood threatened
  - Life –style affected

Information Extracted from Angiography

- Exact site of obstruction
- Length of obstruction
- Number of obstructions
- Distal run-off

MRA: Current Technique

- 3D gradient echo (fast acquisition)
- Gadolinium enhanced
  - 20–40 cc
  - Automated scan delay
- Renal arteries to toes
- Stepping table or bolus chase
- 45-min exam

Limitations of MRI

- Uncooperative patient
- Claustrophobia
- Metal artifact
- Pacemakers/ICDs
- Lack of visualization of calcium

CT Angiography (CTA) of PVD

- Multidetector CT scanner necessary (4+)
  - Many hospitals now have 128 slice
- Iodinated contrast volume similar to conventional angiography
  - 80–150 cc
  - Automated scan delay
- Renal arteries to ankles
- 20 minutes exam
- High power post processing software is crucial

- Large volumes of data are generated via CTA studies and displayed in various formats to refine the analysis of study results
  - Maximum intensity projection-MIP (most common)
  - Shaded surface display
  - 3D Volume rendering

CT Limitations

- With significant and dense calcifications, a false diagnosis of patency can result
- Uncooperative patient
- Pregnancy
- Bad pump
- Inconsistent pedal vessel visualization
- Renal failure/contrast allergy

Digital Subtraction Angiography (DSA)

- Gold standard of arterial imaging
  - Has almost totally replaced conventional cut film angiography

- Compares a pre contrast image with a post contrast image using a computer, and "subtracts" elements common to both
  - Prevents images of objects like bones, etc. from obscuring vascular details
  - Contrast resolution is improved through use of image enhancement software
- Radiation exposure and contrast volumes are lower than conventional angiography
- Images are immediately available for review
- Images are stored in digital format on computerized data storage media
- Interventional procedures can be performed

Suggested Algorithm for Work-up

See Fig. 20.2

Workup: Summary

- Non-invasive vascular lab is first line evaluation in non-acute patients
- ABI is an easy screening test

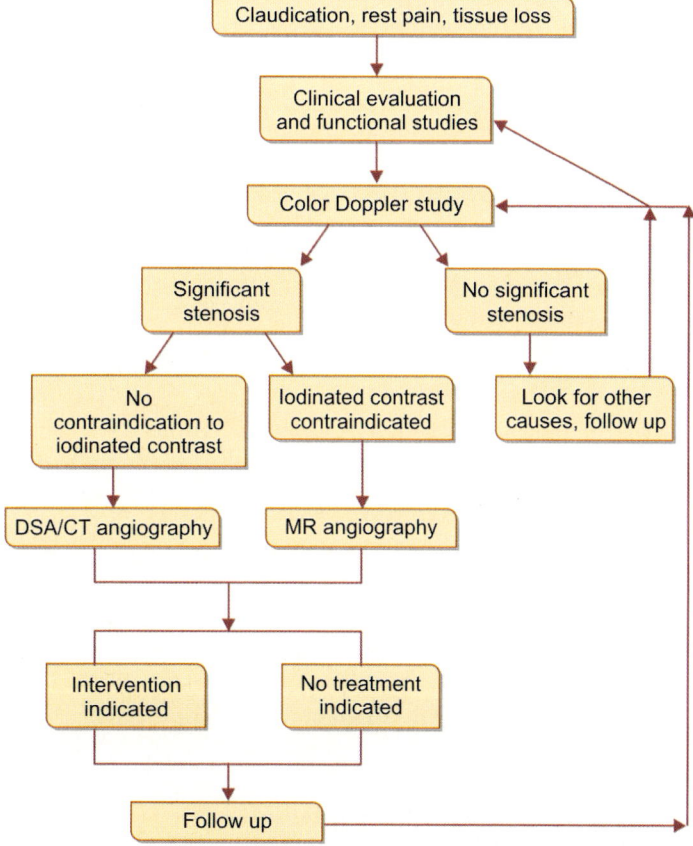

Fig. 20.2: Flowchart showing suggested algorithm for work-up

- Beware of non-compressible vessels in renal failure and diabetes
- Segmental limb pressures can often be combined with Doppler waveform analysis
- MRA is indicated for intervention planning
  - MRA (gadolinium enhanced) provides excellent renal to pedal imaging
  - It surpasses CT for imaging the foot
  - Overestimation of stenosis in small vessels
  - Limited by metal artefacts, magnetic field, and length of study
- CTA indicated for intervention planning
  - CTA provides excellent renal to ankle imaging
  - Pedal imaging is poor
  - Soft tissues and bones are also imaged
  - Small vessel calcification is a limitation

Treatment for PVD

- Life style modification
- Risk reduction
- Drugs
- Per-cutaneous intervention
- Surgery
- Lumbar sympathectomy

Life Style Modification

- Stop smoking
- Exercises just short of pain
- **Buerger's position:** Foot end of the bed raised while sleeping
- Buerger's exercises
- Heel raise to relieve pressure on tendo-achelles
- Weight reduction
- Diet modification

Risk Reduction

- Control of diabetes
- Correction of abnormal lipid profile
- Control of hypertension/ coronary artery disease

Drugs

- **Anti-platelet drugs:** Aspirin or clopidogrel
- Naftidofuryl oxalate can help alter tissue metabolism
- Oxypentafylline
- Prostacyclin

Percutaneous Interventions

- Balloon angioplasty for iliac vessel disease or vessels of leg, upper limb and renal arteries
- Metal Stenting

Operations

- Aorto-femoral bypass
- Femoral-popliteal bypass graft

Material Used

- Dacron graft
- Autogenous vein graft
- Human umbilical vein

Sutures Used

- Prolene suture

Lumbar Sympathectomy

For limb salvage in
- Critically ischemic limb
- Pre gangrene stage
- Adjunct to bypass surgery
- Hyperhidrosis

Table 20.4: Effect of medical treatment

Treatment	Effect
Smoking cessation	10 years mortality decreases from 54% to 18%; at 7 years rest pain drops from 16% to 0%
Antiplatelet agents	22% reduction in vascular events; possible increase in walking distance
Diabetes control	RR = 0.94 (0.8–1.1) for mortality; RR=0.51 (0.01–19.64) for amputation
BP to <140/85 mmHg	RR = 0.87 (0.81–0.94) for mortality; effect on PAD not known
ACE inhibitors	RR = 0.73 (0.61–0.86) for MI, stroke, or CV death
Exercise programs	24% reduction in CV mortality; 150% increase in further walking distance
Cholesterol decrease	RR = 0.81 (0.72–0.87) for MI, stroke, or revascularization; no clinical benefit in PAD
Cilostazol	Significant increase in walking distance

Note: (RR = Risk reduction)

21 | Thoracic Outlet Syndrome (TOS)

Thoracic outlet obstruction (TOS) occurs as a result of compression of subclavian vessels and nerves of the brachial plexus in the region of the thoracic inlet. It is more common in middle aged females. It is also known as Scalenus Anticus syndrome, costoclavicular syndrome or hyper abduction syndrome.

Sites of Obstruction can be at Various Locations (Fig. 21.1)

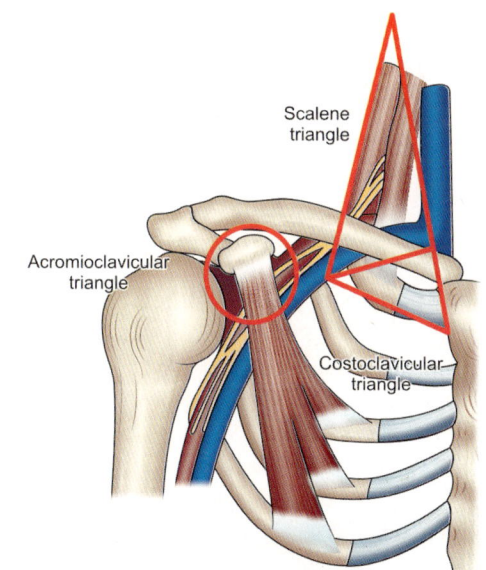

Fig. 21.1: Sites of obstruction in thoracic outlet syndrome

Scalene triangle

Acromioclavicular triangle

Costoclavicular triangle

a. *Inter-scalene triangle* which is bounded by scalenus anticus anteriorly, scalenus medius muscle posteriorly and first rib inferiorly. Subclavian artery and brachial plexus passes through this space.

b. *Inter-costoclavicular space*: It is a narrow space between clavicle and first rib and vein can get compressed in this space.

c. *Sub-coracoid space*: It is a space between coracoid process and pectoralis minor tendon. Artery, nerve and vein can get compressed in this space. During hyper abduction axillary vessels and brachial plexus can bend at 90 degree in this area.

Causes of TOS

- *Cervical rib:* Occurs in 1% of population and produces symptoms in 10% of the population having cervical rib. Symptoms are most commonly seen in thin women with narrow neck in the 3rd or 4th decade. Gradual descent of shoulder girdle due to atrophy of regional muscular is responsible for late onset of symptoms.
- Long transverse process of C7 Vertebrae may act as cervical rib.
- Abnormally high placed first rib
- Scalene anticus muscle hypertrophy may narrow the space in the inter-scalene triangle and cause symptoms.
- Bone dislocation

- Neck hematoma
- Fibrous bands
- Bony tumors

ANATOMY

Subclavian artery and brachial plexus pass through a narrow triangle bounded by:
- Scalenus actinus anteriorly
- Scalenus medius posteriorly
- Base is formed by the first rib

Presentation

Neurogenic (95%)

- Pain in the upper limb on the medial aspect
- Radiation of pain to upper back or neck
- Pain becomes worse by the end of the day due to loss of muscle tone
- Tingling, numbness or paraesthesia
- Wasting of small muscles of the hand

Arterial (4%)

- Compression of the subclavian artery is followed by post stenotic dilatation
- Thrombus may form in the dilated artery due to turbulent blood flow
- Distal embolization can cause distal gangrene of upper limb

Venous (1%)

- Subclavian vein thrombosis may cause limb edema

Examination

- Look for tenderness in the supraclavicular fossa and over the scalenus actinus
- Look for any bony prominence in the supra-clavicular fossa
- Compression of supraclavicular fossa to look for pain and paraesthesiae
- Subclavian bruit can be heard
- *Adson's test*: Patient sits on a stool. Radial pulse is felt in normal sitting posture then patient is asked to take deep inspiration, extend neck backwards and turn chin towards affected side. The test is positive if on deep inspiration, extension of neck and turning the head diminishes the radial pulse because this manoeuvre makes the scalene anterior muscle taut and compresses the subclavian artery.

- *Halsted test (exaggerated military position):* This test is done to elicit costo-clavicular compression. After feeling patients radial pulse in normal posture, patient is asked to throw shoulders backwards and downwards as in exaggerated military posture. This will cause reduction or disappearance of radial as in this posture space between first rib and clavicle is reduced.
- *Wright test:* (Hyper abduction test) patients affected arm is passively hyper-abducted to monitor disappearance or diminution of radial pulse. This occurs due to compression of subclavian artery by tendon of pectoralis minor tendon.
- *Roos test:* Patient abducts the arm to 90 degrees and externally rotate the shoulder. This position is maintained and patient opens and closes the hand rapidly for 3 minutes. Positive test will mean reproduction of symptoms.

Investigations

- Skiagram of the cervical spine and chest
- CT/MRI to exclude cervical disc lesions
- Nerve conduction studies
- Doppler study/Angiogram

Management

- Conservative
  - Rest
- Correction of faulty posture
- Muscle stretching/strengthening exercises
- Short course of analgesics
- Surgery is indicated if
  - Conservative management fails
  - Rapidly progressing sensory or motor symptoms
  - Presence of prolonged nerve conduction velocity
  - Subclavian vein thrombosis
  - Narrowing of subclavian artery

Surgical Approaches

- *Transaxillary approach:* Through transaxillary approach first rib is removed and sympa-thectomy can also be performed. Division of pectoralis minor tendon if it is causing obstruction can also be carried out through this approach.

- *Supra-clavicular approach:* This approach is employed for removal of first rib or to carry out scalenotomy. Scalenotomy means division of scalenus anticus muscle close to the insertion.
- *Infra-clavicular approach:* This approach is employed for division of pectoralis minor tendon.

- *Posterior approach:* The incision is identical to that of upper thoracoplasty. The subclavian vessels and brachial plexus are easily exposed and displaced anteriorly. This approach provides ample exposure for reconstruction of vessels if it is indicated, e.g. post stenotic dilatation of subclavian artery. The cervical rib can also be excised through this approach.

22 | Varicose Veins

Venous disorders involve lower limb most commonly. It is estimated that around 5–7% population of India has varicose veins out of which 0.3 to 1% develop venous ulceration. Chronic venous insufficiency (CVI) leads to ambulatory venous hypertension that can result from venous obstruction or venous reflux. Varicose veins are one of the leading causes of CVI. Varicose veins are defined as dilated tortuous and elongated veins.

Varicose Veins Types

a. *Primary*: It is due to primary pathology of veins. Some patients have family history with abnormality of FOXC2 gene. Probably there is defective connective tissue and smooth muscle in the vein wall which leads to secondary incompetence of valves.
b. *Secondary*: Varicose veins can develop secondary to
   – Deep vein thrombosis
   – Congenital anomaly like Kippel–Trenaunay syndrome or multiple arteriovenous fistulae
   – Pregnancy and pelvic tumors

Anatomy Lower Limb Veins Comprise of

- Deep system of veins which lies below the deep fascia (Carry 90% of blood)
- Superficial system of veins which lies outside the deep fascia (carry 10% blood)
- Perforating veins which pass through the deep fascia joining the superficial to the deep system of veins

Long Saphenous Vein

- Originates at the medial border of the foot
- It passes 1–1.5 inches anterior to the medial malleolus over the distal 1/3rd of the tibia and then along the medial margin of the tibia up to the knee joint
- It is accompanied by the saphenous nerve below the knee joint along the lower 2/3rd of the leg
- At the knee joint it lies 10 cm posterior to the patella
- Travels close to the deep fascia except at the knee joint, where it may become subcuticular
- In the thigh it passes antero-superiorly to reach the saphenous opening which is 3.75 cm below and lateral to the pubic tubercle

Deep Venous System

Deep veins of lower limb arise from three pairs of vena comitantes which accompany anterior tibial, posterior tibial and peroneal arteries. These six veins join together in the popliteal fossa to form the popliteal vein. Popliteal also receives soleal and gastrocnemius veins. Popliteal vein enters sub sartorial canal through adductor hiatus as femoral vein.

Six perforators joining the superficial to deep venous system are located at constant positions which are:

- 2, 4 and 6 inches above the medial malleolus
- Just below the tibia tubercle
- In the adductor (Hunter's) canal of the thigh
- Level of mid-thigh

Short Saphenous Vein

- Arises on the lateral border of the foot by joining of lateral marginal vein and lateral deep venous arch
- Passes behind the lateral malleolus
- Runs up in the midline posteriorly in the intra-fascial compartment
- Pierces the deep fascia in the upper part of the calf, and terminates in the popliteal vein in the midline 4 cm below the popliteal skin crease
- It is accompanied by the sural nerve, lymphatic and popliteal nerve along its course
- Derived anatomically from the posterior axial vein of the lower limb

Factors helping in venous return from the lower limb:

- Negative pressure in the thorax during inspiration to –6mm of Hg, which is transmitted to the great veins.
- Contraction of lower limb muscles compresses the vein and acts as a muscle pump. Normal venous pressure in relaxing phase is 20 mmHg and rises to 80–100 mmHg on muscle contraction.
- *vis a tergo* is produced by arterial pressure which is transmitted to the venous side through the capillary bed.
- Competent valves
- Venae commitantes which lie by the side of the artery are helped by arterial pulsation to propel blood.

VARICOSE VEINS

Varicose veins are defined as the superficial veins which have permanently lost their valvular mechanism and due to resultant venous hypertension in standing position become dilated, tortuous, elongated, palpable and thickened.

Mechanism of Valves

- Valves prevent the reflux of venous blood from distal to proximal and from deep to superficial venous system.

- They are generally absent above the level of the groin.
- Valves can resist pressure of up to 300 mm of Hg.

Pathology

Varicose veins can be primary or secondary (*see* table bottom of the page)

Presentation

- More incidence in females compared to males in western countries however in India male predominance is seen.
- Left limb is more commonly involved than right but reason is not known.
- Long saphenous system is affected in 2/3rd of the cases.
- 80% incidence when both parents are affected, 10% when none are affected

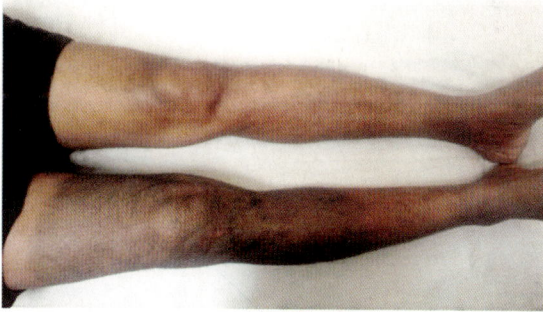

Fig. 22.1: A case of Klippel-Trenaunay syndrome

Symptoms

- Tiredness and aching of calf muscles at the end of the day after prolonged standing
- Heaviness or night cramps
- Unsightly appearance
- Swelling around ankle joint
- Itching, pigmentation, dermatitis around ankle in long standing cases
- Venous ulcer around ankle in long standing cases.

Table 22.1: Classification of varicose veins based on etiology	
Primary	*Secondary*
• Long hours of standing which increase hydrostatic pressure of gravity	• Deep vein thrombosis
• Family history	• Arteriovenous malformation, e.g. Parks Weber syndrome
• Pregnancy	• Hemangiomatous malformation, e.g. Kippel-Trenaunay syndrome
• Ageing	• Pelvic mass or retroperitoneal fibrosis

Complications of Venous Ulcer

- Bleeding from varicose veins due to trauma
- Thrombophlebitis
- Venous hypertension leading to venous ulcer
- Calcification
- Talipes equinovarus deformity of foot
- Eczematoid dermatitis and pigmentation
- Periosteitis of subcutaneous surface of tibia
- Squamous cell carcinoma in long-standing, non healing venous ulcer (Marjolin's Ulcer)

Examination

- Determine which system is involved, i.e. great saphenous or short saphenous or both
- Extent of involvement
- Skin changes, i.e. eczema, discoloration or lipo-dermatosclerosis/ulcer around malleolus
- Trendelenburg's test for patency of sapheno-femoral junction
- Perthe's test for patency of deep veins

Investigations

Color Doppler study of venous system is done for ensuring patency of deep veins and to define the site of incompetent perforators.

Treatment

Management can be
- Conservative
- Sclerotherapy
- Operative management

Conservative Management

See Table 22.2

Conservative Management Includes

- Avoiding prolonged standing
- Crepe bandaging and elastic stockings from toe to thigh, which causes decreased edema, venous volume and reflux and increases venous return.

Table 22.2: Indications and contraindication of conservative management

Indications	Contraindications
• Refusal for surgery	• Arterial insufficiency
• Capillary veins, venous stars (C1)	
• Pregnant patients	
• Waiting for surgery	
• Early cases	

- Limb elevation above the level of heart while lying down

Sclerotherapy

- Injection sclerotherapy first tried by Pravaz in 1851 when he first injected it into an aneurysm.
- In 1853 Chassaignac introduced sclerotherapy in varicose veins.

Method of Compression Sclerotherapy

- Patient is made to recline.
- Vein is filled enough for needle to enter by stroking it down towards the needle.
- 0.5 ml of sclerosant is injected slowly into the vein.
- Injection is retained in the short segment of vein by compression by fingers above and below the site for a minute.
- Local compression is applied.
- Patient is asked to immediately walk around.
- Compression is removed after one week.

Commonly used agents for injection sclero-therapy are:
- 5% monoethanolamine with 2% benzyl alcohol
- 3% sodium tetradecylsulphate in 2% benzyl alcohol
- 25% glycerine with 2% phenol

Complications

- Failure of sclerosis
- Extra-venous injection
- Deep vein thrombosis
- Hypersensitivity
- Skin pigmentation
- Gangrene of distal limb

Ultrasound Guided foam Sclerotherapy

This is an alternative to blind sclerotherapy and can be used to treat the main saphenous trunk. A needle is inserted in the vein to be treated under duplex ultrasound guidance and sclerosant is made in foam by air mixing technique using three way tap. Polidocanol is used rather than sodium tetradecyl sulphate. Foam is monitored under ultrasound scanning as it spreads in the vein. Apex of the saphenous opening is compressed by ultrasound probe to prevent the foam entering the deep veins. The leg is also elevated to prevent foam entering the axial deep veins. These techniques can take care of both long saphenous and short saphe-

Table 22.3: Indication and contraindications of sclerotherapy	
Indications	*Contraindications*
• Varicosity confined below knee and caused by incompetent perforators • Recurrent/residual varicosities post-surgery • Large venous telangiectasia • Dilated branch veins around the knee following early long saphenous incompetence • Refusal for surgery	• Deep venous thrombosis • Sapheno femoral incompetence • Veins in lower 1/3rd of leg • Veins on the foot • Veins in elderly • Veins in fat legs • Immobile patient • Post thrombotic syndrome • Dirty ulcer or extensive eczema

nous venous system. Up to three sittings may be required to completely obliterate the veins. Extravasation of sclerosing agent in subcutaneous tissue should be avoided as it can lead to cutaneous ulceration. The escape of sclerosing agent in deep veins can lead to deep vein thrombosis. Recurrence rates at present are not known.

Surgery

- History of attempts at surgery dates back to nearly 2000 years
- In 1891 Trendelenberg advised ligating long saphenous trunk above the large varices in the thigh
- Stripping was re-established by Linton in 1949
- In 1954, the flexible stripper was invented by T. Myers

Indications: Sapheno-femoral incompetence with varicosities extending up to the thigh

Contraindications: Absence of deep venous system

- Pregnancy
- Patient taking oral contraceptives
- Thrombophlebitis

Types of Surgeries Done

- Flush ligation of sapheno-femoral junction with ligation of all tributaries ending at SFJ
- Stripping of long saphenous up to the knee joint
- Flush ligation of short saphenous vein
- Sub-fascial ligation of perforators

Flush Ligation of Long Saphenous Vein

- Patient lies supine with the table tilted head down to an angle of 15 degrees.
- Curved or Hockey stick incision is made with the outer half lying in the gutter of the groin and inner half curving towards the thigh.
- Alternatively an oblique incision can also be made parallel to the fold of the groin about 7–8 cm long.
- Incision is carried deeper till the superficial fascia is seen, which is then incised
- Gauze is used to separate the fat and exposes the sapheno-femoral junction
- Saphena magna is dissected gently using a Mayos tissue cutting scissors.
- Femoral vein is exposed 1 cm above and below the sapheno-femoral junction.
- The six significant veins joining the termination of saphenous vein are defined and ligated
- The end of the long saphenous vein is ligated with silk and a second ligature is transfixed to avoid hemorrhage. Femoral vein is inspected above and below the junction and long saphenous divided.
- Incision is closed in layers. Biopsy of nodes can be taken if enlarged.

Stripping of Long Saphenous Vein

- Saphenous vein is exposed and flush ligated as above.
- Small tip is passed into the vein at the groin gently.

Table 22.4: Indications and contraindications of surgery	
Indications	*Contraindications*
• Sapheno-femoral incompetence with varicosities extending up to the thigh	• Absence of deep venous system • Pregnancy • Patient taking oral contraceptives • Thrombophlebitis

- A vertical incision is made just below knee and vein exposed.
- The stripper is extruded from the vein and the acorn firmly tied in the vein.
- The stripper is firmly withdrawn with the vein telescoped over it.
- The track is compressed with a large sterile pad for 3 to 5 minutes.
- Incision is closed in layers and bandage applied for seven days.
- Stripping of long saphenous vein is performed up to upper 1/3rd of leg only. Stripping in lower 2/3rd of leg will result in higher chances of injury to saphenous nerve. Other reason for not doing stripping in lower 2/3rd of leg is that perforators in this region do not drain directly in long saphenous vein.

Flush Ligation of the Short Saphenous Vein

- The patient is made to face down and knee flexed by placing a sandbag.
- A 5 cm long transverse incision is made at the level of the knee joint and developed in layers. Sapheno-popliteal junction is marked before surgery by Doppler.
- Deep fascia is identified and incised in the line of skin incision.
- Short saphenous vein is located between the two heads of gastrocnemius.
- The vein is lifted by artery forceps and knee flexed further.
- Dissection is done with a gauze swab up to the sapheno-popliteal junction.
- All branches are identified and ligated.
- Short saphenous is ligated close to the popliteal vein.
- Incision is closed in layers and compression applied.

Complications of surgery

Intraoperative complications:
- Hemorrhage from torn varix
- Division or injury to the common femoral vein
- Sural nerve or saphenous nerve injury

Postoperative complications
- Hematoma and bruising
- Wound infection
- Neuritis
- Lymphedema

- Induration of stripper track
- Lymphedema
- Deep venous thrombosis

Postoperative care
- Maintain firm pressure over the limb
- Regular movement of the operated limb
- Limb elevation above the heart level to reduce venous pressure
- Removal of primary dressing after 7 to 10 days

Sub-fascial Endoscopic Perforator Vein Surgery (SEPS)

Table 22.5: Indications and contraindicaitons of SEPS

Indications	Contraindications
• Chronic venous insufficiency (C4,5,6)	• Secondary varicose veins
	• Arterial insufficiency
	• Deep vein thrombosis

Operating Steps

- 10 mm port is introduced beneath deep fascia 8–10 cm below the tibial plateau 2 cm medial to anterior border of tibia. This port is used as camera port and for insufflations of carbon dioxide gas. 0 degree 10 mm telescope is used.
- Pressure is increased up to 30 mm of Hg. Second 5 mm port is introduced 6–8 cm posterior and inferior to the first port and used as the working port.
- Space is dissected using dissector and perforating veins encountered are clipped and cut. Alternatively, electrocautery and ultrasonic shears can also be applied for ligation.
- The incompetent perforators are identified, transected and coagulated under direct vision.
- All venous channels crossing sub-fascial space from anterior border of tibia till posterior mid line and inferiorly till medial malleolus are ligated.
- At the end of the procedure, incompetent sapheno-femoral junctions and sapheno-popliteal junctions are managed accordingly in the same setting.
- Skin incisions are closed with 3–0 nylon sutures.

Radiofrequency Closure

The intima of smaller veins can be destroyed by heat generation and denaturation of collagen using a probe consisting of a bipolar heat generator. The procedure is performed under ultrasound guidance and position of the probe is confirmed near the sapheno-femoral junction. With the help of a feedback system, temperature in the range of 80–85 degree Celsius is attained. The heated probe is gradually retracted down at a constant rate of 2–3cm/minute. Patient is sedated and local anesthesia instilled along the vein. Radiofrequency closure is suitable for smaller and straighter veins. It must be avoided in presence of dilated veins, veins with aneurysms and in thrombosis of veins.

Endo-venous Laser Therapy

EVLT is similar to radiofrequency closure except that it is a painless procedure and employs diode laser for the destruction of endothelial lining of the target vein. The ultrasound guides the location of probe, which is placed 2 cm distal to the sapheno-femoral junction. The probe is gradually withdrawn and ablates the lumen as it regresses down the vein by boiling the blood present within the lumen. Another added advantage of the procedure lies in the fact that veins of all sizes can be treated with this procedure.

23 Chronic Venous Insufficiency and Varicose Veins (CVI)

- Most common presenting features are
  - Dilated and visible vein in lower limb
  - Non healing ulcer
  - Pain in the legs (venous claudication)
- Duration and onset of symptoms
- Associated symptoms, e.g. calf muscle cramps at night, swelling of legs and ankles increasing at the end of the day and resolving/decreasing the next morning
- Bleeding from dilated veins
- Pain in the dilated veins
- In case of non-healing wound one must exclude peripheral vascular disease (ask about intermittent claudication, rest pain, previous/present gangrene, smoking)
- History of color change of skin or itching of lower limb around the ankle
- Changes in gait (talipes equines may develop in non-healing ulcer as the patient preferentially walks on the toes)
- History of pain and redness over the dilated veins may be suggestive of superficial thrombophlebitis
- Any history suggestive of deep vein thrombosis such as acute onset swelling of thigh and calf, pain or any risk factor for the same. Especially in post-partum period in female patients
- Occupation should be mentioned (especially if the job involves long hours of standing or strenuous exercise, e.g. barbers, conductors, athletes)
- *Family history:* Important in case of congenital conditions such as Klippel-Tenaunay and Park-Weber syndrome. Suspect if:
  - Cutaneous hemangiomas
  - Pulsatile veins (arterialization of veins)
  - Limb lengthening
  - No history of trauma to the thigh
- *Past history:* History of previous varicosities or any intervention for the same

SCHEME OF EXAMINATION

Local Examination

Inspection

- In standing position
- Talk about the visible dilated veins present on the medial/lateral/posterior side and their extent in effect describing the affected system, i.e. the long saphenous, short saphenous systems or both
- Any visible swellings or visible cough impulse in the groin (saphena varix)
- Reticular veins/Telangiectasias
- Describe ulcers if any
  - Scar marks/discoloration

Palpation

- Elongated, tortuous and palpable veins which are non-tender, non-pulsatile

- Thickening of skin
- Calf tenderness
- Palpable cough impulse in the groin
- Arterial pulsations
- Measurement of limb length

Tourniquet Tests

- To rule out sapheno-femoral junction incompetence, perforators in the thigh and patency of deep veins.
- Perform the FEGAN'S TEST prior to the tourniquet test to get an idea about the location of possible perforators.

Brodies-Trendelenburg Test

- Patient is recumbent
- Raise the legs to empty the veins
- Occlude SFJ by tourniquet/thumb pressure approx 3.75 cm below and lateral to pubic tubercle
- Ask the patient to stand
- Three possibilities
  - Normal/Negative test—veins fill gradually by capillary inflow over 45–60 seconds
  - Immediate filling of veins despite sustained pressure—denotes perforator incompetence. If the pressure is removed subsequently and the veins become more distended then there is possible SFJ incompetence
  - Rapid filling after removal of thumb—SFJ incompetence

Three tourniquet test

- For mid-thigh and adductor canal perforators
- Patient is recumbent
- Raise the legs and empty the veins
- Three tourniquets are tied at the SFJ, just below the mid-thigh and just above the knee
- Ask the patient to stand
- Three possibilities
  - *Filling of leg veins:* Implies that the leg perforators are incompetent.
  - *Lowermost tourniquet opened:* If the segment fills then the adductor canal perforator is incompetent.
  - *Mid-thigh tourniquet opened:* If the intervening segment fills then the mid-thigh perforator is incompetent.

Multiple tourniquet test

- Is usually not done as it is quite cumbersome and difficult to perform due to the variable position of the perforators.

Modified Perthes' test for patency of deep veins

- Patient remains standing
- Tourniquet is tied around the mid-thigh, tight enough to occlude the superficial veins (Ideally a BP cuff with a width which is two-thirds the circumference of the limb should be used)
- Patient is asked to jump on tiptoes 30 times
- If patient complains of a bursting pain in the calf and there is visible dilatation of the veins then obstruction of the deep venous system is suspected
- Perthes' test was originally described by the German surgeon, George Perthes. It is also known as the Delbet-Mocquot test. It was modified by Ochsner and Mahorner.

Schwartz test

- Is a palpatory confirmation of valvular incompetence.
- One finger is placed over the vein at the maximally dilated point
- Tap with a finger distally
- Feel for a thrill with the proximally placed finger
- Now reverse the action tap proximally and feel distally
- The test is positive only when the thrill is felt bidirectionally or from above downward.

Morrissey test

- Indicates incompetent veins between the right atrium and the leg veins and is positive in severe incompetence of the SFJ
- Patient is recumbent
- Raise the legs till the varicose veins are empty
- Patient is asked to cough and saphenous opening is watched for an impulse.

Auscultation

- Check for any bruit to rule out arterialization

How to State the Diagnosis

Varicose veins <state the system: GSV/SSV/Both> with Chronic venous insufficiency <state the class according to CEAP classification>

CEAP Classification

Classification of chronic lower extremity venous disease

C–Clinical Classification (C 0 to 6)

- **Class 0:** No visible/palpable signs of venous disease
- **Class 1:** Telangiectasia/reticular veins/ malleolar flare
- **Class 2:** Varicose veins
- **Class 3:** Edema without skin changes
- **Class 4:** Skin changes ascribed to venous disease (pigmentation/eczema/lipodermatosclerosis)
- **Class 5:** Skin changes (i.e. class 4) with healed ulceration
- **Class 6:** Skin changes (i.e. class 4) with active ulceration (Fig. 23.1)

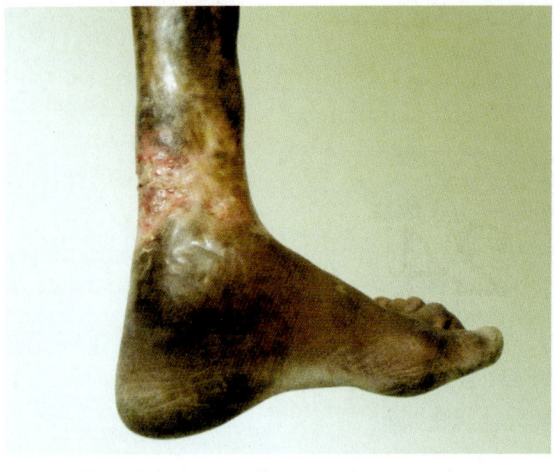

Fig. 23.1: A case of recurrent venous ulcer

Subcategories

- **'a':** Asymptomatic
- **'s':** Symptomatic (associated with lower extremity aching/pain/skin irritation)

E–Etiologic Classification

- E – Congenital
- P – Primary
- S – Secondary

A–Anatomic Classification

- S – Superficial venous system
- D –Deep veins
- P – Perforators

P–Pathophysiologic Classification

- R – Reflux
- O –Obstruction
- R, O–Reflux and obstruction

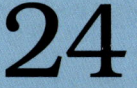

24 | Nerve Injuries

NEURON

- It is the structural unit of nervous system
- **Neuron consist of:**
  - Body of the cell
  - Dendrite(receiving processes) which may be multiple or single
  - Axon which is single and is discharging process. Axon can be myelinated or non myelinated
- In myelinated fibers conduction is faster than in unmyelinated
- Somatic fibers are myelinated
- Autonomic nerve fibers are unmyelinated

Structure of Peripheral Nerve

- *Endoneurium*: Formed by Schwann cell basement membrane and collagen fibers. Covers single myelinated fiber or no. of unmyelinated fibers
- *Perineurium*: Covers group of nerve fibers known as fascicles.
- *Epineurium*: Outer most sheath of nerve

Response of a Nerve to Injury

- Wallerian degeneration in distal part of nerve if axon disrupted
- Regeneration of axons in proximal part of nerve at the rate of 1–2 mm/day
- Monitored by Tinel's sign clinically.

Frequency of Nerve Injuries

- Data taken from a trauma population in Canada indicates that 2–3% of patients have a major nerve injury
- In New South Wales, Australia, 2% of patients were reported to have a major nerve injury.

Etiology

- Trauma
  - Blunt trauma
  - Penetrating wound
- Iatrogenic wrong site injections, e.g. axillary nerve or sciatic nerve can be damaged.
- Associated with certain fractures, e.g. fracture humerus giving rise to radial nerve injury, supracondylar fracture leading to ulnar nerve injury
- During operation
- Acute compression due to tight plaster cast

Pathophysiology

- Demyelination of axons distal to injury
- Axonal degeneration distal to division. This is also called Wallerian degeneration.
- Disruption of the sensory and/or motor function of the injured nerve
- Recovery of function occurs after
  - Remyelination
  - Axonal regeneration
  - Reinnervation of the sensory receptors, muscle end plates, or both

Clinical

- Loss of muscle function
- Loss of sensation to the affected nerve's sensory distribution
- Causalgia pain

Tinel's Sign

- Tap along the course of nerve distal to proximal
- Transient tingling sensation in the distribution of injured nerve
- Positive sign – regeneration is progressing
- Positive in type 2 and 3 injuries
- Absent in type 4 and 5 injuries

Classification of Nerve Injury

- Seddon in 1943
- Sunderland in 1951

Seddon Classification

- Neurapraxia
- Axonotmesis
- Neurotmesis

First-Degree Injury or Neurapraxia

- Temporary conduction block
- Demyelination of the nerve at the site of injury
- Electrodiagnostic study results are normal, above and below the level of injury
- No denervation or muscle changes
- Complete recovery may take up to 12 weeks.

Second-Degree Injury or Axonotmesis

- More severe trauma or compression. Axons disrupted
- Wallerian degeneration distal to the level of injury
- Proximal axonal degeneration to at least the next node of Ranvier
- Electrodiagnostic studies
  - Denervation changes in the affected muscles
  - Motor unit potentials (MUPs) in cases of reinnervation
- Axonal regeneration at the rate of 1 mm/day or 1 inch/month
- Monitored with an advancing Tinel's sign
- Endoneurial tubes intact, so recovery is complete
- Axons reinnervate their original motor and sensory targets

Third-Degree Injury

- Injury more severe than second-degree injury
- Axons and endoneurial tube disrupted
- Electrodiagnostic studies
  - Denervation changes
  - Fibrillations in the affected muscles
- Endoneurial tubes are not intact
- Recovery is mismatched, incomplete, mixed

Fourth-Degree Injury

- Large area of scar at the site of nerve injury
- Precludes any axons from advancing distal to the level of nerve injury
- No improvement in function is noted
- Surgery to restore neural continuity
- Axons, endoneurium, perineurium disrupted, but epineurium intact

Fifth-Degree Injury

- Complete transection of the nerve
- Requires surgery to restore neural continuity
- Endo, Peri and Epineurium disrupted

Sixth-Degree Injury

- Introduced by Mackinnon
- Mixed nerve injury that combines the other degrees of injury
- Some fascicles of the nerve are working normally
- Other fascicles may be recovering
- Other fascicles may require surgical intervention to permit axonal regeneration

Indications for Surgery

- Closed injuries with no evidence of recovery at 3 months
- Open injury (i.e. laceration)
- Crush injury

Investigations

- Nerve conduction studies
- Electromyography
- Muscle fibrillations – evidence of denervation
- Reinnervation is noted by the presence of motor unit potentials

Treatment

- *Open injuries*: Surgical repair
- *Closed injuries*: Conservative management initially, if no recovery in 3 months then exploration

Carpal Tunnel Syndrome (CTS)

- Compressive neuropathy of the median nerve at the wrist in carpal tunnel

Carpal Tunnel: Anatomy

- Located at the base of the palm
- Bound on 3 sides by carpal bones
- Anteriorly transverse carpal ligament

Contents

- Median nerve
- Flexor tendons
- Synovial sheaths

Pathophysiology

- Hypertrophy or edema of the flexor synovium
- Pain secondary to nerve ischemia

Frequency

- Overall prevalence of CTS is 2.7%
- Most frequently encountered peripheral compressive neuropathy
- Estimated lifetime risk 10%

Mortality/Morbidity

- Early in the course neurologic findings are reversible
- If untreated
  - Thenar atrophy
  - Chronic hand weakness
  - Numbness in the median nerve distribution

Age/Sex Distribution

- More prevalent in females
- Most common in middle-aged persons

History

- Intermittent "pins-and-needles" paresthesia
- Pain worse at night

Physical Examination

- Weakness of thumb abduction
- Sensory hyperalgesia along the palmar aspect of the index finger
- Phalen's sign
  - Hyperflexion of the wrist for 60 seconds leads to paresthesia in the median nerve distribution
- Sensitivity and specificity 68% and 73%
- Tapping the volar wrist over the median nerve leads to paresthesia
- Shaking or flicking one's hands gives relief
- Loss of 2-point discrimination in the median nerve distribution
- Abductor pollicis brevis atrophy

Etiology

- Inflammation of the flexor tendon sheath
- Edema from trauma of any type
- Pregnancy or oral contraceptive-related edema
- Acromegaly
- Rheumatoid arthritis
- Gout or pseudogout
- Hypothyroidism

Investigations

- Electromyographic (EMG) and nerve conduction studies
  - Determination of the site and severity of nerve compression
- Magnetic resonance imaging (MRI) when
  - Clinical picture is confusing
  - Nerve conduction studies are equivocal

Treatment

- Wrist immobilization with a splint
- Nonsteroidal anti-inflammatory drugs (NSAIDs)
- A corticosteroid with lidocaine injection
- Surgery
  - Surgical release of the transverse carpal ligament
  - Long-term success rate of 90%

Brachial Plexus Injuries (Upper Lesions)

- These are caused by the excessive displacement of the head to the opposite side
- Depression of the shoulder on the same side
- This causes excessive traction or tearing of C5 and C6 roots of the plexus

Nerves to be Affected

- The suprascapular nerve
- The nerve to the subclavius
- The musculocutaneous nerve
- Axillary nerve
- All muscles with nerve fibers derived from C5 and 6 roots and will therefore be functionless

Muscles to be Paralyzed

- Supraspinatus (abductor of shoulder)
- Subclavius (depresses the clavicle)
- Infraspinatus (lateral rotator of shoulder)
- Biceps brachii (flexor of elbow)
- Coracobrachialis (flexor of shoulder)
- Deltoid (abductor of shoulder)
- Teres minor (lateral rotator of shoulder)

Erb-Duchenne Palsy

- The limb hangs limply by the side likened to a waiter or porter hinting for a tip.
- There will be a loss of sensation down the lateral side of the arm.

Brachial Plexus Injuries (Lower Lesions)

- Loss of sensation will occur along the medial side of the arm
- Lower lesions can also be produced by a presence of a cervical rib or malignant metastases from the lungs in the lower deep cervical lymph nodes
- Are usually traction injuries caused by excessive abduction of the arm
- The first thoracic nerve is usually torn
- The hand has a clawed appearance caused by hyperextension of metacarpophalangeal joints and flexion of interphalangeal joints.

25 Soft Tissue Sarcoma (STS)

- It accounts for less than 1% of all adult malignancies and 7–8% of pediatric malignancies.
- The tumors most commonly metastasize by hematogenous route to lungs. Soft tissue sarcomas which also metastasize to lymph nodes are epitheloid sarcoma, clear cell sarcoma, angiosarcoma, lymphosarcoma, rhabdomyosarcoma and malignant fibrous histiocytoma (MFH).
- The most common mesenchymal tumor is Ewing's sarcoma; but as it is a bone tumor it is not considered under STS.
- The most common extremity tumor in adult is MFH followed by liposarcoma and leiomyosarcoma.
- The most common retroperitoneal sarcoma is liposarcoma.
- In children, the most common extremity sarcoma is the rhabdomyosarcoma.
- The investigation of choice for establishing the diagnosis is core cut tissue biopsy. If core cut biopsy yields negative result repeatedly then incisional biopsy is preferred.
- In incisional biopsy of an extremity tumor, the incision should be longitudinal so that during definitive surgery the previous incision can be included in the resection. During incisonal biopsy adequate hemostasis should be achieved and flaps should be minimally raised to prevent hematogenous dissemination of the tumor cells. Drain placement should be avoided.
- Excision biopsy is indicated only if the tumor size is <3 cm and if it is superficial to the deep fascia.
- In radiological imaging, MRI is preferred for the extremity and trunk tumor as it provides exact anatomical delineation. On T1 weighted images, the tumor appears as low signal intensity and on T2 weighted imaging; it appears as heterogenous high signal intensity lesion.
- CECT abdomen is preferred in cases of retroperitoneal and visceral sarcomas as it defines involvement of the contiguous structures and vascular involvement. MRI is less accurate in this perspective.
- Ultrasonography is useful only for guiding core cut biopsy and for the assessment of recurrence.
- Only in myxoid liposarcoma of the extremity, CECT abdomen and pelvis is indicated to assess for metastases.
- HRCT chest is indicated if there is a suspicious lesion on chest X-ray, tumor size more than 5 cm and if it is a high grade tumor
- The histopathological classification of STS are as follows:
  1. Sarcomas with no malignant potential
     a. Well differentiated liposarcoma
     b. Dermatofibrosarcoma protuberans
  2. Sarcomas with intermediate malignant potential

a. Myxoid liposarcoma
b. Extraskeletal chondrosarcoma

3. All other sarcomas are associated with high recurrence

- The staging system as per the 7th AJCC is as follows:

A. Grade: G1- low; G2 and G3- high

B. T1-tumor size ≤ 5 cm
   T2-tumor size > 5 cm
   The tumor is further divided into 'a' and 'b' based on whether the tumor is superficial or deep to deep fascia respectively. The retroperitoneal and visceral sarcomas are considered 'b' lesions.

C. Lymph node involvement
   N0 – no involvement and N1 – lymph node involvement present

D. Metastasis
   M0– absent and M1 – present

Staging

1. **Stage Ia:** T1a/b G1 N0 M0
   Stage Ib: T2a G1 N0 M0
2. **Stage IIa:** T1a/b G2/3 N0 M0
   Stage IIb: T2a G2/3 N0 M0
3. **Stage IIIa:** T2b G2/3 N0/1 M0
4. **Stage IV:** Any T Any G Any N M1

- The basic management of soft tissue sarcoma consists of surgery followed by radiotherapy
- Surgery typically consists of wide excision with a normal margin of 2 cm. The excision may demand en-bloc removal of vessels and bones which needs to be reconstructed later on
- The radiotherapy can be delivered in the form of external beam RT, brachytherapy or intensity modulated RT
- The role of chemotherapy in STS is only in cases of recurrent high grade disease and in case of systemic disease
- The drug of choice for chemotherapy is doxorubicin
- The treatment plan as per staging is as follows:
  - **Stage I:** Surgery and follow-up
  - **Stage II:** Surgery with or without radiotherapy
  - **Stage III:** Surgery with radiotherapy with or without chemotherapy
  - **Stage IV:** Chemotherapy followed by surgery and radiotherapy based on response

Section III

26 Premalignant Conditions of Oral Cavity

Lesions Which are Definitely Premalignant

1. Leukoplakia
2. Erythroplakia
3. Chronic hyper-plastic Candidiasis

Lesions having Higher than Normal Incidence of Malignancy

1. Oral sub mucus fibrosis
2. Syphilitic glossitis
3. Sideropenic dysphagia

Lesions having Doubtful Association

1. Oral lichen planus
2. Discoid lupus erythrematosis
3. Dyskeratosis congenita

LEUKOPLAKIA

WHO has defined leucoplakia as any white patch or plaque in oral cavity which cannot be characterized clinically or pathologically to any other lesion.

Sites of Leukoplakia

1. Oral cavity (commonly seen on tongue)
2. Larynx
3. Perianal region
4. Glans penis
5. Vulva

Etiology

Chronic irritation of mucosa due to

1. Sharp tooth or ill fitting denture
2. Smoking
3. Sepsis
4. Spirits
5. Spices
6. Syphilis
7. Vitamin deficiency

There may be idiopathic leukoplakia without any source of irritation except tobacco consumption.

Epidemiology

a. It is present in less than 1% of individuals.
b. It is potentially a malignant condition with a malignant transformation rate ranging from 0.6 to 20%. Most of the malignant changes occur within the fissures. Warning signs of malignant change in leukoplakia are:
   i. Local thickening
   ii. Bleeding
   iii. Area of redness
   iv. Pain in the lesion
c. Majority of cases occur in the fifth to seventh decade of life. Approximately 80% of patients are older than 40 years.
d. More common in men than in women, with a male-to-female ratio of 2:1.

Pathology

Macroscopically it appears as thickened grey white plaque with cracks or fissures. Plaque is difficult to rub off.

Microscopically

1. There is hyperplasia of superficial layers of the squamous epithelium
2. Hyperkeratosis, swelling and vacuolation of cells of the middle layer
3. Hyperplasia and hyperchromasia of the basal layers
4. Dyskeratosis

Four stages of leukoplakia:
1. **Stage 1:** Thin grey transparent patch on tongue
2. **Stage 2:** Thin patch becomes white and opaque with development of cracks and fissures over it later on
3. **Stage 3:** There is nodule formation due to hyperplasia or there is development of smooth, red shiny patches due to desquamation of epithelium
4. **Stage 4:** There is appearance of carcinoma. Malignant change usually occurs in fissures. It should be suspected if there is local thickening, bleeding or pain

Clinically it can appear as uniform homogenous white plaque with low potential of malignancy. It can also appear as specked or nodular leukoplakia with high malignant potential.

Warning Signs of Malignancy in Leukoplakia

1. Development of nodules in a previous homogenous white patch
2. Development of ulcer or erosion in to the lesion
3. A lesion which feels harder at periphery
4. Leukoplakia at floor of the mouth or at under the surface of tongue are highly suspicious

Treatment

a. Removal of underlying cause. If patient stops smoking leukoplakia will disappear in 60% of cases
b. Biopsy of suspicious lesions should be taken
c. Small lesions can be treated with surgical excision with primary closure or by Carbon dioxide laser excision
d. Larger defects resulting from excision will need grafting

ERYTHROPLAKIA

It is a bright red velvety plaque in the oral cavity with irregular outline and nodular surface. The incidence of malignancy is 17 fold higher than leukoplakia.

Treatment

Treatment is total excision by surgery or by Carbon dioxide laser. Resected specimen should be sent for careful pathological examination.

27 Oral Cavity Cancer

Oral cavity cancer accounts for 30 percent of head and neck cancers in India. Buccal mucosa cancer is very common in India and constitutes 42% of all oral cavity cancers in contrast to the US where it forms only 5% of all oral cancers. High incidence of buccal mucosa cancer is due to habit of chewing betel nut with tobacco and keeping a quid in the oral cavity for a long time.

Anatomy

Oral Cavity Extends from

- Anteriorly the junction of skin to vermilion junction of the anterior lips
- Posteriorly the junction of the hard and soft palates above and the line of circumvallate papillae below

It Includes Following Structures

- Lip
- Anterior 2/3 of tongue
- Buccal mucosa
- Floor of mouth
- Lower gingiva
- Retromolar trigone
- Upper gingiva
- Hard palate

Lymph Drainage of Oral Cavity

Recent studies have shown that lymphatic spread from oral cavity cancer in untreated neck occurs due to embolic spread rather than through permeation of lymphatic channels. This concept raises a question mark on concept of en block dissection of primary tumor and lymph bearing area. Lymph spread occurs in a step wise fashion and lower cervical and posterior cervical lymph nodes are rarely involved in oral cavity cancer

- *First station nodes*: Buccinator, jugulo-digastric, submandibular and submental
- *Second station nodes*: Parotid, jugular and the upper and lower posterior cervical nodes

Factors Affecting Lymph Node Involvement in Oral Cavity Cancer

Larger tumor, more posterior location of tumor and the less well differentiated tumor are more likely to have lymph node metastasis

Epidemiology

- Sixth most common cancer in the world
- Largely preventable
- In India
  - Commonest malignant neoplasm
  - 30–40% of all cancers

Etiology/Risk Factors

- *Tobacco consumption*: 90 percent of oral cavity cancers can be directly attributed to smoking. The relative risk of oral cavity cancer is seven times in comparison to non smokers.
- *Use of alcohol*: Alcohol acts as an irritant, solvent for carcinogen and promoter for

carcinogenesis. Risk of developing oral cavity cancer is six times in comparison to non drinkers. The risk of developing oral cavity cancer is 38 times more for patients who consume both alcohol and tobacco.
- Use of alcohol and tobacco produces a field defect due to chronic carcinogen exposure. The entire mucosa of upper aero digestive tract is at risk
- Use of areca (betel) nut
- Leucoplakia
- Erythroplakia
- Submucous fibrosis
- Consumption of foods rich in nitrites and nitrosamines
- Retroviruses, Adenoviruses or the Epstein-barr virus (EB virus)
- Herpes simplex viruses (HSV) and the Human papilloma viruses (HPV)
- The risk of second malignancy after successful treatment of oral carcinoma is 3.7 percent every year and increases to 24 percent at ten years.

Pathology

A. More than 90 percent are squamous cell carcinomas. The squamous cell carcinoma can be exophytic, ulcerative or a combination of both. The exophytic growth is less aggressive.
B. Microscopic types:
   - Basaloid type
   - Verrucous type presents as exophytic growth has a more favorable prognosis with less chances of metastasis.
   - Sarcomatoid type presents as bulky poly-poidal rapidly growing mass and has a very poor prognosis
   - Poorly differentiated carcinoma

Staging

TNM Classification
- Primary tumor (T)
  - **TX:** Primary tumor cannot be assessed
  - **T0:** No evidence of primary tumor
  - **Tis:** Carcinoma *in situ*
  - **T1:** Tumor 2 cm or less in greatest dimension
  - **T2:** Tumor more than 2 cm but not more than 4 cm in greatest dimension
  - **T3:** Tumor more than 4 cm in greatest dimension
  - **T4:** Tumor invades adjacent structures

- Regional lymph nodes (N)
  - **NX:** Regional lymph nodes cannot be assessed
  - **N0:** No regional lymph node metastasis
  - **N1:** Metastasis in a single ipsilateral lymph node, 3 cm or less in greatest dimension
  - **N2:** Metastasis in a single ipsilateral lymph node, more than 3 cm but not more than 6 cm in greatest dimension; or in multiple ipsilateral lymph nodes, none more than 6 cm in greatest dimension; or in bilateral or contralateral lymph nodes, none more than 6 cm in greatest dimension
  - **N3:** Metastasis in a lymph node more than 6 cm in greatest dimension
- Distant metastasis (M)
  - **MX:** Distant metastasis not assessed
  - **M0:** No distant metastasis
  - **M1:** Distant metastasis present

Mode of Spread

1. *Local spread:* Local spread to adjacent structures like soft tissue, bones, and neurovascular structures.
2. *Lymph nodes spread:* First halt is lymph nodes in the supraomohyoid triangle.
3. Distant metastasis is rare and occurs in advanced cases or in recurrent cases. It generally occurs in lungs or bones.

Mandible Involvement

It generally starts through dental socket or through dental pulp and reaches the root of tooth. From root of tooth cancellous portion of mandible is involved. After this spread occurs through mandibular canal.

Clinical Features

a. Indurated mass that bleeds on touch
b. Non healing ulcer
c. Slurring of speech
d. Tooth extraction socket that fails to heal
e. Persistent gingival inflammation
f. Loosening of tooth
g. Trismus or ankylosis
h. Pain is a late feature
i. Orocutaneous fistula
j. Lymph nodes in the neck
k. Weight loss

AJCC Stage Groupings

Stage 0:   Tis, N0, M0
Stage I: T1, N0, M0
Stage II: T2, N0, M0
Stage III: T3, N0, M0; T1, N1, M0; T2, N1, M0;
                 T3, N1, M0
Stage IVA: T4, N0, M0; T4, N1, M0; Any T, N2,
                 M0
Stage IVB: Any T, N3, M0
Stage IVC: Any T, Any N, M1

Preoperative Clinical Examination in a Case of Oral Cavity Carcinoma

1. Complete examination of oral cavity along with status of oral hygiene and teeth
2. Presence of precancerous lesions like sub mucous fibrosis and leukoplakia is noted
3. Tumor itself is described in detail, e.g. size of tumor, type (ulcerative, proliferative or infiltrative), involvement of adjacent structures, e.g. skin, bone, lymph nodes, trismus are all documented
4. Neck is carefully examined for lymph node enlargement

Investigations in Case of Oral Cavity Cancer

1. Punch biopsy from primary lesion and fine needle aspiration cytology from palpable lymph nodes. If the lesion appears to be verrucous type then a biopsy by knife needs to be taken.
2. **Imaging:** Oblique and occlusive views of the mandible and ortho-pantogram (OPG) to rule out mandible involvement especially antral or alveolar involvement. CT scan is useful in doubtful cases of mandible involvement or to rule out extension of disease in infra-temporal fossa. Indications of CT are:
   a. Patient with trismus
   b. For antral tumors
   c. Assessment of pterygoid fossa
   d. To evaluate metastatic disease of neck
   e. Clinically negative neck
   f. Patients with large nodes

Abdominal ultrasonography is done to rule out liver metastasis. Chest X-ray is done for pulmonary metastasis.

MRI is useful in knowing the extent of soft tissue involvement or perineural involvement.

Treatment Option

- Surgery alone
- Radiation therapy alone
- Combination of these

Stage Wise Treatment

1. *Treatment for T1 and T2 lesion:* Surgery and radiotherapy gives equally good results. Any of the two methods can be utilised. Combined modality is not necessary. Choice of treatment depends upon skill and experience of clinician treating the case and the facilities available at the institution.

Radiotherapy (RT): Prior to starting radio-therapy all broken and loose teeth need to be removed and wound after teeth removal should be allowed to heal before starting radiotherapy. Broken teeth should be removed before RT as the teeth become brittle after RT and there are chances of osteonecrosis of the jaw. RT is given by telecobalt machine in the dose of 6000 cg delivered in 6 weeks. For further boost at the primary site radioactive iridium wire can be implanted (brachy therapy). Advantages of RT are good cosmetic and functional results. Drawbacks of RT are dental problems, dryness of mouth due to radiotherapy induced atrophy of salivary glands and post irradiation fibrosis leading to delayed trismus.

Surgery: It involves wide excision of lesion carried out intraoral. Raw area can be covered by split skin graft. Benefit to patient is short duration of treatment in comparison to RT. Drawbacks include shrinkage and fibrosis of graft in postoperative period leading to fibrosis and trismus. Sometimes it may be difficult to obtain a clear margin at the base.

Surgery is preferable over radiotherapy in following situations
   a. If there is concomitant submucus fibrosis
   b. In presence of mandibular involvement
   c. Verrucous carcinoma as it is relatively radio resistant due to less vascularity
   d. T1 lesions as a results of surgery are functionally better
   e. If there is history of previous irradiation
   f. Multiple primary tumors
   g. Extensive premalignant changes in surrounding areas

h. Adenocarcinoma or melanoma

i. Lesions in lower gingivo-buccal sulcus

Laser Excision: This is a recent alternative for early oral cavity cancer in which carbon dioxide or diode laser is used. The tumour can be excised with a wide margin and clear base. The resultant raw area is left open to heal by epithelisation. There is minimum blood loss and postoperative pain. A more satisfactory histo-pathological examination of laser excised tissue can be carried out in comparison to cautery excised tissue. An advantage of laser therapy includes very short treatment time, no dental problem, no dryness of mouth and no trismus.

2. *Surgery for T3 and T4 Lesions:* Surgery is primary modality of treatment for T3 and T4 lesions as RT is not curative in these cases. RT is only used as palliative treatment for unresectable and recurrent lesions.

Criteria for unresectability are:

1. Involvement of tonsil, hard palate or soft palate

2. Extensive involvement of skin in the form of fungation

3. Involvement of pterygoid muscles or infra-temporal fossa

4. Lymph nodes involvement which are fixed

5. Patient unfit to undergo major resection and reconstructive procedures as surgery is likely to last for more than 6 hours.

Extent of Surgery in T3 and T4 Lesions

In order to achieve curative resection a wide margin with 2 cm of healthy mucosa should be excised along with the tumor. If it is difficult to achieve clear wide margin superiorly, upper teeth are removed along with the mucosa of upper alveolus and alveolar bone. The mucosal flap is sutured to the mucoperiosteum of the hard palate. To obtain clear margin posteriorly tonsils can be removed. The resected margin should include all precancerous lesions. It is essential that pathologist comments on the status of cut margins.

Mandibular Involvement in Buccal Mucosa Cancer

Routes of mandibular involvement:

1. Direct invasion of mandible by primary tumor

2. Mandible can be involved from occlusive surface, periodontal membrane and the dental canal

3. Once it reaches the mandibular canal it spreads widely within bone

4. Infra-temporal fossa can be involved through the peri-neural lymphatics

5. In elderly patients' vertical height of horizontal ramus of mandible is less as these patients are edentulous, so that mandibular canal comes near the occlusive surface and near the lower border thus there is early mandibular involvement without much chances of marginal mandibulectomy.

Types of mandibular resection in oral cavity cancer:

1. The segmental resection of mandible is carried out in following situations:

   a. The clinical and radiological involvement of mandible

   b. To facilitate wide margin resection

   c. To facilitate reconstruction

   d. In lesions involving full thickness of cheek

As disease rarely involves the posterior segment of ascending ramus, so it is possible to perform a segmental resection of mandible without removing a L shaped piece of bone comprising head, neck, posterior border and insertion of medial pterygoid muscles.

Marginal mandibulectomy: In this procedure the alveolar part is removed preserving the lower border. It results in loss of teeth but without malocclusion and facial contour without cosmetic deformity. It is a good operation for lesions of the floor of the mouth or tongue. The line of excision extends below the mylohyoid muscle thus en block excision of the floor of the mouth is achieved. Marginal mandibulectomy has little role in T3 or T4 lesions as in these cases one is likely to cut through the involved soft tissue.

Extent of Lymph Node Dissection

In cases of node negative cancer supra-omohyoid dissection is done which involves removal of nodes from level 1 to level 3. The specimen is submitted for frozen section. A complete neck dissection is done only if lymph node shows metastatic disease on frozen section. The classical radical neck dissection is preserved for extensive neck disease, i.e. large or multiple nodes, fixed nodes, nodes in the lower third of the deep cervical chain, nodes in the posterior triangle and recurrence in the neck after RT.

Chemotherapy

Effective chemotherapy drugs are Methotrexate, 5 Fluorouracil (5FU), Cisplatin and Bleomycin. Chemotherapy may have a role in palliative settings, or given as neoadjuvant chemotherapy or as an adjuvant therapy after surgery.

28 Salivary Gland Diseases

Various salivary gland diseases are:
- Development disorders
- Functional disorders
- Obstructive disorders
- Non-neoplastic disorders
- Neoplastic disorders

DEVELOPMENT DISORDER

Congenital absence of one or more of salivary glands, usually involving parotid gland can occur rarely.

Sometimes duct atresia involving submandibular duct involving floor of mouth due to failure to canalize during development can occur and the newborn infant presents with swelling of the submandibular gland on the affected side.

Ectopic salivary tissue can be seen in the lymph nodes within the neck or at the angle of mandible below the inferior dental canal. The later condition is also known as Stafne's bone cyst and usually occurs due to invagination of ectopic lobe of submandibular salivary gland in to mandibular bone on lingual aspect.

Accessory lobe involving parotid gland is seen in 20 percent of cases and arises from horizontal component of parotid duct over its course on the surface of masseter muscle.

FUNCTIONAL DISORDERS

Sialorrhea

- The term sialorrhea means increase in salivary flow

- It can occur due to
  - Local causes like painful oral ulcers
  - Due to post extraction
  - Post-surgery wounds
  - It can be due to dentures/appliances
- It has varied aetiology resulting from neurological disorders ranging from psychosis, Bell's palsy, Parkinson's disease stroke or cerebral palsy, rabies and mercury or iodine toxicity.

Xerostomia

- It means decrease in saliva flow leading to dry mouth. Normal salivary flow decreases with age in both sexes and in postmenopausal females.
- It can also be a feature of chronic anxiety or depression.
- It can also occur in dehydration.
- Anti-muscarinic drugs like atropine, tricyclic antidepressants, or sympathomimetic drugs like ephedrine or iso-prenaline can cause xerostomia.
- Its causes also include mumps, sarcoidosis, Sjögren's syndrome, lupus, post-irradiation.

OBSTRUCTIVE DISORDERS

Stone Formation (Sialolithiasis)

- 80% occur in submandibular gland
- 10% in parotid gland, 7% in sublingual gland and rest in the minor salivary gland

- Majority of stones occur in the submandibular gland because secretions are viscid, contain more mucus and high content of bicarbonate. Submandibular gland has non-dependent drainage as the submandibular duct has a long and curved course and lies below the level of its opening in floor of mouth thus predisposing to stasis. In contrast parotid duct has a straight course and secretions are more serous in nature and have less viscosity.
- Multiple occurrence in same gland is common.

Submandibular Stones

Diagnosis

- 80% of submandibular stones are radiopaque and can be seen on plain X-ray
- In contrast majority of parotid gland stones are radiolucent and cannot be detected on plain X-ray
- Pain and sudden enlargement of gland while eating. Onset of swelling and pain is rapid and usually occurs within 1 minute of meals and the swelling subsides within 1 hour of finishing meals. Pain can be referred to side of the tongue due to irritation of lingual nerve it hooks around duct and sometimes there is tooth ache
- Later on pain becomes continuous and swelling becomes constant. This is thought to occur due to irreparable damage to salivary gland
- There can be discomfort and swelling in the floor of mouth due to impacted stone
- Enlarged submandibular gland can be palpated with the upper border lying beneath the horizontal ramus of the mandible
- Orifices of the Wharton duct on either side of the frenulum of the tongue may be red and edematous or may show grey colored stone impacted at the duct end
- Pressure on the gland may produce discharge from the duct orifice
- Course of the duct is felt for any stone (firm or hard lump)
- Occlusal radiograph (80%) oblique lateral view or posterior occlusal view may reveal the stone

Treatment

- Can be removed transorally if in duct and easily palpable
- If in gland and gland is damaged, then gland should be removed.

Parotid Lithiasis

Diagnosis

- Based on history
- Swelling during meals
- Bimanual palpation of painful gland
- 40% non-radiopaque
- Most parotid stones are multiple

Treatment

- Stones in extraglandular portion of the duct can be removed transorally
- Intraglandular stones removed from extraoral approach

NON-NEOPLASTIC DISORDERS

Acute Sialadenitis

- Viral-Mumps
- Bacterial
  - Swelling, dehydration, xerostomia leading to failure of secretion with ascending infection
  - *Staphylococcus aureus, streptococcus pyogenes*, most common infective organism
- Painful swelling parotid gland, overlying skin red, shiny and tense, pus from parotid duct
- Treatment
  - Pus culture
  - Appropriate antibiotic
  - Supportive therapy
    ◊ Fluids
    ◊ Heat
    ◊ Salivary stimulants

Chronic Sialadenitis

- Chronic recurrent parotitis
- Age 3–6
- Caused by *Streptococcus viridans*
- May spontaneously heal during puberty

NEOPLASTIC DISORDERS

Incidence

- Relatively uncommon
- 2% of head and neck neoplasms
- It comprises of 1.2 percent of all neoplastic disease
- All salivary gland tumors present as slowly growing masses present for several years

- Even the malignant salivary gland neoplasm are slow growing and pain is not a reliable indicator of malignancy as the benign tumor can present with pain and aching sensation due to distension of the capsule of involved gland or due to element of out flow obstruction
- Reliable signs of malignancy are
  - Facial nerve involvement in case of parotid gland
  - Induration and/or ulceration of the overlying skin or mucosa
  - Regional lymph nodes involvement

Investigations of Salivary Gland Tumors

- CT and MRI are either equally helpful in case of parotid or submandibular tumor. These imaging modalities will accurately delineate the tumors, will confirm that they are actually arising from salivary gland. These investigations will also confirm if the swelling is well localized (suggestive of benign disease) or diffuse and invasive (suggestive of malignancy). These investigations will also define the relation of tumor with surrounding structures thus help in planning future surgery.
- Open surgical biopsy is absolutely contraindicated. Open biopsy is only indicated if there is infiltration or ulceration of overlying skin. For tumors of minor salivary gland especially on palate open incisional biopsy is indicated as at these sites there are very high chances of malignancy and biopsy can be obtained without opening other tissue planes.
- FNAC (Fine needle aspiration cytology) is a safe alternative to open biopsy for major salivary gland. There is no risk of needle seedling if the needle used is 18 gauge or more.

Classification of Salivary Gland Tumors (WHO Classification 1991–Simplified)

- Adenoma
  - Pleomorphic adenoma
  - Warthin's tumor
- Carcinoma
  - Acinic cell tumor
  - Mucoepidermoid carcinoma
  - Adenoid cystic carcinoma
  - Adenocarcinoma
  - Squamous cell carcinoma
  - Undifferentiated carcinoma
  - Carcinoma in pleomorphic adenoma
- Non epithelial tumors
  - Hemangioma
  - Lymphangioma
  - Neurofibroma
  - Neurilemoma
- Malignant lymphoma
- Unclassified and allied conditions

GLAND WISE DISTRIBUTION

- 75% occur in parotid gland and only 15% are malignant.
- 10% occur in the submandibular gland and 1/3rd of these are malignant.
- 15% occur in the minor salivary glands and nearly half of them are malignant.
- Tumor in sublingual gland are rare(0.3%) and nearly all of them are malignant.

Malignancy

- Sublingual 90%
- Submandibular 30%
- Parotid 15%
- Minor salivary gland 50%

Clinical Classification

- Benign (seldom recurrent)
  - Adenolymphoma (Wharthin's tumor)
  - Oxyphil adenoma (Oncocytoma)
  - Other types of monomorphic adenoma
- Benign (often recurrent)
  - Pleomorphic adenoma (mixed tumor)
  - Mucoepidermoid tumor (low-grade)
  - Acinic cell tumor (same)
- Malignant
  - Carcinoma in pleomorphic adenoma
  - Adenoid cystic carcinoma
  - Acinic cell tumor
  - Mucoepidermoid tumor (high-grade)
  - Squamous carcinoma
  - Adenocarcinoma, other types
  - Undifferentiated carcinoma

Pleomorphic Adenoma

- Most common of all salivary gland neoplasms
  - 70% of parotid tumors

- 50% of submandibular tumors
- 45% of minor salivary gland tumors
- 6% of sublingual tumors
- 4–6th decades
- F:M = 3 – 4:1
- Slow-growing, painless mass
- *Parotid*: 90% in superficial lobe, mostly in tail of gland
- *Minor salivary gland*: Lateral palate, sub mucosal mass

Histopathology

- Gross pathology
  - Smooth
  - Well-demarcated
  - Solid
  - Cystic changes
  - Myxoid stroma
- Histology
  - Mixture of epithelial, myopeithelial and stromal components
  - *Epithelial cells*: Nests, sheets, ducts, trabeculae
  - *Stroma*: Myxoid, chrondroid, fibroid, osteoid
  - No true capsule
  - Tumor pseudopods

Treatment

- Complete surgical excision
  - Parotidectomy with facial nerve preservation
  - Submandibular gland excision
  - Wide local excision of minor salivary gland
- Avoid enucleation and tumor spillage

Warthin's Tumor

- Also known as papillary cyst adenoma lymphomatosum. It is benign monomorphic cystic tumour containing epithelial and epithelial lined multiple cystic spaces and lymphoid tissue.
- It commonly arises in parotid gland, rare in submandibular gland.
- Arises from terminal ductule of parotid gland. It may also arise from periparotid lymph node which has incorporated parotid tissue during its development.
- 6–10% of parotid neoplasms
- 10% bilateral or multicentric
- *Presentation*: Slow-growing, painless mass

Histopathology

- Gross pathology
  - Encapsulated
  - Smooth/lobulated surface
  - Cystic spaces of variable size, with viscous fluid, shaggy epithelium
  - Solid areas with white nodules representing lymphoid follicles
- Histology
  - Papillary projections into cystic spaces surrounded by lymphoid stroma
  - *Epithelium*: Double cell layer
    ◊ Luminal cells
    ◊ Basal cells
- *Stroma*: Mature lymphoid follicles with germinal centers

Oncocytoma

- *Rare*: 2–3% of benign salivary tumors
- 6th decade
- M:F = 1:1
- *Parotid:* 78%
- *Submandibular gland:* 9%
- *Minor salivary glands:* Palate, buccal mucosa, tongue
- Presentation
  - Enlarging, painless mass
- Technetium-99m pertechnetate scintigraphy shows hot activity
  - Mitochondrial hyperplasia

Histopathology

- Gross
  - Encapsulated
  - Homogeneous, smooth
  - Orange/rust color
- Histology
  - Cords of uniform cells and thin fibrous stroma
  - Large polyhedral cells
  - Distinct cell membrane
  - Granular, eosinophilic cytoplasm
  - Central, round, vesicular nucleus
- Electron microscopy
  - Mitochondrial hyperplasia
  - 60% of cell volume

Mucoepidermoid Carcinoma

- Most common salivary gland malignancy
- 5–9% of salivary neoplasms

- Parotid 45–70% of cases
- Palate 18%
- 3rd–8th decades, peak in 5th decade
- More common in females
- Presentation
  - *Low-grade:* Slow growing, painless mass
  - *High-grade:* Rapidly enlarging, +/– pain
  - Minor salivary glands: may be mistaken for
    ◊ Benign or inflammatory process
    ◊ Hemangioma
    ◊ Papilloma
- Gross pathology
  - Well-circumscribed to partially encapsulated to unencapsulated
  - Solid tumor with cystic spaces
- Histology
  - Low grade
    ◊ Mucus cell > epidermoid cells
    ◊ Prominent cysts
    ◊ Mature cellular elements
  - Intermediate grade
    ◊ Mucus = epidermoid
    ◊ Fewer and smaller cysts
    ◊ Increasing pleomorphism and mitotic figures
  - High-grade
    ◊ Epidermoid > mucus
    ◊ Solid tumor cell proliferation
    ◊ Mistaken for squamous cell carcinoma
    ◊ Mucin staining
- Treatment
  - Influenced by site, stage, grade
  - Stage I and II
    ◊ Wide local excision
  - Stage III and IV
    ◊ Radical excision
    ◊ +/– neck dissection
    ◊ +/– postoperative radiation therapy

Adenoid Cystic Carcinoma

- Overall 2nd most common malignancy
- Most common in submandibular, sublingual and minor salivary glands
- M = F
- 5th decade
- Presentation
- Asymptomatic enlarging mass
- Pain, paresthesias, facial weakness/paralysis

- Gross pathology
  - Well-circumscribed
  - Solid, rarely with cystic spaces
  - Infiltrative
- Histology
  - Cribriform pattern
    ◊ Most common
    ◊ "Swiss cheese" appearance
  - Tubular pattern
    ◊ Layered cells forming duct-like structures
    ◊ Basophilic mucinous substance
  - Solid pattern
    ◊ Solid nests of cells without cystic or tubular spaces
- Treatment
  - Complete local excision
  - Tendency for perineural invasion: facial nerve sacrifice
  - Postoperative XRT
- Prognosis
  - *Local recurrence:* 42%
  - *Distant metastasis:* Lung
  - *Indolent course:* 5-year survival 75%, 20-year survival 13%

Acinic Cell Carcinoma

- 2nd most common parotid and pediatric malignancy
- 5th decade
- F > M
- Bilateral parotid disease in 3%
- Presentation
  - Solitary, slow-growing, often painless mass
- Gross pathology
  - Well-demarcated
  - Most often homogeneous
- Histology
  - Solid and microcystic patterns
    ◊ Most common
    ◊ Solid sheets
    ◊ Numerous small cysts
  - Polyhedral cells
  - Small, dark, eccentric nuclei
  - Basophilic granular cytoplasm
- Treatment
  - Complete local excision
  - +/– postoperative XRT

- Prognosis
  - *5-year survival:* 82%
  - *10-year survival:* 68%
  - *25-year survival:* 50%

Adenocarcinoma

- Rare
- 5th to 8th decades
- F > M
- Parotid and minor salivary glands
- Presentation
  - Enlarging mass
  - 25% with pain or facial weakness
- Histology
  - Heterogeneity
  - Presence of glandular structures and absence of epidermoid component
  - Grade I–III
- Treatment
  - Complete local excision
  - Neck dissection
  - Postoperative XRT
- Prognosis
  - *Local recurrence:* 51%
  - *Regional metastasis:* 27%
  - *Distant metastasis:* 26%
  - 15-year cure rate:
    - ◊ Stage I = 67%
    - ◊ Stage II = 35%
    - ◊ Stage III = 8%

Malignant Mixed Tumors

- Carcinoma ex-pleomorphic adenoma
  - Carcinoma developing in the epithelial component of pre-existing pleomorphic adenoma
- Carcinosarcoma
  - True malignant mixed tumor—carcinomatous and sarcomatous components
- Metastatic mixed tumor
  - Metastatic deposits of otherwise typical pleomorphic adenoma

Carcinoma Ex-Pleomorphic Adenoma

- 2–4% of all salivary gland neoplasms
- 4–6% of mixed tumors
- 6–8th decades
- Parotid > submandibular > palate
- Risk of malignant degeneration

- 1.5% in first 5 years
- 9.5% after 15 years
- Presentation
  - Long-standing painless mass that undergoes sudden enlargement
- Gross pathology
  - Poorly circumscribed
  - Infiltrative
  - Hemorrhage and necrosis
- Histology
  - Malignant cellular change adjacent to typical pleomorphic adenoma
  - Carcinomatous component
  - Adenocarcinoma
  - Undifferentiated
- Treatment
  - Radical excision
  - Neck dissection (25% with lymph node involvement at presentation)
  - Postoperative XRT
- Prognosis
  - Dependent upon stage and histology

Squamous Cell Carcinoma

- 1.6% of salivary gland neoplasms
- 7–8th decades
- M:F = 2:1
- Must rule out
  - High-grade mucoepidermoid carcinoma
  - Metastatic squamous cell carcinoma to intraglandular nodes
  - Direct extension of squamous cell carcinoma
- Gross pathology
  - Unencapsulated
  - Ulcerated
  - Fixed
- Histology
  - Infiltrating
  - Nests of tumor cells
  - Well differentiated
    - ◊ Keratinization
  - Moderately-well differentiated
  - Poorly differentiated
    - ◊ No keratinization
- Treatment
  - Radical excision
  - Neck dissection
  - Postoperative XRT

- Prognosis
  - *5-year survival:* 24%
  - *10-year survival:* 18%

Undifferentiated Carcinoma

- Lymphoepithelial malignancy
  - *Eskimos:* Parotid gland, F > M, familial
  - *Asians:* Submandibular, M > F
- Large-cell
  - Bimodal peaks
  - M > F
  - Parotid gland
- Small-cell
  - 6–7th decades
  - M:F = 1.6:1
  - Parotid gland

Management of the N0 Neck

- Recurrence in the neck = low likelihood of salvage
- *Parotid:* Clinical neck disease, 16%
  - N– disease = 74% 5-year survival
  - N+ disease = 9% 5-year survival
- Submandibular: clinical neck disease, 8%
  - N- disease = 41% 5-year survival
  - N+ disease = 9% 5-year survival
- Increased risk of occult neck metastasis
  - High-grade malignancies
  - Advanced primary tumor stage (T3–T4)
  - High risk histology
    ◊ Undifferentiated, squamous cell carcinoma, adenocarcinoma, high-grade muco-epidermoid, salivary duct carcinoma
  - Tumor size > 3 cm
  - Patient > 54 years of age
  - Facial paralysis
  - Extracapsular, perilymphatic spread
- Neck dissection
  - Advantages
    ◊ Pathologic staging
    ◊ Improved counselling and prediction of prognosis
  - Disadvantages
    ◊ Longer OR time, increase in complications, increased cost
    ◊ Functional deficits, cosmetic effects

- Type
  ◊ *Parotid:* levels II-IV
  ◊ *Submandibular:* levels I-III
- Radiation therapy
  - Advantage
    ◊ Avoids surgical sequlae
  - Disadvantages
    ◊ Radiation effect on normal tissue
    ◊ Radiation induced malignancies
  - **Proponents argument:** The same factors that increase the risk of occult neck disease also increase the risk for local recurrence and necessitate postoperative XRT to the primary, so it is reasonable to treat the neck with XRT as well.

Role of Fine-Needle Aspiration Biopsy

- Efficacy is well established
- Accuracy = 84 – 97%
- Sensitivity = 54 – 95%
- Specificity = 86 – 100%
- Safe, well tolerated
- Opponents' argument
  - Doesn't change management
  - Surgery regardless of reported diagnosis
  - Obscuring final pathologic diagnosis
  - Frequency of "inadequate" sampling, requires multiple biopsies, prolongs course until definitive treatment, increases cost
- Proponents' argument
  - Important to distinguish benign vs. malignant nature of neoplasm
  - Preoperative patient counselling
  - Surgical planning
  - Differentiate between neoplastic and non-neoplastic processes
  - Avoid surgery in large number of patients

Cell of Origin of Tumors

Bicellular Theory

- Intercalated ducts
  - Pleomorphic adenoma
  - Warthin's tumor
  - Oncocytoma
  - Acinic cell
  - Adenoid cystic
- Excretory ducts
  - Squamous cell
  - Mucoepidermoid

Multicellular Theory (Fig. 28.1)

- Striated duct—oncocytic tumors
- Acinar cells—acinic cell carcinoma
- Excretory Duct—squamous cell and mucoepidermoid carcinoma
- Intercalated duct and myoepithelial cells—pleomorphic tumors

Contradictory Evidence

- Luminal cells are readily capable of replication
- Acinar cells participate in gland regeneration
- Immunohistochemical staining of S-100 protein
  - Present in many salivary gland neoplasms
  - Not present in normal ductal cells

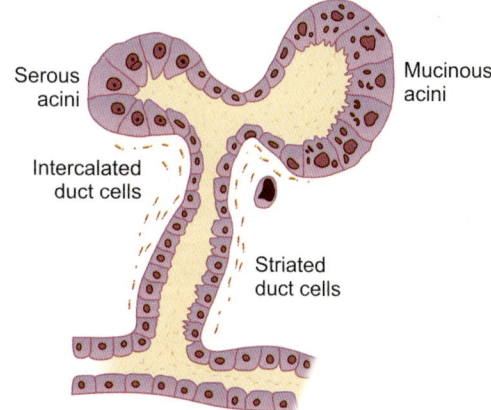

Fig. 28.1: Structure of the salivary gland

29 Swellings of Jaw

ANATOMICAL CHARACTERISTICS OF JAW BONES

a. Jaw bones are mesodermal in origin with membranous ossification
b. Jaw bones have cartilage at places like pre-maxilla, symphysis mentis and condylar process
c. Mandible and maxilla contain epithelial elements like embedded tooth germs in their substance not found in any other bone
d. There are pleuripotent cells in the region of lamina dura
e. Upper jaw contains maxillary sinus lined by columnar epithelium
f. Epithelium of the cheek and floor of the mouth are intimately fixed to the mucoperiosteum of the gum

Jaw Tumor can Arise from

a. *Mucoperiosteum:* Swelling arising from alveolar margin of jaw is known as **Epulis.**

   The Epulis can be fibrous, granulomatous, myeloid, sarcomatous or carcinomatous.

b. *From tooth germ:* These swellings are known as **odontomes**. These can be odontogenic developmental cysts or odontogenic tumors. The odontogenic developmental cyst can be dental cyst, dentigerous cyst or keratocyst. Odentogenic tumors are odentomas or amelo-blastoma.

c. *From maxillary antrum:* It can be carcinoma or sarcoma
d. From bone, e.g. osteoclastoma

Classification of Jaw Swellings

Epulis

Definition: It is a discrete and localised swelling arising from the alveolar margin of jaw. The term epulis means upon the gum. So epulis is a swelling situated upon the gum. It can originate from:

a. Bone
b. The periosteum
c. Mucous membrane
d. Junction of periodontal membrane with alveolar mucosa

Types of Epulis

- *Fibrous epulis:* It is a fibroma and consists of fusiform cells with many new blood vessels and arises as a result of chronic irritation. Initially present as soft, red swelling which later on becomes firm and pink as more collagen is deposited in the central mass. It arises from the periosteum at the neck of incisor or premolar teeth.
- More common in females in the age group of thirties.
- Present as slowly growing polypoidal swelling in response to local irritation from sharp margin of teeth or carious cavity. As it grows it separates the teeth and ultimately loosens them.

- It may undergo malignant changes, e.g. fibro-sarcoma.
- Excision is the treatment of choice. Adjacent tooth or teeth and resection of wedge of bone with its root must be performed to avoid recurrence.

Granulomatous Epulis

It is also known as false epulis or pregnancy epulis or pyogenic granuloma. It is a mass of granulation tissue around a carious tooth. Similar condition found in pregnancy is known as gingivitis gravidarum which is a temporary condition that occurs due to hormonal changes and regresses after child birth. It is present as bright red or pink colored swelling which is soft, vascular and bleeds easily on touch. Often associated with a carious tooth, poor oral hygiene and offensive smell of mouth due to infection of the epulis. Draining lymph nodes may be enlarged or tender. The treatment is extraction of carious tooth and replacement of ill-fitting denture if any. Good oral hygiene should be maintained. The granulation tissue is scraped and sent for histopathology. The mass of granulation tissue is excised by electrocautery.

Myeloid Epulis

It is a purple pedunculated mass and is actually an osteoclastoma arising from underlying bone. *Microscopically it consists of multinucleated giant cells with fibrocellular tissue in stroma.*

It is present as a firm mass arising due to expansion of the marginal bone under cover of the mucoperiosteum, but the mucosa over the gum is hyperemic edematous, and soft to touch. Swelling is usually plum colored due to high vascularity. It is more rapidly growing tumor in comparison to other types of epulis. The adjoining teeth are loosened or separated.

X-ray shows a typical soap bubble appearance.

Treatment is curettage with filling of the residual cavity with cancellous bone chips in case of small swelling. In case of large epulis radical excision of the bone should be performed.

Carcinomatous Epulis

It is an epithelioma of the gum arising from the mucous membrane of the alveolar margin. It is an infiltrating tumor which at a later stage can fungate to give rise to an ulcerated mass. It may present as a lump or an ulcer which can be painful. Soon it may invade the bone and regional lymph nodes are very commonly involved. Biopsy is performed to confirm the diagnosis.

Treatment is adequate excision of growth along with adequate margin of healthy tissue which means excision of maxilla in upper jaw and excision of mandible in lower jaw. Radiotherapy can be tried in selected cases.

Diagnosis

- Complete history
  - Pain, loosing of teeth, dental malocclusion, localised jaw swellings and delayed tooth eruption
- Thorough physical examination
  - Inspection, palpation, percussion, auscultation
- Plain radiographs
  - Panorex, dental radiographs
- CT for larger, aggressive lesions
- Obtain histopathological/cytological diagnosis
  - FNA – To rule out vascular lesions, inflammatory lesions
  - Excisional biopsy – smaller cysts, unilocular tumors
  - Incisional biopsy – larger lesions prior to definitive therapy

Odontogenic Cysts

- Inflammatory
  - Radicular
  - Para-dental
- Developmental
  - Dentigerous

Dental or Radicular Cyst

- Most common (65%)
- Arises from epithelial cell rests of Malassez
- It is the response to inflammation to chronically infected tooth and necrotic pulp. The continued irritation stimulates the nests of cells to proliferate. The centre of the mass gets necrosed, liquefied and gets converted in to the cyst. This type of cyst is usually lined by stratified squamous epithelium. The contents may be fluid or semisolid and usually contain cellular debris, cholesterol crystals and foreign body giant cells.

- The cyst usually appears at the root of normally erupted teeth which is chronically infected or carious
- Commonly seen in middle age persons
- More commonly occurs in upper jaw and may attain large size to encroach upon maxillary antrum. It eventually open in to it
- With enlargement of cyst there is resorption of adjacent bone thus leading to expansion of jaw. It may fill the maxillary antrum and then it should be differentiated from carcinoma of the antrum
- When the bone is thinned there will be eggshell crackling and fluctuation will be present if bone is completely destroyed
- Radiographic findings
  - Pulp less, non-vital tooth
  - Small well-defined periapical radiolucency
- Treatment — extraction of causative carious teeth and root canal treatment. The cyst is approached intraorally. The cyst wall is curetted and whole epithelial lining is removed. The soft tissue is pushed in to obliterate the residual cavity and wound is sutured.

Paradental Cyst

- Associated with partially impacted 3rd molars
- Result of inflammation of the gingiva over an erupting molar
- 0.5 to 4% of cysts
- Radiology — radiolucency in apical portion of the root
- Treatment — enucleation

Dentigerous (Follicular) Cyst

- Most common developmental cyst (24%)
- This is a swelling arising in connection with and containing unerupted permanent teeth
- Lesion arises from the follicle of the developing teeth. Follicle contains inner epithelial lining and outer connective tissue covering
- The cyst is solitary and multilocular
- Lining of the cyst is usually fibrous but can be stratified squamous or columnar
- Contents of cyst are thick and viscid with cholesterol crystals and unerupted teeth
- The cyst displaces teeth deeper in to the jaw and prevents it from erupting. The tooth may lie obliquely free in the cyst cavity or may be embedded in the cyst wall

- Cyst enlarges with expansion of bone and displacement of teeth to which cyst is attached
- Radiographic findings
  - Unilocular radiolucency with well-defined sclerotic margins
- Histology is non-keratinizing squamous epithelium
- *Clinical features:* Commonly seen in young adults and children. It may involve the lower or upper jaw. Commonly occur in association with lower third molar or premolar teeth
- Present with painlessly growing swelling with missing teeth at the site of cyst
- *Treatment:* Total excision of cyst via intraoral approach. Other options are enucleation of cyst or decompression if total excision is not possible

Odontogenic Keratocyst

- 11% of jaw cysts
- May mimic any of the other cysts
- Most often in mandibular ramus and angle
- Radiographically
  - Well-marginated, radiolucent
  - Multilocular in nature
- Histology
  - Thin epithelial lining with underlying connective tissue (collagen and epithelial nests)
- High frequency of recurrence (up to 62%)
- Complete removal difficult and satellite cysts can be left behind
- Treatment
  - Depends on extent of lesion
  - Small – simple enucleation, complete removal of the cyst wall
  - Larger – enucleation with/without peripheral ostectomy
- Long term follow-up required (5–10 years)

Odontogenic Tumors

- Ameloblastoma
- Calcifying epithelial odontogenic tumor
- Adenomatoid odontogenic tumor

Ameloblastoma

- Most common odontogenic tumor which is benign, but locally invasive low grade malignant epithelial tumor with a high rate of recurrence if not removed adequately, but does not have any tendency to metastasize.

- Most commonly arise from embryonic enamel organ of tooth. It can also arise from displaced dental epithelial remnants.
- It is clinically and histologically similar to basal cell carcinoma
- Most commonly occurs in the 4th and 5th decades
- The tumor enlarges slowly and produces destruction and enlargement of mandible. Once the outer cortex is thinned out tumour ulcerates.
- Spread is mainly local without any lymphatic or blood borne spread. However, endobronchial spread is rarely seen. This apparently arises from ulceration of overlying intraoral mucous membrane over the enlarging membrane with inhalation of fragmented or detached tumor in to the bronchial tree.
- Subtypes of ameloblastoma
  - Multi-cystic (86%)
  - Uni-cystic (13%)
- Classical radiographic findings are:
  - Classically seen as multilocular radiolucency of posterior mandible which is well-circumscribed and known as soap-bubble appearance
  - Unilocular often confused with odontogenic cysts
- Histology
  - Classic–sheets and islands of tumor cells, outer rim of ameloblasts is polarized away from basement membrane
  - Centre looks like stellate reticulum

If squamous differentiation (1%) seen — diagnosed as ameloblastic carcinoma.

Clinical Features of Ameloblastoma

- Commonly seen in females in any age group above 11 years of age, but common in 4th and 5th decade
- Painless progressive swelling in the lower jaw at or near its angle or in the molar region
- Irregular lobulated surface of the swelling leads to distortion of face and ugly deformity. Swelling grows more towards the cheek with normal medial or lingual side

- On palpation there is egg shell crackling
- There is marked protrusion of mandible or malalignment of teeth or malocclusion of teeth. There are no missing teeth
- No regional lymph nodes palpable

Treatment of Ameloblastoma

According to growth characteristics and type
- Unicystic
  - Complete removal
  - Peripheral ostectomies if extension occurs through cyst wall
- Classic infiltrative (aggressive)
  - Mandibular — adequate normal bone around margins of resection
  - Maxillary — more aggressive surgery, 1.5 cm margins
- Ameloblastic carcinoma
  - Radical surgical resection (like squamous cell carcinoma)
  - Neck dissection for lymph node metastasis.

Adenomatoid Odontogenic Tumor

- Associated with the crown of an impacted anterior tooth
- Painless expansion
- Radiographic findings
  - Well-defined expansile radiolucency
  - Root divergence, calcific flecks ("target")
- Histology
  - Thick fibrous capsule, clusters of spindle cells, columnar cells (rosettes, ductal) throughout
- Treatment – enucleation, recurrence is rare

Related Jaw Lesions

- Giant cell lesions
  - Central giant cell granuloma
  - Brown tumor
  - Aneurysmal bone cyst
- Fibro-osseous lesions
  - Fibrous dysplasia
  - Ossifying fibroma
- Condensing osteitis
- Plastic-like reactive proliferation

30 Thyroid Gland

- **1816** – Prout successfully treats goiter with iodine
- **1835–40** – Graves and von Basedow describe *"Merseburg triad"* of goiter, exophthalmos, and palpitations
- **1886** – Horsley postulates thyroid hyper-secretion as the cause of Graves' disease
- **1891** – Murray cures myxedema with hypodermic extract of sheep thyroid
- **1915** – Kendall crystallizes thyroxine
- **1929** – TSH identified
- **1950** – Duffy associates X-ray therapy with thyroid cancer
- **1970's** – FNA comes into vogue

History of Thyroid Surgery

- Thyroid surgery was condemned for years as heroic and butchery so much so in 1850 French Academy of Medicine proscribed any thyroid surgery
- Till mid 1800's there were only 106 documented cases of thyroid surgery
- There was high mortality of 40% mainly due to exsanguination and sepsis
- 1870's-80's – Billroth from Vienna emerged as the leader in thyroid surgery as he achieved mortality rate of 8% in thyroid surgery and showed need for RLN preservation

- Von Eiselber defined need for parathyroid preservation in thyroid surgery and gave emphasis on speed of surgery
- Kocher from Bern further improved thyroid surgery
  - By decreasing mortality from 2.4 (1889) to 0.18% in 1900
  - He laid emphasis on meticulous technique
  - He performed 5000 cases till his death in 1917
  - He was awarded nobel prize in 1909 for his efforts
- Halstead was a student of Kocher and Billroth. When he returned to the US in 1880 and started working at Hopkins with Cushing, Osler, Welch laid groundwork for thyroid specialists Mayo, Lahey, Crile.

Anatomy

- Endocrine organ
- Attached to front and sides of trachea and larynx
- Consists of right and left lobes
- Pyramidal lobe
- Isthmus joining two lobes overlying 2nd and 3rd tracheal rings
- **Blood supply:** Superior and inferior thyroid arteries
- **Venous drainage:** Superior, middle and inferior thyroid veins
- Nearby structures
  - Recurrent and external laryngeal nerves
  - Parathyroid glands

- Trachea/larynx
- Esophagus/pharynx
- Carotid sheath with its structures

Embryology

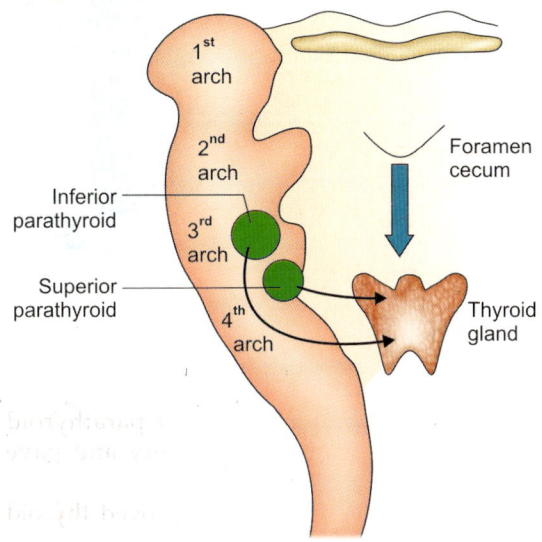

Fig. 30.1: Development of the thyroid and parathyroids

- Develops from foramen cecum
- Passes anterior to hyoid to resting position in neck
- May find thyroid tissue from tongue to anterior mediastinum

Evaluation of Thyroid Swelling

Thyroid swelling can be:
- Diffuse smooth enlargement of whole gland
- Multi-nodular enlargement
- Solitary nodular goitre

Differential Diagnosis
Diffuse Enlargement

- Physiological goitre in adolescent persons
- Colloid goitre in endemic areas
- Primary or Graves' disease
- Riddle's thyroiditis

Multi-nodular Goitre

- Non-toxic multi-nodular goitre in iodine deficiency areas or in persons who are using non iodised salt

- Toxic multi-nodular goitre (Plummer's disease)
- Follicular carcinoma developing in long standing multi-nodular goitre

Solitary Nodule

- Dominant nodule (part of MNG) other nodules are not palpable
- Papillary carcinoma
- Follicular carcinoma
- Anaplastic carcinoma
- Medullary carcinoma
- Follicular adenoma
- Hemorrhage in necrotic nodule
- Hashimoto's thyroiditis

Epidemiology

- *Nodules in thyroid are very common, whereas cancer is not so common*
- *Goal is to minimize "unnecessary" surgery but not miss any cancer*
- Incidence of thyroid nodule increases with age
- During autopsy in 9th decade 80% of women and 65% men had thyroid nodules
- Estimated 5–15% of nodules are cancerous
- Although thyroid cancer is more common in women, a nodule in a man is more likely to be malignant

Pregnancy

- Increases risk of developing thyroid nodules as there is increased renal iodide excretion and basal metabolic rate
- Ultrasound detected nodules in thyroid case commonly seen in
  - 9.4% nulliparous women
  - 25% women previously pregnant

Radiation

- Therapeutic XRT for malignancy raises risk for thyroid cancer and appears to be dose-dependent. Expected radiation risk is 7.7 at 100 cGy. Maximum risk is approximately 30 years after exposure. Thyroid nodules in a radiated patient have 35–40% chance of malignancy. Thyroid malignancy in a radiated patient is not more aggressive than spontaneously occurring cancer, but radiation exposure is only an unequivocal environmental cause of thyroid cancer

- Childhood exposure to radiation
  - Younger age – greater risk
  - Thyroid suppression therapy may help to decrease risk
  - I-131: risk of leukemia with high doses

Pediatric Age Group

- Nodule more likely to be cancer in adults. Currently incidence is approximately 20%
- 10% thyroid cancer occurs before 21 years of age
- Thyroid malignancy accounts for 1.5–2.0% of all pediatric malignancies and more likely to present with neck metastasis
- Most common cause of thyroid enlargement in children is chronic lymphocytic thyroiditis
- Medullary thyroid carcinoma is also common in pediatric age group
  - Is associated RET proto-oncogene (chromosome 10) mutation

Miscellaneous

- Higher rate of nodules found in patients
  - Who have hyperparathyroidism
  - Are undergoing hemodialysis

History

- Age less than 20 or greater than 60 is more likely to be malignant
- A nodule in a man is more likely to be cancer
- Exposure to radiation increases risk of malignancy
- Symptoms of hyper- or hypo functioning of thyroid
- Rapid enlargement of a mass
- Breathlessness, hoarseness and dysphagia
- Family history of medullary thyroid carcinoma
- Family history of other thyroid carcinoma
- History of Hashimoto's thyroiditis as these patients are more likely to develop thyroid lymphoma
- Pain indicates thyroiditis or malignancy infiltrating local structures or hemorrhage in to a necrotic nodule

History Elements Suggestive of Malignancy

- Progressive enlargement
- Hoarseness
- Dysphagia
- Dyspnea
- High-risk (family history, radiation)
- Not very sensitive/specific

Rapid Increase in Size in Days

- Hemorrhage in necrotic nodule
- Anaplastic carcinoma
- Thyroiditis

Causes of Dyspnea in Goitre

- Long-standing MNG — tracheomalacia or tracheal compression leading to collapse of tracheal rings
- Malignant thyroid leading to infiltration in lumen of trachea
- Involvement of bilateral recurrent laryngeal nerve
- Congestive heart failure in hyperthyroidism
- Retrosternal extension

Examination

- Stethoscope, glass of water, tendon hammer should be ready before starting examination
- Introduce yourself
- *Position:* Patient seated, palpate from behind
- Privacy
- Light
- *Exposure:* Neck and anterior chest

Overview of Method

- *General inspection:* Around the bed, patient
- *Hands:* Acropachy, sweaty palms, tremor
- *Pulse:* There will be tachycardia with increase in sleeping pulse rate
- *Face:* Peaches and cream complexion
- *Eyes:* Eye disease and eye signs
- *Neck:* Thyroid, trachea and lymph nodes
- *Legs:* Pretibial myxoedema, reflexes

General Inspection

- Thin/fat
- Muscle wasting
- Nervous/agitated
- Under-clothed and sweaty in hyperthyroidism
- Overdressed but cold in hypothyroidism
- Hoarseness of voice due to myxoedema or recurrent laryngeal nerve involvement (RLN)/fatigable voice (due to external laryngeal nerve involvement)
- Stridor on tracheal compression

Hands

Thyroid acropathy: Clubbing, digital swelling, periosteal new bone

Sweaty palms
Pulse: Rate, rhythm, sleeping pulse rate

Eye Disease

Examine: from front, above and the side
Lids:

- *Lid retraction:* One can see the white sclera above the upper border of cornea
- *Lid lag:* Upper lid will lag behind the eye ball if patient is asked to follow the examiner's finger which is placed in front of the patient and moved up and down. Patient is instructed not to move the head, but to look at the finger.

Eyes: Exophthalmos, proptosis, ophthalmoplegia, periorbital swelling.
Conjunctivae: Chemosis, ocular injection
Optic Nerve: Optic neuropathy
Exophthalmos: Sclera visible above and below the eye
Proptosis: On looking from above, eyeball protrudes forward beyond supraorbital ridge
Ophthalmoplegia: Inferior oblique is the first muscle to get involved.
Chemosis and ocular injection.

Neck

Inspection

- Stand in front of the patient
  - Visible?
  - Enlarged?
  - Symmetrical?

WHO Grading of Goitre

- **Grade 1:** Palpable but not visible
- **Grade 2:** Visible with neck extended
- **Grade 3:** Visible in neutral position of neck

Also Observe

- Scars
- Observe swallow
- Observe patient sticking tongue out (thyroglossal cyst)

Palpation

- Stand behind patient
- Thumbs on occiput
- Flex neck slightly
- Palpate
- Size
- Tenderness

- Surface
- Consistency
- Discrete nodules
- Moves on swallowing?
- *Lymph nodes:* Thyrohyoid membrane, angle of jaw
- Palpate trachea
  - Central?
  - *Berry sign:* Look for carotid pulsation at level of upper border of thyroid cartilage along anterior border of SCM.

Physical Findings Suggestive of Malignancy

- Fixation
- Adenopathy
- Fixed cord
- Induration
- Stridor

Percussion

- Percuss for a retrosternal goitre
- Pemberton's test

Auscultation

- Thyroid bruit

Legs

- Pretibial myxoedema
- Quadriceps reflexes

Investigations
Laboratory Investigations

- Confirm status of thyroid biochemical estimation
  - TSH estimation
  - If abnormal then T3, T4 estimation
- Thyroid antibody profile — Graves' disease, Hashimoto's thyroiditis
- Thyroglobulin
  - Post-treatment test to detect recurrence of malignancy
- Serum calcitonin — only in cases of medullary carcinoma of thyroid
- RET proto-oncogene

Ultrasound of Thyroid

- Thyroid vs non-thyroid swelling
  - Good screen for thyroid presence in children
- Cystic vs solid
- Localization for FNA
- May distinguish solitary nodule from multinodular goitre

- Can detect small nodules
- Vascular invasion (carotid/internal jugular vein)
- Enlarged lymph nodes

Findings Suggestive of Malignancy

- Presence of halo
- Irregular border
- Presence of cystic and solid components
- Presence of calcifications
- Heterogeneous echo pattern
- Extra-thyroidal extension
- No findings are definitive

Fine Needle Aspiration Cytology of Thyroid

- Has become standard first-line test for diagnosis
- Safe, efficacious, cost-effective
- Allows pre-operative diagnosis and therefore planning
- Can diagnose
  - Colloid goiter
  - Papillary carcinoma
  - Anaplastic and medullary carcinoma
- Best tool for determining pathology other than surgical excision
- Can be as high as 80% sensitive and 95% specific
- Operator dependent in obtaining adequate amount of tissue
- Should not be relied on if negative in patient with previous neck irradiation
- Interpreting report
  - *Benign:* 90–95% likelihood it is benign
  - *Indeterminate/suspicious:* If it is follicular neoplasm the patient is taken for hemi-thyroidectomy and frozen sections. If frozen section report is follicular carcinoma total thyroidectomy is performed
  - *Insufficient/inadequate specimen:* Do it again (and again)
  - *Malignant:* Patient planned for surgery
- Procedure
  - 25-gauge needle
  - Multiple passes
  - Ideally from periphery of lesion
  - Reaspirate after fluid drawn
  - Immediately smeared and fixed
  - Papanicolaou stain common

FNAC of papillary carcinoma
- **NG:** Nuclear grooves
- **IC:** Intranuclear inclusions

Pitfalls of FNAC

- Sampling error in
  - Small (<1 cm) nodules
  - Large (>4 cm) nodules
- Hashimoto's versus lymphoma
- *Follicular neoplasms:* It cannot differentiate between follicular adenoma and follicular carcinoma
- In fluid only cysts not very useful
- Somewhat dependent on the skill of the cyto-pathologist

Nuclear Medicine – Thyroid scan

- Indication
  - For toxic SNG undergoing surgery
  - Toxic MNG undergoing surgery
  - Follow up of carcinoma thyroid

Technetium 99m

- Most commonly used isotope
- **99m:** "m" refers to metastable nuclide
- Decay product of Molybdenum-99
- Long half-life before decaying into Tc-99
- Administered as pertechnate (TcO^{4-})
- Images can be obtained quickly
- "One-Stop" evaluation
- Hot nodules need follow up iodine scan
- Discordant nodules higher risk of malignancy

Iodine

- ^{127}I
  - Only stable isotope of iodine
- ^{123}I
  - Cyclotron product
  - Half-life 13.3 hours
  - Expensive, limited availability
  - Low radiation-exposure to patient
- ^{131}I
  - Fission product
  - Half-life 8 days
  - Cheap, widely available
  - Better for metastasis (diagnostic and thera-peutic) (high radiation exposure)
- ^{125}I
  - No longer used
  - Long half-life (60 days); high radiation exposure with poor visualization

Thallium-201

- Expensive, role poorly defined
- Can detect (but not treat) metastasis

- Not trapped or organified – mechanism unclear
  - Potassium analogue
- Potential advantages:
  - Not necessary to be off thyroid replacement
  - Patients with large body iodine pool (e.g. recent CT with contrast) or hypofunctioning gland
  - Can sometimes image medullary carcinoma

Gallium-67

- Generally lights up inflammation
  - Hashimoto's thyroidits
- Uses in thyroid imaging limited in
  - Anaplastic Carcinoma
  - Lymphoma

Other Imaging Agents

- ^{99m}Tc Sestamibi
  - Concentrates in mitochondria
  - Better for Hurthle cell neoplasm
- ^{99m}Tc Pentavalent DMSA
- Radioiodinated MIBG
- Developed for medullary (APUD derivative)
- Radiolabeled monoclonal antibodies

Interpretation of Results

- Most authors feel that hot nodule in hyperthyroid patient has low malignancy risk
- Nodule in clinically hyperthyroid patient may be cold nodule against background of Graves, so scan may help

Other Investigations

- Indirect laryngoscopy to look for the movement of vocal cords. This is important for medicolegal purposes as there can be asymptomatic paresis of one vocal cord due to previous viral infections
- X-ray neck soft tissue
  - It is mandatory before thyroid surgery to rule out any pathology in cervical spine as the neck is hyperextended during thyroid surgery. If there is any pathology in cervical spine hyperextension of neck should be avoided.
  - May show:
    ◊ Tracheal deviation
    ◊ Calcifications (suggest papillary or medullary)
- Serum calcium as base line

31 Benign Thyroid Disease

- Benign non toxic conditions
  - Diffuse goitre
  - Multi-nodular goitre
  - Solitary nodular goitre (Follicular adenoma)
- Benign toxic conditions
  - Toxic multi-nodular goitre
  - Graves' disease
  - Toxic adenoma
- Inflammatory conditions
  - Chronic (Hashimoto's) thyroiditis
  - Sub-acute (De Quervain's) thyroiditis
  - Riedel's thyroiditis

TOXIC MULTI-NODULAR GOITRE

Goitrogenesis

- Iodine deficiency results in decreased levels of thyroid hormones (hypothyroidism)
- Decreased T3 and T4 circulating levels lead to increased TSH which causes hypertrophy of thyroid (diffuse non toxic goitre)
- Some follicles may become autonomous and will have greater intrinsic growth and functional capability (multi-nodular goitre)
- Follicles continue to grow and function despite decreasing TSH (toxic multi-nodular goitre)

Presentation

- Usually picked up on routine physical exam or as incidental finding

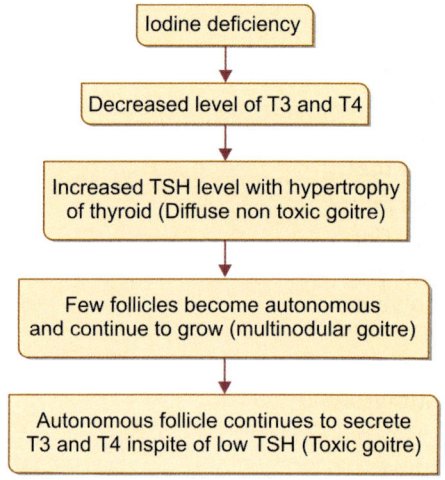

Fig. 31.1: Pathogenesis of toxic multinodular goitre

- Patients may have clinical or subclinical thyrotoxicosis
- Patients may have compressive symptoms: tracheal, vascular, esophageal, recurrent laryngeal nerve

Treatment of Diffuse or Multi-nodular Goitre

- Suppressive therapy in euthyroid states
- *Antithyroid medications:* Propylthiouracil and methimazole in diffuse toxic goitre
- I-131 in selected case of toxic MNG
- Surgical therapy if compressive symptoms, for cosmetic reason or in toxic MNG

GRAVES' DISEASE

- Most common form of thyrotoxicosis commonly seen in young females
- Autoimmune etiology with familial predisposition
- Thyroid receptor stimulating antibody unique to Graves' disease; other autoantibodies present (TgAb, TPOAb)
- Affects females five times more often than males

Presentation

- *Thyrotoxicosis:* Palpitations, nervousness, easy fatigability, diarrhea, excessive sweating, intolerance to heat, weight loss
- Eye signs
- Diffuse goitre

Graves' Ophthalmopathy

- *Class one:* Spasm of upper lids with thyrotoxicosis (Lid retraction)
- *Class two:* Peri-orbital edema and chemosis
- *Class three:* Proptosis (exophthalmos)
- *Class four:* Extraocular muscle involvement
- *Class five:* Corneal involvement
- *Class six:* Loss of vision due to optic nerve involvement

Treatment

- Antithyroid drugs
  - May require prolonged therapy
- Radioactive iodine
  - May worsen ophthalmopathy unless followed by steroids
- Surgery
  - Make patient euthyroid prior to surgery
  - Potassium iodide two weeks prior to surgery can decrease the vascularity of the gland and to make thyroid firm.

Thyrotoxicosis and Thyroid Storm

- *Acute thyrotoxicosis:* Beta-blockers, barbiturates, cholestyramine
- *Thyroid storm:* Manage aggressively with beta-blockers, calcium channel blockers, PTU, methimazole, sodium iodide, digitalis or diuretics for heart failure, fluid and electrolyte management

TOXIC ADENOMA

- Autonomously functioning thyroid nodule hyper-secreting T3 and T4 resulting in thyrotoxicosis (Plummer's disease)
- Almost never malignant
- Manage with anti-thyroid drugs followed by either I-131 or surgery

Chronic Thyroiditis

- Also known as Hashimoto's disease
- Probably the most common cause of hypothyroidism
- *Autoantibodies include:* Thyroglobulin antibody, thyroid peroxidase antibody, TSH receptor blocking antibody
- Painless goitre in a patient who is either euthyroid or mildly hypothyroid
- High incidence of permanent hypothyroidism
- May have periods of thyrotoxicosis in initial period
- Treat with levothyroxine

Sub-acute Thyroiditis

- Also known as De Quervain's thyroiditis
- Most common cause of thyroid pain and tenderness
- Acute inflammatory disease most likely due to viral infection
- Transient hyperthyroidism followed by transient hypothyroidism; permanent hypothyroidism or relapses are uncommon

Treatment

- *Symptomatic:* NSAIDs or glucocorticoids
- Beta-blockers indicated if there are signs of thyrotoxicosis
- Levothyroxine may be given during hypothyroid phase

Riedel's Thyroiditis

- Rare disorder usually affecting middle-aged women
- Likely autoimmune aetiology
- Fibrous tissue replaces thyroid gland
- Patients present with a rapidly enlarging hard neck mass
- Has to be differentiated from anaplastic carcinoma

32 | Thyroid Malignancies

- Accounts for 3 percent of all malignancies in the US. Occult carcinoma in 6–35% of glands at autopsy (usually 4–10 mm)
- About 48,000 cases in the US every year
- About 1740 deaths occurred due to thyroid malignancy in the US in 2011
- Accumulated annual incidence has been reported to be 3.7 cases per 1,00000 population
- The female to male sex ratio is 3:1

Aetiology

a. Irradiation of thyroid under age of 5 increases incidence of papillary carcinoma
b. Short latency aggressive papillary cancer is associated with ret/PTC3 oncogene
c. Less aggressive papillary cancer are associated with RET/PTC1 oncogene
d. Incidence of follicular carcinoma is high in endemic goiter area probably as a result of TSH stimulation
e. Malignant lymphoma develops in autoimmune thyroiditis

Histopathology

Histological subtype showing relative incidence of primary thyroid tumour:
- Papillary – 60%
- Follicular – 20%
- Medullary – 5%
- Anaplastic – 10%
- Lymphoma – 5%

Papillary Carcinoma

- Most common
- 30% have node metastasis at diagnosis
- Radiation related
- Contain mixture of papillary and colloid filled follicles
- Histologically tumor shows papillary projections
- Histologically, psammoma bodies distinguish from benign adenoma
- Tumor may be multifocal or multi-centric involving one lobe or both lobes. Multifocal tumor is generally due to lymphatic spread in the rich intra-thyroidal lymph plexus
- Spread is mainly to lymph nodes. Blood borne spread is uncommon and only occurs if tumor has spread beyond the capsule of thyroid gland
- Papillary cancer less than 1cm in diameter is known as micro-carcinoma and has excellent prognosis
- "Orphan Annie eyed " nuclei are characterized by pale empty nuclei.

Follicular Carcinoma

- 20% of malignancies
- Distinguished from normal follicular adenomas by invasion of capsule or blood vessels
- FNA inadequate for diagnosis

- Hurthle cell tumor is a variant of follicular neoplasm in which oxyphil cells predominate histologically. They are associated with poor prognosis

Medullary Carcinoma

- 5–10% of cases
- Arise from the C cells which produce calcitonin
- Diagnosis based on elevated calcitonin levels and cold thyroid nodule

Anaplastic Carcinoma

- < 10%
- Highly aggressive with local extension at time of diagnosis

- No suitable therapy
- Prognosis <1 year from diagnosis

Treatment

For all malignancies, once the diagnosis has been confirmed by FNAC, the imaging of neck is done by CT or MRI. Total thyroidectomy is done for tumors more than 2 cm or those with nodal involvement or distant metastasis. Functional selective dissection of involved nodes is performed. If the tumor is less than 2 cm in diameter hemi-thyroidectomy is carried out. Some group of surgeons carry out total thyroidectomy and central compartment node dissection in all patients.

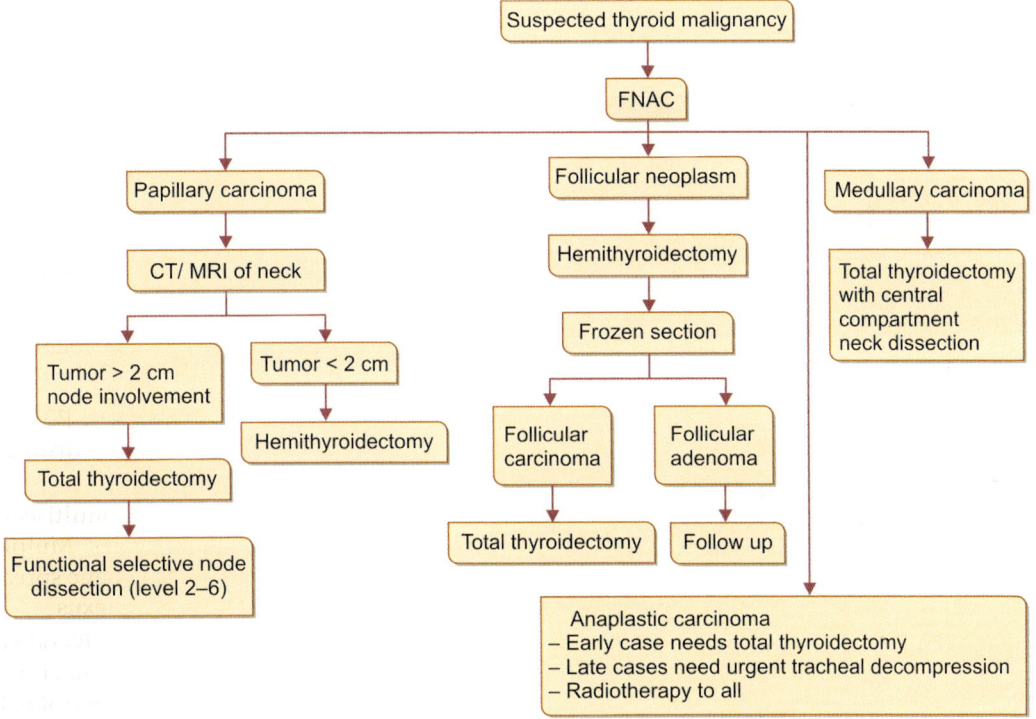

Fig. 32.1: Flowchart for management of thyroid neoplasms

33 Hyperparathyroidism

TYPES

- Primary
  - Incidence
    ◊ 1:550 in females >40 years
    ◊ 1:2000 in males >40 years
  - Etiology
    ◊ Sporadic-adenoma (80%), hyperplasia (12%)
    ◊ Part of MEN
    ◊ Post radiation
- Secondary
  - Chronic renal failure
  - Malabsorption
- Tertiary

Clinical Features

- Renal
  - Stones (25–30%)
  - Nephrocalcinosis (5–10%)
  - Hypertension
- Bone disease
  - Osteitis fibrosa cystica
  - Subperiosteal resorption
  - Osteoclastomas (brown tumor)
- GI disturbances
- Emotional disturbances
- Articulation/soft tissue manifestations
  - Chondrocalcinosis
  - Pseudogout
  - Vascular/cardiac calcification
  - Skin necrosis
- Neuromuscular

Physical examination is unremarkable.

Investigations

Biochemical

- Hypercalcemia
- Hypophosphatemia
- S. parathormone
  - Measured by IRMA or ICMA assay
  - Increased in 85–90% cases
  - False positive in patients on lithium or thiazides
- *Chloride:* Phosphate ratio >33
- Urine calcium >50 mmol/24 hours

Radiology

- Skull
- Phalanges
- Jaw
- Clavicle

Management

Conservative

- For secondary hyperparathyroidism

Drugs

- Estrogens increase cortical bone density
- Bisphosphonates
- Calcimimetics, e.g. R568

Surgery

- Mainstay of the treatment

Indications

- Overt manifestations
- S. calcium >12 mg/dl
- Marked hypercalciuria >400 mg/dl
- Markedly reduced bone density
- Parathormone >500 pg/ml
- Enlarged parathyroid on imaging
- Osteitis fibrosa cystica
- Age >50 years

Pre-operative Localization

- Indications
  - Recurrent or persistent hyperparathyroidism
  - Unilateral neck exploration
  - Recurrence of parathyroid carcinoma
- Ultrasound
  - Sensitivity 36–76%
- CT Scan
  - Sensitivity 46–76%
  - Good for ectopic/mediastinal glands
  - Drawbacks
    ◊ Metallic clips – artefacts
    ◊ Difficult for intrathyroid glands
    ◊ Differentiation from lymph nodes
- MRI
  - Sensitivity 50–78%
  - Does not differentiate between fat and parathyroid
  - Expensive
- Radio-isotope scan (^{99m}Tc Sestamibi scan)
- Angiography/venous sampling

Pre-Operative Preparation

- Serum calcium should be reduced if >15 mg/dl
  - Increasing urinary calcium excretion
  - Inhibition of bone resorption
  - Dialysis

MULTIPLE ENDOCRINE NEOPLASIA

MEN Type I

- Autosomal dominant
- Causative gene on chromosome 11q13
  - Hyperparathyroidism 90% (Multiglandular)
  - Multiple neuroendocrine tumors of pancreas usually gastrinoma (75%)
  - Pituitary tumors (>30%), usually prolactinoma
- Disease is multiglandular

MEN Type II

- Gene on 10q

MEN Type IIa

- Medullary thyroid cancer (100%)
- Pheochromocytoma (50%)
- Hyperparathyroidism (25%) — single gland disease

MEN Type IIb

- Marfanoid feature
- Multiple mucosal ganglioneuromas

34 Evaluation of a Patient with Neck Mass

EMBRYOLOGY

Brachial System

- **Branchial system:** 6 pairs of pharyngeal arches separated by endodermally lined pouches and ectodermally lined clefts
- Each arch consists of a nerve, artery and cartilaginous structures
- The remaining neck musculature gains contributions from cervical somites
- First branchial arch:
  - Maxillary and mandibular (Meckel's) process regress to leave the malleus and incus
  - Ossification around Meckel's cartilage gives rise to the mandible, sphenomandibular ligament and anterior malleolar ligaments
  - Muscles—temporalis, masseter, pterygoids, mylohyoid, ant belly of digastric, tensor tympani, tensor veli palatine
  - Pouch
- Eustachian tube, middle ear
- Temporal bone
  - Cleft
- External auditory canal/tympanic membrane
- Second branchial arch
  - Reichert's cartilage contributes to the superstructure of the stapes, the upper body and lesser cornu of the hyoid, the styloid process and stylohyoid ligament
  - Muscles—platysma, muscles of facial expression, posterior belly of digastric, stylohyoid, and stapedius

- Nerve—7th cranial nerve
- Artery—stapedial artery
- Third branchial arch
  - Lower body of the hyoid and greater cornu
  - Muscles—stylopharyngeus, superior and middle pharyngeal constrictors
  - Nerve—9th cranial nerve
  - Artery—common carotid and proximal portions of the internal and external carotid
  - Third branchial pouch
- Inferior parathyroids
- Thymus gland and thymic duct
- Fourth and sixth branchial arches fuse to form the laryngeal cartilages
- Fourth arch
  - Muscles—cricothyroid, inferior pharyngeal constrictors
  - Nerve—superior laryngeal nerve
  - Artery—right subclavian, aortic arch
  - Fourth pouch—superior parathyroid glands and parafollicular thyroid cells
- Sixth branchial arch
  - Muscles—Remaining/intrinsic laryngeal musculature
  - Nerve—Recurrent laryngeal nerve
  - Artery—Pulmonary artery and ductus arteriosus
- Epipericardial ridge
  - Mesodermal elements of the sternocleidomastoid, trapezius, and lingual and infrahyoid musculature

- Nerve—hypoglossal and spinal accessory nerve
- Cervical sinus of His

Thyroid Gland
- Endoderm of the floor of mouth between the 1st and 2nd archs
- Descends as a bilobed diverticulum from the foramen cecum around the 4th week to rest by the 7–8th week.

Triangles of the Neck

Anterior Triangle
- **Medial:** Midline
- **Lateral:** Posterior border of sternocleido-mastoid muscle
- **Superior:** Lower border of mandible

Submental Triangle
- **Medial:** Midline
- **Lateral:** Anterior belly of digastric muscle
- **Inferior:** Hyoid bone

Submandibular Triangle
- **Medial:** Anterior belly of digastric muscle
- **Lateral:** Posterior belly of digastric muscle
- **Superior:** Inferior border of mandible

Carotid Triangle
- **Supero-medial:** Posterior belly of digastric muscle

- **Lateral:** Posterior border of sternocleido-mastoid muscle
- **Medial:** Midline

Posterior Triangle
- **Medial:** Posterior border of sternocleido-mastoid muscle
- **Lateral:** Anterior border of trapezius muscle
- **Inferior:** Middle 1/3 of clavicle

Divided in two by posterior belly of omohyoid muscle:
- Postero-superior triangle
- Antero-inferior triangle

Diagnosis
- Location
  - **Congenital masses:** Consistent in location
  - **Metastatic masses:** Key to primary lesion
  - Midline neck masses
    - ◊ Thyroid nodules
    - ◊ Cervical lymphadenopathy
    - ◊ Thyroglossal duct cyst
    - ◊ Thymus gland anomalies
    - ◊ Plunging ranula
  - Lateral neck masses
    - ◊ Branchial cleft anomalies
    - ◊ Laryngoceles
    - ◊ Dermoid and teratoid cysts

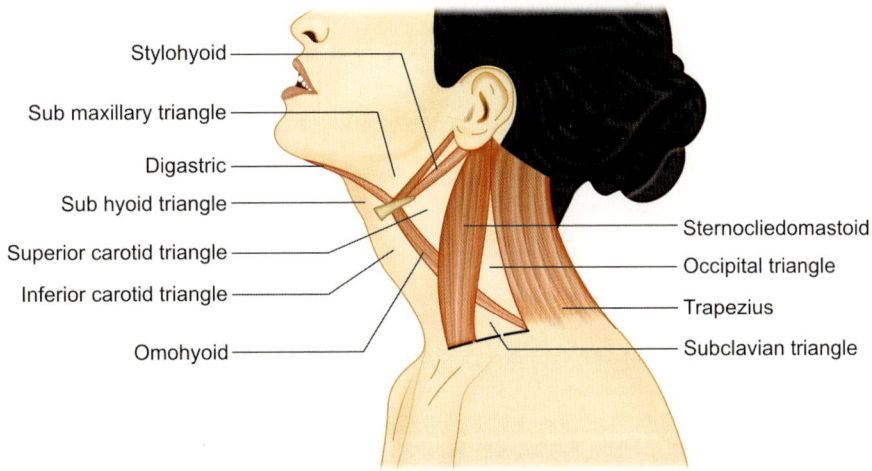

Fig. 34.1: Anatomical classification of triangles of the neck

- History
  - Developmental time course
  - Associated symptoms (dysphagia, otalgia, voice)
  - Personal habits (tobacco, alcohol)
  - Previous irradiation or surgery
- Physical examination
  - Complete head and neck exam (visualize and palpate)
  - Emphasis on location, mobility and consistency

Investigations

Fine Needle Aspiration Biopsy

- Standard of diagnosis
- Indications
  - Any neck mass that is not an obvious abscess
  - Persistence after a 2 week course of antibiotics
- Small gauge needle
  - Reduces bleeding
  - Seeding of tumor – not a concern
- No contraindications except vascular tumor
- Proper collection required
- Minimum of 4 separate passes
- Skilled cytopathologist essential
- On-site review best

Computed Tomography

- Distinguish cystic from solid
- Extent of lesion
- Vascularity (with contrast)
- Detection of unknown primary (metastatic)
- Pathologic node (lucent, >1.5 cm, loss of shape)
- Avoid contrast in thyroid lesions.

Magnetic Resonance Imaging

- Similar information as CT
- Better for upper neck and skull base
- Vascular delineation with infusion

Ultrasonography

- Less important now with FNAB
- Solid versus cystic masses
- Congenital cysts from solid nodes/tumors
- Noninvasive (pediatric)

Radionuclide Scanning

- Salivary and thyroid masses
- Location — glandular versus extra-glandular

- Functional information
- FNAB now preferred for thyroid nodules
  - Solitary nodules
  - Multinodular goiter with new increasing nodule
  - Hashimoto's with new nodule

Nodal Mass Workup in the Adult

- Any solid asymmetric mass must be considered a metastatic neoplastic lesion until proven otherwise
- Asymptomatic cervical mass — 12% are cancers with 80% of these being squamous cell carcinoma
- Ipsilateral otalgia with normal otoscopy, there should be direct attention to tonsil, tongue base, supraglottis and hypopharynx
- In unilateral serous otitis — direct examination of nasopharynx should be done
- Panendoscopy
  - FNAB positive with no primary on repeat exam
- Directed biopsy
  - All suspicious mucosal lesions
  - Areas of concern on CT/MRI
  - None observed — nasopharynx, tonsil (ipsilateral tonsillectomy for jugulodigastric nodes), base of tongue and piriformis fossa
- Synchronous primaries present in 10 to 20% of cases
- Unknown primary
  - Primary can be in 40%
  - Without suggestive findings on CT or panendoscopy yield is 20%
  - Tonsillar fossa is the cause in up to 80% cases
- Open excisional biopsy with frozen section
  - Only if complete workup negative
  - Occurs in ~5% of patients
  - Be prepared for a complete neck dissection in case of squamous cell carcinoma on frozen section
  - Inflammatory or granulomatous — culture
  - Lymphoma or adenocarcinoma — close wound and further work up.

Primary Tumor

- Thyroid mass
- Lymphoma
- Salivary tumors

- Lipoma
- Carotid body and glomus tumors
- Neurogenic tumors

Thyroid Masses

- Leading cause of anterior neck masses
- Children
  - Most common neoplastic condition
  - Male predominance
  - Higher incidence of malignancy
- Adults
  - Female predominance
  - Mostly benign
- Lymph node metastasis
  - Initial symptom in 15% of papillary carcinomas
  - 40% with malignant nodules
  - Histologically (microscopic) in >90%
- FNAB has replaced radionuclide scanning
  - Decrease number of patients with surgery
  - Increased number of malignant tumors found at surgery
  - Unsatisfactory aspirate — repeat in 1 month

Lymphoma

- More common in children and young adults
- Up to 80% of children with Hodgkin's have a neck mass
- Signs and symptoms
  - Lateral neck mass only (discrete, rubbery, nontender)
  - Fever
  - Hepatosplenomegaly
  - Diffuse adenopathy
- FNAB — first line diagnostic test
- If suggestive of lymphoma — open biopsy
- Full workup — CT scans of chest, abdomen, head and neck; bone marrow biopsy

Salivary Gland Tumors

- Any enlarging mass anterior/inferior to ear or at the mandible angle is suspected to be of salivary gland origin
- Benign
  - Asymptomatic except for mass
- Malignant
  - Rapid growth, skin fixation, cranial nerve palsies
- Diagnostic tests
  - FNAB

  ◊ Shown to reduce surgery by 1/3 in some studies
  ◊ Delineates intra-glandular lymph node, localized sialadenitis or benign lympho-epithelial cysts
  ◊ May facilitate surgical planning and patient counselling
  ◊ Accuracy >90% (sensitivity: ~90%; specificity: ~80%)
  - CT/MRI — deep lobe tumors of parotid gland intra vs. extra-parotid tumor
- Be prepared for total parotidectomy with possible facial nerve sacrifice

Carotid Body Tumor

- Rare in children
- Pulsatile, compressible mass
- Mobile side to side but not upward or downward
- Clinical diagnosis, confirmed by CT angiography
- Treatment
  - Irradiation or close observation in the elderly
  - Surgical resection for small tumors in young patients
    ◊ Hypotensive anesthesia
    ◊ Preoperative measurement of catecholamines

Lipoma

- Soft, ill-defined mass
- Usually >35 years of age
- Asymptomatic
- Clinical diagnosis — confirmed by excision

Neurogenic Tumors

- Arise from neural crest derivatives
- Include schwannoma, neurofibroma, and malignant peripheral nerve sheath tumor
- Increased incidence in NF syndromes
- Schwannoma most common in head and neck

Congenital and Developmental Mass

- Epidermal and sebaceous cysts
- Branchial cleft cysts
- Thyroglossal duct cyst
- Vascular tumors

Epidermal and Sebaceous Cysts

- Most common congenital/developmental mass
- Older age groups
- Clinical diagnosis
- Elevation and movement of overlying skin
- Skin dimple or pore
- Excisional biopsy confirms

Dermoid and Teratomatous Cysts

- Developmental anomalies composed of different germ cell layers
- Isolation of pleuripotent stem cells or closure of germ cell layers within points of failed embryonic fusion lines
- Classified according to composition
- Dermoid cyst
  - Mesoderm and ectoderm
  - Midline, para-median, painless masses that usually do not elevate with tongue protrusion
  - Commonly misdiagnosed as thyroglossal duct cysts.
  - Treatment is simple surgical excision
- Teratoid/Teratomatous cyst and teratoma
  - All three germ cell layers — Endoderm, mesoderm and ectoderm
  - Larger midline masses, present earlier in life
  - 20% associated with maternal polyhydramnios
  - Unlike adult teratomas, they rarely demonstrate malignant degeneration
  - Surgical excision

Thyroglossal Duct Cyst

- Most common congenital neck mass (70%)
- 50% present before age 20
- Midline (75%) or near midline (25%)
- Usually just inferior to hyoid bone (65%)
- Elevates on swallowing/protrusion of tongue
- It is important to differentiate thyroglossal duct cyst from Ectopic thyroid tissue
- Treatment is surgical removal (Sistrunk's operation) after resolution of any infection. It involves excision of cyst along with the tract and middle of hyoid bone

Vascular Tumors

- Lymphangiomas and hemangioma
- Usually within 1st year of life

- Hemangiomas often resolve spontaneously, while lymphangiomas remain unchanged
- CT/MRI may help define extent of disease
- Treatment
  - Lymphangioma — surgical excision for easily accessible or lesions affecting vital functions; recurrence is common
  - Haemangioma — surgical excision reserved for those with rapid growth involving vital structures or associated thrombocytopenia that fails medical therapy (steroids, interferon)

Ranula

- *Simple ranula:* Unilateral oral cavity cystic lesion
- *Plunging ranula:* Pierce the mylohyoid to present as a paramedian or lateral neck mass
- *Cyst aspirate:* High protein, amylase levels
- CT scan/MRI
- Treatment is intraoral excision to include the sublingual gland of origin

Laryngoceles

- Congenitally formed from an enlarged laryngeal saccule
- Classified as internal, external, or both
- Internal
  - Confined to larynx, usually involves the false cord and aryepiglottic fold
  - Hoarseness and respiratory distress or neck mass
- External and combined laryngoceles
  - Soft, compressible, lateral neck mass that distends with increase in intralaryngeal pressures
  - Extends through the thyrohyoid membrane at the entrance of the superior laryngeal nerve
  - CT scan is useful in delineation
- 1–3% of Laryngoceles will harbor an underlying laryngeal carcinoma
- All adult patients should undergo direct laryngoscopy at the time of surgical intervention.

Sternomastoid Tumor of Infancy (Pseudotumor)

- Firm mass of the sternocleidomastoid muscle, chin turned away and head tilted towards the mass

- Tumor is actually a hematoma with subsequent fibrotic replacement
- Ultrasound helps in diagnosis
- Physical therapy is very successful
- Myoplasty of the sternocleidomastoid muscle only if refractory to physiotherapy

Inflammatory Disorders

- Lymphadenitis
- Granulomatous lymphadenitis

Lymphadenitis

- Very common, especially within 1st decade
- Tender node with signs of systemic infection
- Directed antibiotic therapy with follow-up
- FNAB indications (pediatric)
  - Actively infectious condition with no response
  - Progressively enlarging
  - Solitary and asymmetric nodal mass
  - Supraclavicular mass (60% malignancy)
  - Persistent nodal mass without active infection.

Lymphadenopathy

- Equivocal or suspicious FNAB in the pediatric nodal mass requires open excisional biopsy to rule out malignant or granulomatous disease.

Granulomatous Lymphadenitis

- Infection develops over weeks to months
- Minimal systemic complaints or findings
- Common etiologies
  - TB, atypical TB, cat-scratch fever, actino-mycosis, sarcoidosis
  - Firm, relatively fixed node with involvement of skin
- Typical *M. tuberculosis*
  - More common in adults
  - Posterior triangle nodes
  - Rarely seen in our population
  - Usually responds to anti-TB medications
  - May require excisional biopsy for further workup
- Atypical *M. tuberculosis*
  - Pediatric age groups
  - Anterior triangle nodes
  - Brawny skin, induration and pain
  - Usually responds to complete surgical excision or curettage
- Cat-scratch fever (Bartonella)
  - Pediatric group
  - Preauricular and submandibular nodes
  - Spontaneous resolution with or without antibiotics

35 | Penetrating Neck Trauma

TYPES OF WEAPONS

As shown by formula ($K = 1/2\ mv^2$), velocity is more important than mass in the amount of energy carried by a weapon.

Therefore, two basic types of weapons — low and high velocity.

- Low velocity — knives, ice picks, glass
- High velocity — handguns, shotguns, shrapnel.

Guns

Three Basic Types

- Low velocity (handguns) ~ 400ft/lb
- High velocity (rifles) ~ 3000ft/lb
- Shotguns — energy and impact varies with distance

Ballistics

Deviation from straight line motion stabilizes bullets in flight. Various forms of these motions are:

- Yaw
- Precession
- Nutation

It also lends to decreased predictability of trajectory.

Cavitation: Tissue flows forward and outward and creates a temporary vacuum cavity that sucks in contaminants and transmits a shock wave. Entry and exit wounds are small.

Anatomy

First divided into zones in a paper from Monson et al. cook county hospital 1969

- **Zone I** – Clavicles to cricoid
- **Zone II** – Cricoid to angle of the mandible
- **Zone III** – Angle of the mandible to base of the skull

Zone I

- Inferior trachea and esophagus
- Vessels of the root of the neck: The brachiocephalic trunk, the subclavian arteries, the common carotid arteries, the thyrocervical trunk and the corresponding veins, thoracic duct, thyroid gland, spinal cord.

Zone II

- The larynx, hypopharynx
- *Vessels:* Common carotid arteries, the internal and external carotid arteries, the internal jugular veins
- Cranial nerves 10, 11, and 12, and the spinal cord

Zone III

- The pharynx
- *Vessels:* Carotid arteries, the vertebral arteries, the internal jugular veins

Neck Exploration – Incisions

Zone II/III Injuries

- "Hockey stick incision"
- Open in layers
- Retract the SCM laterally
- Methylene blue to aid in visualizing leaks
- Mandibulotomy or mandibular subluxation for zone III

Zone I

- Left anterior thoracotomy or left posterolateral thoracotomy for left zone I
- Midline sternotomy with extension to the right supraclavicular region for right zone I

Incidence

- Most common site of injury is aerodigestive tract (20%)
- Internal jugular vein was the most commonly injured vessel followed by carotid

Mortality

- Mortality has decreased over the years
- Most still due to exsanguination

Initial Management

- Airway — Intubation vs. surgical airway
- Breathing
- Circulation — IV access, immediate exploration
- Examination — Determine weapon trajectory

Signs of Injury

Vascular

Shock, profuse bleeding, evolving stroke, expanding hematoma, hemoptysis, hematemesis, unequal pulses, bruits or thrills

Larynx/Trachea

Subcutaneous emphysema, hoarseness, respiratory distress, stridor

Esophagus

Neck pain, blood in saliva, fever, odynophagia

Management of the Stable Patient

The Old Standard

- If platysma is breached — immediate neck exploration including laryngoscopy, esophagoscopy

- Based on war time experiences
- Fogelman et al. (1956) showed that immediate neck exploration led to better outcomes for vascular injuries
- Led to high rate of negative neck explorations in > 50%
- Arteriogram slowly began to gain acceptance as screening tool before exploration, especially for zone 1 and 3 injuries as vascular injuries in these zones are difficult to detect on explorations

Arteriogram

- Zone I and Zone III vascular injuries are difficult to visualize by physical exam, making arteriogram useful in these patients
- Flint et al. (1973) reported absence of physical findings in 32% of patients with major zone I vascular injury
- Arteriogram can be followed by embolization

A Newer Algorithm

- Mandatory exploration is not always necessary
- 63% of the patients can be managed by the observation
- Entire study population had a mortality of 1.5%, similar to those in more rigorous treatment protocols
- Similar results obtained in other large studies with similar protocols
- Arteriogram in asymptomatic patients with zone I injury is mandatory

CT Scan

- Metallic markers at the skin entry sites, skin violation, subcutaneous fat stranding, soft tissue air or hematoma, vertebral fracture, contrast extravasation, missile location can aid in identifying weapon trajectory and structures at risk
- Should only be used in stable patients

Duplex Ultrasonography

- Requires the presence of reliable technician and radiologist
- 100% sensitivity in detecting arterial injury, using arteriography as the gold standard

Management of Vascular Injuries

- *Common carotid:* Repair preferred over ligation in almost all cases. Saphenous vein graft may be used. Shunting is rarely necessary. Thrombectomy may be necessary.
- *Internal carotid:* Shunting is usually necessary
- *Vertebral:* Angiographic embolization or proximal ligation can be used if the contralateral vertebral artery is intact.
- *Internal jugular:* Repair vs. ligation.

Management of Esophageal Injury

- Best detected by combination of esophagoscopy and esophagogram in symptomatic patients
- Injection of air or methylene blue in the mouth may aid in localizing injuries
- Close wounds in a watertight 2 layered fashion
- Controlled fistula with T-tube or exteriorization of low non-repairable wounds
- Small pharyngeal lesions above arytenoids can be treated with oral restriction and observation for 5–7 days
- All patients should be nil per oral for 5–7 days

Management of Laryngeal/Tracheal Injury

- Diagnosed through direct laryngoscopy for suspicious wounds
- Immediate tracheotomy for suspected laryngeal injury
- Entry incision in the cricoid cartilage, extending in the midline to the thyroid membrane, and meticulously close mucosal lacerations, using advancement flaps if necessary, or rarely grafts
- Wire vs. miniplate fixation of cartilaginous fractures

Points to Remember

- Mandatory neck exploration is no longer considered acceptable
- Remember ABC for initial management
- Physical examination is probably the most useful diagnostic tool
- Intervention should be directed to sites of possible injury
- Non-invasive diagnostic modalities should be considered

36 | Lymphadenopathy

There are more than 600 lymph nodes in the body. Lymphatics are present in all organs except in brain, eyes, bone marrow and cartilage.

It can be defined as any abnormality in the size, consistency or character of lymph nodes. Any lymph node more than 1 cm in size is taken as abnormal except in the inguinal area.

- It is concerning to the patient and physician due to the possibility of underlying malignancy.

Pathological Basis of Lymph Node Enlargement

Lymph node enlarges due to the following factors operating in isolation or in combination:

a. In response to antigen there is increase in the number of benign lymphocytes and macrophages. This is known as reactive hyperplasia of lymph nodes.

b. There may be infiltration of inflammatory cells in to lymph nodes in acute or chronic infections. This is known as lymphadenitis.

c. There may be malignant proliferation of lymphocytes or macrophages leading to lymphoma development.

d. There may be metastatic deposits in the lymph nodes leading to metastatic lymph node enlargement.

e. Lymph nodes may enlarge due to deposition of metabolic laden macrophages in it as seen in various lipid storage disorders.

Lymph nodes enlargement at following site is most likely to be malignant:

a. Supraclavicular lymph nodes

b. Paraumbilical lymph nodes

c. Epitrochlear lymph nodes

Inguinal lymph nodes are more likely due to inflammatory pathology.

Lymphadenopathy can be localized or generalized. Localized lymphadenopathy means involvement of one group of lymph nodes. Generalized means involvement of two or more non contiguous group of lymph nodes.

Broad Categories of Lymphadenopathy can be Summarized as

- Malignancies
- Infections
- Autoimmune disorders
- Miscellaneous and unusual conditions
- Iatrogenic causes

Important points in History

- Age and duration
  - Incidence of malignancy rate increases with age

- Many healthy children have palpable lymph-node enlargement due to infectious or benign aetiology
- Any lymphadenopathy lasting for <2 weeks or >1 year with no progressive increase in size has a very low likelihood of being neoplastic
- Rare exception to this statement can be :
  ◊ Low-grade Hodgkin's/ Non-Hodgkin's lymphomas
  ◊ Chronic lymphocytic leukemia
- History of exposures
  - Animal insect bite infectious contacts, chronic use of medications. Travel-related exposures and immunization status
  - History of tobacco, alcohol, ultraviolet radiation exposure raises suspicion for metastatic carcinoma
  - Occupational exposures to silicon or beryllium can also present with lymph node enlargement
  - *Sexual history and orientation:* AIDS can present with progressive generalized lymphadenopathy
  - Medications like allopurinol, atenolol, captopril, carbamazepine, gold, hydralazine, penicillin and phenytoin can cause lympha-denopathy

- Associated symptoms
  - Constitutional symptoms
    ◊ Fever, fatigue, malaise with atypical lymphocytosis suggests mononucleosis syndromes
    ◊ Significant fever, night sweats, unex-plained BW loss >10% of normal body weight are suggestive of "B" symptoms of Hodgkin's lymphoma
    ◊ Arthralgia, muscle weakness, unusual rash raises suspicion of autoimmune diseases such as rheumatoid arthritis, SLE, or dermatomyositis

Physical Examination

- Head and neck lymph nodes(LN)
- Axillary LN
- Inguinal LN
- Abdominal examination for liver and spleen enlargement, ascites
- Examination of local drainage area of enlarged lymph nodes

Lymph Nodes of the Head and Neck and the Regions that they Drain

- Supraclavicular nodes are the most likely to be malignant and should always be investigated, even in children.

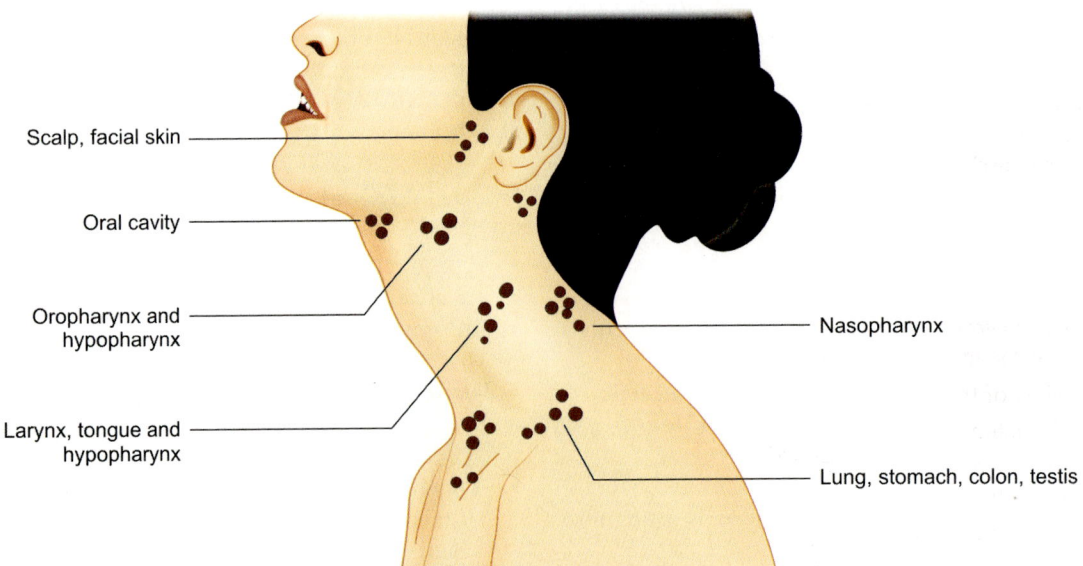

Scalp, facial skin

Oral cavity

Oropharynx and hypopharynx

Larynx, tongue and hypopharynx

Nasopharynx

Lung, stomach, colon, testis

Fig. 36.1: Lymph node drainage of the neck

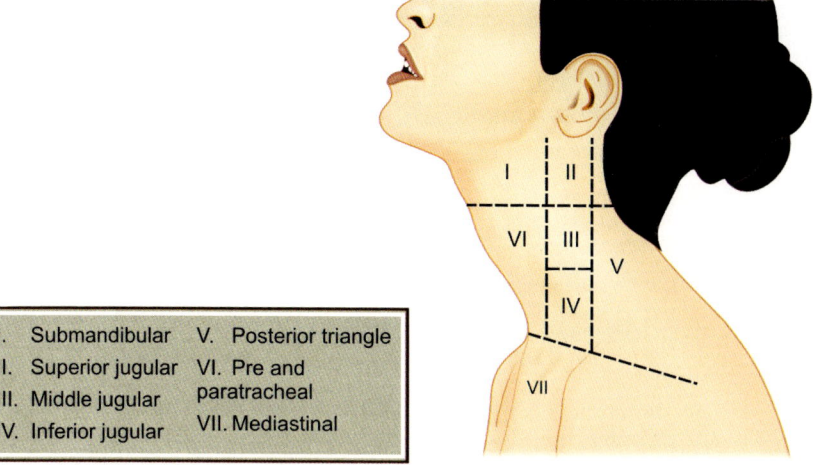

I. Submandibular   V. Posterior triangle
II. Superior jugular   VI. Pre and
III. Middle jugular   paratracheal
IV. Inferior jugular   VII. Mediastinal

Fig. 36.2: Various levels of lymph nodes of the neck

Table 36.1: Drainage area and pathologies associated with various lymph nodes of the head and neck

Lymph nodes enlarged	Drainage area	Infections	Malignancy
Pre-auricular	Scalp, skin mycobacterial infections	Scalp infection, squamous cell carcinomas	Lymphomas, head and neck
Posterior cervical	Scalp, neck, upper thoracic skin	Scalp infection, mycobacterial infections	Skin neoplasms, lymphomas, head and neck squamous cell carcinomas
Supraclavicular	Gastrointestinal tract, genitourinary tract, respiratory system	Mycobacterial/fungal infections	Abdominal/thoracic neoplasms, thyroid/laryngeal diseases
Submandibular	Oral cavity	Mononucleosis, upper respiratory bacterial/viral infections, mycobacterial infections, toxoplasma, cytomegalovirus, dental disease, rubella	Squamous cell carcinoma of head and neck, lymphomas, leukemias
Anterior cervical anterior neck	Larynx, tongue, oropharynx, viral infections	Mononucleosis, upper respiratory bacterial/ leukemias Mycobacterial infections, toxoplasma, cytomegalovirus, dental disease, rubella	Squamous cell carcinoma of head and neck, lymphomas

Axillary Lymph Nodes and the Structures that they Drain

- Most of the cases are nonspecific or reactive
- Persistent lymphadenopathy is less common
- Breast adenocarcinoma often metastasizes initially to axillary nodes
- Ante-cubital or epi-trochlear lymphadenopathy can suggest lymphoma or melanoma of the extremity

Inguinal Lymph Nodes and the Structures that they Drain

- It is common, with nodes enlarged up to 1 to 2 cm in diameter in many healthy adults, but there is low suspicion of malignancy.
- Benign reactive lymphadenopathy and infection are the most common aetiologies.
- Although some tumors, such as Hodgkin's lymphomas, penile/vulvar SCC, melanoma in

Table 36.2: Drainage area and pathologies associated with various lymph nodes of the upper limb

Lymph nodes enlarged	Drainage area	Infections	Malignancy
Infra-clavicular			Highly suspicious for Non-Hodgkin's lymphoma
Axillary	Breast, upper extremity and thoracic wall	Skin infection, trauma, Cat-Scratch disease, sarcoidosis, syphilis, leprosy, brucellosis, leishmaniasis	Breast adenocarcinoma, skin neoplasms, lymphomas, leukemias, soft tissue
Epitrochlear	Ulnar forearm, hand	Skin infections	Lymphoma, skin malignancies

Table 36.3: Drainage area and pathologies associated with various lymph nodes of the lower limb

Lymph nodes enlarged	Drainage area	Infections	Malignancy
Horizontal node group	Lower abdomen, external genitalia (skin), anal canal, lower half of vagina, lower extremity	Benign reactive lymphadenopathy, sexually transmitted diseases, skin infections	Lymphomas, squamous cell carcinoma of the penis, vulva and anus, skin neoplasms, soft tissue/Kaposi's sarcoma

this area, may present with inguinal lymphadenopathy but it is not a typical presenting finding in either case.

Generalized Lymphadenopathy

- When lymphadenopathy is found in two or more distinct anatomic regions
- More likely to result from serious infections, autoimmune diseases, and disseminated malignancies
- Patient should be fully investigated to rule out serious problems
- Generalized adenopathy infrequently occurs in patients' with neoplasms, but it is occasionally seen in patients with leukemias and lymphomas or advanced disseminated metastatic solid tumors.

Nodal Character and Size

- Hard and painless nodes have higher suspicion of malignancy or granulomatous disease
- Viral infection typically produces hyperplastic nodes that are bilateral, mobile, non-tender, and well demarcated
- Palpable supraclavicular, iliac or popliteal nodes of any size and epitrochlear nodes larger than 5 mm are considered abnormal
- Increasing size and persistence over time are of greater concern for malignancy

Diagnosis and Management

- *The first step:* Reviewing patients' medications, considering unusual causes of lymphadenopathy,

and reconsidering the risk factors for neoplasm. If a diagnosis is not suggested, and the patient is deemed low risk for neoplasm, the regional lymphadenopathy can be safely observed.

- It is suggested that non-inguinal lymphadenopathy lasting more than one month merits specific investigation.
- Fine needle aspiration cytology (FNAC) should be done in all cases of lymphadenopathy if lymph nodes appear to be significant on clinical examination or if associated with abnormality in drainage area or if there are systemic signs and symptoms.

Lymph Node Biopsy

Lymph node biopsy is indicated only if the repeated FNAC is inconclusive or if the diagnosis of lymphoma is suspected or if tissue is required for specialised tests like immunohistochemistry or special staining. The diagnosis of lymphoma cannot be made on FNAC.

- Once biopsy has been chosen, ideally the largest, most suspicious, and most accessible node is selected, taking into account differing diagnostic yields by site
- Inguinal nodes offer the lowest yield, and supraclavicular nodes have the highest
- Excisional biopsy remains the diagnostic procedure of choice.

37 Breast: Anatomy and Benign Diseases

- Breast is a modified sebaceous gland lying on the subcutaneous tissue over pectoral fascia
- Palpable limit of the extent of breast
  - Vertical from 2nd to 6th ribs inclusive
  - Horizontal from side of sternum to mid-axillary line

    However, the thin layer of breast tissue usually extends from beyond the palpable limits up to costal margin inferiorly, posterior axillary line laterally and up to mid sternum medially. While performing a total mastectomy for carcinoma one should take care to remove whole of the breast which is extending beyond the palpable limit
- 2/3 of the breast lies on pectoralis major, 1/3 lies on serratus anterior
- Breast lies in the subcutaneous tissue and is separated from muscle by deep fascia
- Axillary tail of spencer is part of breast
  - Extends from the outer part of the breast and reaches upto 3rd rib in the axilla
  - This portion of breast lies under deep fascia
  - Comes in direct contact with axillary lymph nodes

Architecture of the Breast

Acini
↓
Lobules
↓
Lobes

- Arranged in a radiating fashion like spokes of wheel
- Converge on nipple
- Each lobe is drained by a collecting duct
- 10–15 collecting ducts
- Each collecting duct drains a segmental system of smaller ducts and lobules

Lobule
↓
Ductule
↓
Subsegmental duct
↓
Segmental duct
↓
Lactiferous sinus
↓
Collecting duct

- Larger ducts are the site of duct papilloma and duct ectasia
- From distal ducts arise fibroadenoma, cysts, and sclerosing adenosis

Blood Supply

- Lateral thoracic artery – branch of 2nd part of axillary artery
- Perforating branches of the internal mammary artery via 2nd, 3rd and 4th intercostal spaces
- Lateral branches of 2nd, 3rd and 4th intercostal arteries

Venous Drainage

- Axillary vein
- Internal mammary vein
- Intercostal vessels

Lymphatic Drainage

Lymphatics of the Skin Except Nipple and Areola

- Pass in radial direction
- End in surrounding nodes
  - Outer side — axillary nodes
  - Upper part — supraclavicular nodes
  - Inner part — internal mammary nodes

Lymphatics of the Nipple and Areola

- Subareolar plexus of Sappey which communicates with the lymphatics of the breast.

Lymphatics of the Breast Parenchyma

- 75% drain into axillary lymph nodes
- 25% from the medial and lateral portions of the breast drain into internal mammary nodes

Axillary lymph nodes are arranged in 5 sets

- *Anterior* — along the lateral thoracic veins, under anterior axillary fold. Axillary tail of Spence lies in close contact with these lymph nodes
- *Posterior* — along the posterior axillary fold in relation to the subscapular vessels
- *Lateral* — along the upper part of humerus in relation to the axillary vein
- *Central* — in the fat of the upper part of axilla in relation to the intercostobrachial nerve
- *Apical set* — also called infraclavicular lymph nodes.

Investigations of Breast Diseases

Mammography (Usually done in patients more than 35 years)

- It is soft tissue X-ray of the breast.
- It is done by placing the breast in direct contact with the ultrasensitive film and exposing it to low voltage, high amperage X-rays.
- Dose of radiation is 0.1 rad.
- Two views are taken
  - Cranio-caudal view
  - Medio-lateral view

- Uses
  - Breast screening to detect carcinoma breast at an early stage
  - To detect tumor which are not clinically palpable (<0.5 cm)
  - For evaluation of opposite breast in proven cases of carcinoma of one breast
  - Follow-up of cases of breast carcinoma treated with breast conservation.

Ultrasonography

- Particularly useful in young women less than 35 years of age with dense breast in whom mammograms are difficult to interpret
- To distinguish cystic from solid lesions
- Can be used to detect impalpable breast lumps

Magnetic Resonance Imaging (MRI)

- To distinguish scar from recurrence in patients who have had previous breast conservative surgery for breast cancer
- For imaging breasts of patients with implants
- Screening tool in high risk breast cancer patients
- Evaluation of axilla in recurrent disease

Fine Needle Aspiration Cytology (FNAC)

- It is a technique to obtain cells for examination
- Using 21G needle and 10 ml syringe, without releasing the negative pressure in the syringe
- Aspirate is then smeared onto a slide which is air dried

Biopsy of Breast Lesions

- Tru-cut needle biopsy
- Excision biopsy is done if repeated trucut biopsy negative
- Incision biopsy is done only in fungating lesion.

Triple Assessment of a Lump

- For every breast lump, diagnosis should be made by a combination of clinical assessment, mammography/ultrasonography and a tissue sample taken either for cytological or histopathological analysis
- Accuracy of diagnosis is 95%

Nipple Discharge

- Physiological discharge — milky discharge following pregnancy or lactation
- Pathological discharge

Nipple Discharge
Milky
• Lactation
• Galactocele
Non-milky
Blood
• Ductal carcinoma
• Ductal papilloma
• Duct ectasia
• Paget's disease
• Fibroadenosis
Serous
• Early pregnancy
Thick creamy
• Duct ectasia
Purulent (yellow)
• Breast abscess
Various shades (brown, green, black)
• Fibroadenoma
• Duct ectasia

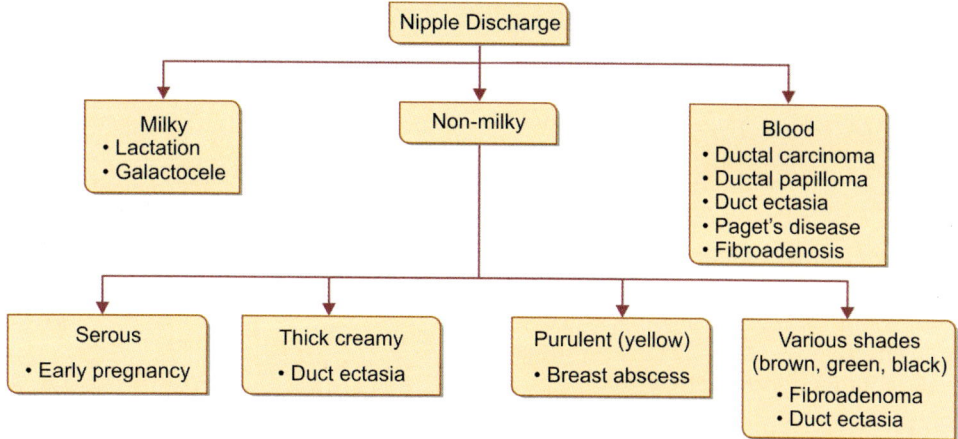

Fig. 37.1: Flowchart showing etiology of nipple discharge

Management of Nipple Discharge

Management of nipple discharge (after Headley Atkins)
With lump
Triple assessment
Manage accordingly
Without lump
Localized to one duct
Removal of duct (microdochectomy) and histopathological examination
Many ducts
Examine discharge for occult blood
Blood positive
Blood negative
Above 40 years
• Simple mastectomy and histopathological examination
• Total excision of ducts and histopathological examination
Below 40 years
Observe
Discharge may disappear
Localizes to one duct
Lump appears
Microdochectomy
Lump excision

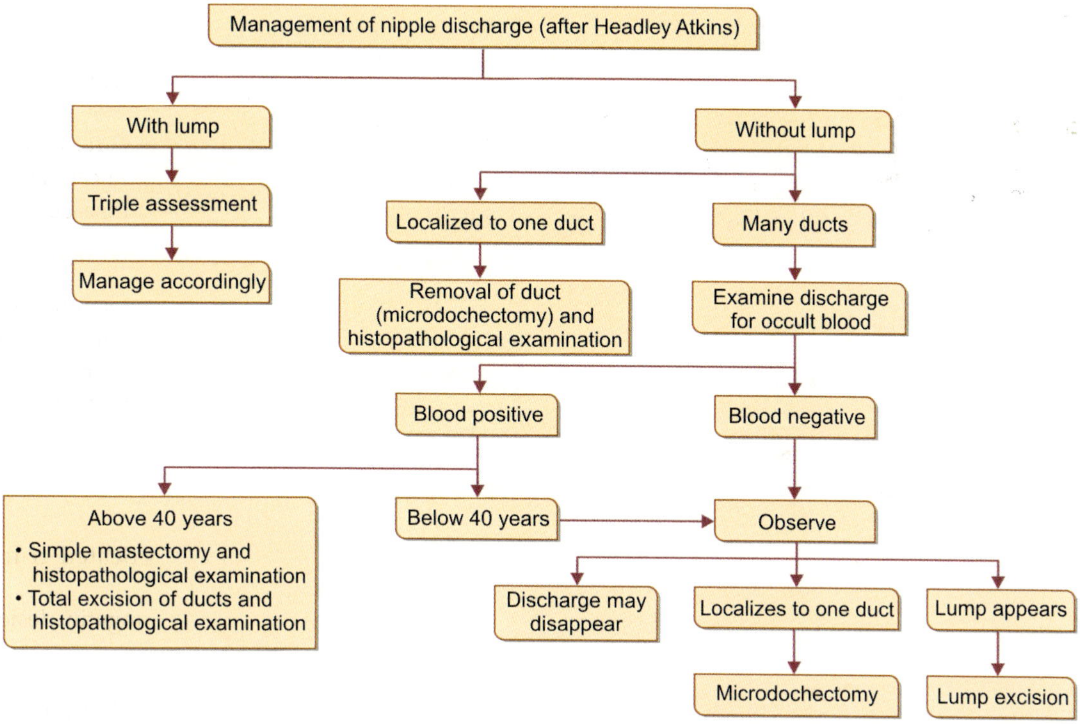

Fig. 37.2: Flowchart showing management of nipple discharge

Breast Abscess

Classification

- According to severity of onset
  - Acute
  - Subacute
  - Chronic
- According to their position
  - Premammary, e.g. subareolar
  - Intramammary
  - Retromammary
- Acute intramammary abscess is most common. It accounts for 85% of breast abscesses.

Etiology

- >90% occur in lactating breast
- Most common during first lactation
- Infecting organism is *Staphylococcus*, which enters the breast from infant's throat either along the milk duct or through a crack in the nipple
- Abscess occurs more frequently during
  - First month of lactation
  - When child is >6 months old and is developing teeth. Teeth cause trauma to the nipple which acts as a portal of entry for the organisms

Clinical Features

Stage of Cellulitis

- Breast is swollen, congested and painful. It is associated with fever.

Stage of Localization and Abscess Formation

- Toxins released by *Staphylococci* cause tissue necrosis and abscess spreads to adjacent tissues. Since abscess is deep seated, fluctuation is a late sign. However, overlying skin shows edema and tense induration.

Treatment

Stage of Cellulitis

- Conservative treatment
- Support to breast, local heat, analgesia
- Antibiotics, e.g. cloxacillin or erythromycin
- Infected breast should be emptied of milk using a breast pump. Feeding should be from the opposite breast only.

If the patient does not respond to antibiotics, repeated aspirations (may be ultrasound guided) under antibiotic cover are performed. This often leads to disappearance of abscess, hence avoids incision and drainage.

Incision and Drainage

- If no response within 48 hours of antibiotics
- If there is an area of tense induration after emptying the breast of milk
- Fluctuation is a late sign.
- Usually indicated if there is marked skin thinning or redness of overlying skin as in late cases.

38 Breast Cancer

- Most common cancer in women
- In India it is second to cancer cervix
- 23.2 per 100,000 population in India
- In the US, one out of 11 females will develop carcinoma breast during life time
- Tumor clinically palpable when >1 cm
  - Needs 30 tumor doubling time from single cell to attain this size
  - Average tumor doubling time 109 days
  - Takes 8–9 years to attain 1 cm size
- *Female:* Male ratio 150:1

Risk Factors

Hormonal

- Excessive exposure of estrogens unopposed by progesterone
  - Early menarche
  - Late menopause
  - Null parity
  - Late first pregnancy
  - Patient with estrogens secreting tumor of ovary
  - Obesity
- Consumption of animal fat and protein

Pathology

- *In situ* carcinoma
  - Ductal
  - Lobular
- Invasive carcinoma
  - Stellate type
  - Circumscribed type
  - Others — medullary, mucoid, tubular, inflammatory, Paget's disease of nipple

Ductal Carcinoma *in Situ*

- Confined to ducts
- No invasion of basement membrane

Presentation

- Lump
- Thickening near nipple
- Nipple discharge
- Can be detected on mammography — clustered microcalcification

Subtypes

- Comedo — poor prognosis
- Solid
- Cribriform plate
- Micropapillary

Treatment

- Single focus — wide excision
- Multifocal — mastectomy

Lobular Carcinoma *in Situ*

- Arises in acini of breast lobules
- Cannot be detected on mammography

- It has no malignant potential itself but patients with lobular carcinoma *in situ* are more prone to develop invasive ductal carcinoma.

High Risk Group for Development of Breast Cancer

- Females with juvenile papillomatosis of breast
- Patients with ataxia telangiectasia
- Males with Klinefelter's syndrome
- Family history of breast cancer
- Previous history of breast cancer
- Radiation exposure before 30 years

Stellate Type Invasive Ductal Carcinoma

- Irregular edge
- No capsule
- Hard consistency due to dense stroma
- Infiltrate into surrounding breast tissue
- Gritty sensation on cutting
- Both cut surfaces take concave shape due to elastic content

Circumscribed Type Invasive Ductal Carcinoma

- Well defined
- Multilobular
- Grows in pushing fashion

Genetic Factors

- Patients with mutated BRCA1 and BRCA2 genes
- Overexpression or mutation of p53 gene

Histopathology of Breast Cancer

- *In situ* cancer can be of ductal, lobular or Paget's disease of the nipple (which can have associated component of invasive ductal carcinoma)
- Invasive carcinoma—80%
- Invasive lobular carcinoma—10 %
- Uncommon histopathological types—10%
  - Medullary
  - Tubular
  - Mucinous
  - Papillary
  - Squamous
- Invasive ductal carcinoma (NOS)—80 %

Diagnosis

- Core needle biopsy/ FNAC to confirm the diagnosis

Table 38.1:	
Advantage of core needle biopsy over FNAC	*Advantage of FNAC*
Can differentiate in situ from invasive carcinoma	Less invasive/ traumatic
Differentiate subtypes of carcinoma	No local anaesthesia required
Differentiate lobular from ductal carcinoma	Economical
Differentiate giant fibroadenoma from sarcoma	No cut required
Application of hormone receptor assay	

TNM Classification

Primary Tumor

- TX   Tumor cannot be assessed (Previously excised) or completely disappeared after chemotherapy
- T0   No evidence of tumor clinically but detected on screening mammography
- Tis   *In situ* carcinoma
- T1   2 cm or less
- T2   >2 cm but <5 cm
- T3   >5 cm
- T4a   Extension to chest wall (chest wall includes ribs, intercostal muscles or serratus anterior, but not pectoralis major muscle)
- T4b   Peau d'Orange
        Ulceration of skin
        Satellite skin nodule
- T4c   Both T4a and T4b

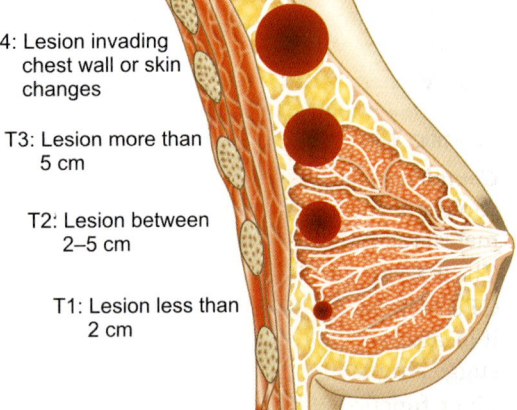

T4: Lesion invading chest wall or skin changes

T3: Lesion more than 5 cm

T2: Lesion between 2–5 cm

T1: Lesion less than 2 cm

Fig. 38.1: T staging of breast cancer

Regional Lymph Node

- NX Regional lymph nodes cannot be evaluated
- N0 Regional lymph nodes free from disease
- N1 Metastasis to movable ipsilateral regional lymph nodes
- N2a Metastasis to ipsilateral axillary lymph nodes fixed to each other or other structures
- N2b Involvement of internal mammary lymph detected on clinical examination as parasternal mass or on X-ray chest or CT chest, but not on lymphoscintigraphy.
- N3a Involvement of infra-clavicular lymph nodes
- N3b Involvement of both ipsilateral axillary and internal mammary group of lymph nodes
- N3c Involvement of superaclavicular lymph nodes

Distant Metastasis

- MX Distant metastasis cannot be assessed
- M0 No distant metastasis present
- M1 Distant metastasis including metastasis to ipsilateral supraclavicular lymph nodes

TNM Group Staging

Stage I	T1	N0	M0
Stage IIA	T0/T1	N1	M0
	T2	N0	M0
Stage IIB	T2	N1	M0
	T3	N0	M0
Stage IIIA	T0–2	N2	M0
	T3	N1/N2	M0
Stage IIIB	T4	Any N	M0
Stage III C	Any T	N3	M0
Stage IV	Any T	Any N	M1

Metastatic Work Up

- *Complete blood count (CBC):* An abnormal CBC should prompt evaluation of bone marrow for metastatic disease
- Chest X-ray (PA view) for all patients
- CT chest/abdomen reserved for stage III diseases if localizing symptoms or abnormal lab values suggesting liver involvement
- Liver function test including alkaline phosphatase (ALP). Elevated levels of liver enzymes or ALP along with Gamma GGT suggest liver secondaries. Elevated ALP alone with or without calcium suggests bone secondaries
- Bone scan in stage III, localizing symptoms or isolated abnormal ALP
- FDG-PET scan role still evolving but may be useful to detect occult metastasis but not a standard of care
- Evaluation of cardiac systolic function by echocardiography or MUGA scans before and during treatment with anthracylines-based chemotherapy or during herceptin therapy as both are potentially cardiotoxic drugs
- Mammography for the opposite breast and for the same breast if BCS is being planned

Role of MRI in Breast Cancer

- It can be used as a problem solving tool in the setting of equivocal imaging (Mammogram or USG) findings or equivocal physical examination findings, when breast cancer is suspected, but cannot be established by conventional methods
- In the evaluation of patients who have previously under gone excision biopsy for breast cancer and no lump is palpable
- Evaluation of axillary node metastasis and unknown primary: MRI can detect ipsilateral breast cancer in 75 to 86 percent of cases when clinical examination and mammographic examination is normal
- In monitoring response to neo-adjuvant chemotherapy in locally advanced breast cancer. Earliest response to chemotherapy is decrease in the contrast enhancement of tumor even before decrease in size

Chemoprevention by Tamoxifen

Subgroup of patients who can be benefited with chemoprevention by tamoxifen to reduce breast cancer risk

- Patients with history of lobular carcinoma *in situ*
- Patients with atypical ductal or lobular hyperplasia
- Premenopausal women with mutation in either BRCA1 or BRCA2 gene
- Premenopausal women >35 with 5 yrs risk of developing breast cancer >1.66% (On Gail model)

Prognostic Factors

- Age of patient — young patient has poorer prognosis
- Size of tumor
- Lymph node metastasis
- Grade of tumor
- Tumor with lymphovascular invasion
- High S-phase fraction
- Aneuploidy/Polyploidy
- Tumor with poor nuclear grade
- Tumor with over expression of HER-2 (*erb B2*) gene
- Tumor with mutated p53 gene
- More microvessels in tumor
- Presence of type IV collagenase, cathepsin D, plasminogen activator

Treatment

Early Breast Cancer

- Appropriate surgery followed by adjuvant chemotherapy and radiotherapy if indicated
- Aim of adjuvant chemotherapy
  - To take care of occult micrometastasis and to have survival benefit

Indications of Adjuvant Chemotherapy

- All node positive patients irrespective of menopausal status or ER status.
  - CAF × 6 cycles
  - Taxane plus anthracycline based regimen (AC × 4 followed by Paclitexal × 4)
- Node negative and ER positive if they fall in high risk like
- High grade
- HER2 gene amplification
- Size more than 2 cm
- Young age < 45 years
- Node negative and ER –ve patients if more than 1cm or less than 1cm if HER2 +ve, high grade, or lymph vascular invasion present
- Adjuvant chemotherapy for node –ve patients can be
  - AC × 4 cycles
  - CAF × 6 cycles
  - Oral or IV CMF (Bonadonna regimen) 6 – 8 cycles
  - Role of taxane in node negative cancer not clear
  - Adjuvant trastuzumab therapy

- In patients whose tumor over express HER2 as assessed by FISH or are designated 3+ by IHC
  - Suggested regimen (AC × 4 followed by weekly paclitaxol × 12 cycles and trastuzumab for 1 years)

Appropriate Surgery can be

- Modified radical mastectomy
- Breast conservation surgery (BCS) (excision of lump along with 2 cm of tumor free margin all around + axillary lymph node staging)

Contraindications of BCS

- Two or more primary tumors in different quadrants (Multi-centric disease)
- Extensive malignant appearing micro calcifications on mammography
- Persistent positive inspite repeat re-excision surgery after BCS
- Previous breast or mantle irradiation
- Pregnancy
- H/o collagen vascular disease
- Patients who are positive for BRCA1 or BRCA2 mutation
- Tumor more than 5 cm
- Central quadrant tumor

Adjuvant Chemotherapy (Summary)

- Premenopausal
  - Irrespective of ER/PR status → CAF six cycles to all
  - In HER2 neu +ve → herceptin + paclitaxel based chemotherapy
- Postmenopausal:
  - ER+/PR+ → hormone therapy
  - ER– /PR– → CAF six cycles

Indication for Radiotherapy in Early Breast Cancer

- After BCS, radiotherapy to the remaining breast tissue in all cases
- Radiotherapy to the chest wall to avoid local recurrence if :
  - Positive tumor margins in resected specimen
  - Lympho-vascular invasion present
  - Tumor > 5 cm in size
  - **Lymph nodes:** > 4 positive LN present Radiation field should also include supra-

clavicular nodes and upper internal mammary nodes

- In young premenopausal patients with ER –ve tumor
- Aim of RT is to decrease loco regional recurrence there is no increase in survival by RT
- RT should be given after completing adjuvant chemotherapy as concurrent chemotherapy increases the side effects of radiotherapy

Locally Advanced Breast Cancer

- Neo adjuvant chemotherapy (6 cycles, assess response at 3 cycles)
  - CAF (2nd line is paclitaxel based)
- Followed by surgery:
  - MRM (Role of BCS in locally advanced disease after down staging is still evolving) and radiotherapy to the chest wall in all cases

Advanced Breast Disease/ Metastatic Breast Disease

- ER+/ PR+ → hormone therapy
- ER–/PR–
- Failed hormone therapy

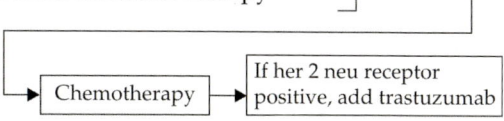

- Nottingham Prognostic Index (NPI)
  - (Tumor size in cm X0.2) + lymph node stage (1 = no nodes, 2 = 1 to 3 nodes, 3 = 4 or more nodes)+ grade(1, 2 or 3)
  - Excellent if NPI <2.4
  - Good if NPI <3.4
  - Moderate 1 if NPI <4.4
  - Moderate 2 if NPI <5.4
  - Poor if NPI >5.4

39 Empyema Thoracis

DEFINITION

- It is defined as accumulation of pus in the pleural cavity.
- It is derived from the Greek word *"empyein"*, which means: pus-producing.

Criteria for Diagnosis of Empyema

- Frank pus on tapping, organisms presence on culture or gram staining or all the tests positive for $pH<7.2$, glucose level of fluid <400 mg/L, LDH above 1000 IU/ml, protein level >3 gm/ml and WBC count >15000 cells/cc
- Physical and radiological signs along with relevant clinical pictures

Stages in Empyema

- Exudative phase
- Fibrinopurulent stage
- Organizational stage

Exudative Stage

- Focus of infection in lungs leads to increased permeability of visceral pleura
- Exudate fluid in pleural cavity with normal pH glucose level, however, leucocytes may be seen.
- Visceral pleura remains elastic
- Dimensions of thoracic cavity maintained

Fibrinopurulent Stage

- Much larger fluid collection
- Obvious frank pus in pleural cavity
- Contains many polymorphs, leucocytes, bacteria and cellular debris
- Fibrin deposition on both visceral and parietal pleura
- Formation of loculations in the fluid in pleural cavity
- Low glucose and low pH
- High LDH levels

Organizational Stage or Consolidative Phase

- Growth of fibroblasts from both surfaces
- Sheet of inflammatory tissue gradually compress the underlying tissue
- Contraction of affected hemithorax
- Mediastinal shift to same side
- Elevation of diaphragm
- Narrowing or crowding of rib spaces
- Inelastic membrane is produced which is known as pleural peel or cortex

Historical Perspective

- Known since the time of hippocrates who described open drainage
- Greek physicians described placement of indwelling tubes and irrigation
- Evarts Graham from the US in 1918 advanced understanding of empyema, differentiated between pneumococcal and streptococcal empyema and also described principles of management which are valid even in the present era

Graham's Principles of Treatment for Empyema

- Avoidance of open drainage in acute stage
- Prevention of chronic empyema by the rapid sterilization and obliteration of the infected cavity
- Careful attention to the nutrition of the patient

Types of Empyema

- Primary if there is no evidence of surgical intervention or no history of trauma to chest
- Secondary if history of surgical intervention or trauma present to thorax

Etiology

- Production of pus from infection of structures surrounding the pleural space
  - From lung
  - From mediastinum
  - Infection from below diaphragm

Infection from Lung

- Pneumonia (most common)
- Lung abscess
- Bronchiectasis
- Trauma to the lung

From Mediastinal

- Rupture of esophagus
- From infection of head and neck leading to mediastinitis

Infection below the Diaphragm

- Liver abscess rupture in to pleural cavity
- Subphrenic abscess

Others

- Post traumatic
- Iatrogenic
- Post-operative
- Blood spread

Organisms

- The most common:
  - *Staphylococcus aureus* (90% of causes in infants and children)
  - *Streptococcus pneuomoniae*
  - *H. influenzae*
  - Tubercular

Clinical Stages

- *Acute stage:* Within the first 2 weeks of the onset
- *Chronic stage:* After 2 weeks or with the formation of the thick peel and loculations

Causes of Chronicity

- Inadequate tube drainage of empyema
- Chronic pulmonary disease (tuberculosis or fungal infection)
- Immunosuppressed patients
- Presence of foreign body within the pleural space

Clinical Features

Signs

- Fever, tachycardia, patient looks toxic
- Dyspnea
- Cough and expectoration
- Pleuritic chest pain
- Easy fatiguability
- Loss of weight
- Night sweating
- Sometimes patient may be virtually asymptomatic
- Increased respiratory rate
- Decreased movement of hemithorax
- Dullness on percussion
- Diminished breath sounds
- Displacement of mediastinum to opposite side in acute stage

Complications

- Rupture into the lung
- Bronchopleural fistula
- Spread to the subcutaneous tissue
- Empyema necessitans
- Septicemia and septic shock

Investigations

- Chest X-ray
- CT scan in case of chronic empyema to rule out pathology of lung.
- Ultrasonography assists in aspiration of pus

Diagnosis

- Diagnosis is confirmed by thoracocentesis; frank pus or merely cloudy fluid may be aspirated from the pleural space. The pleural fluid typically has a leukocytosis, low pH (<7.20), low glucose (<60 mg/dL), a high LDH (lactic dehydrogenase), elevated protein and may contain infectious organisms.

Management

- Diagnostic thoracocenetesis of pus
  - If thin pus → closed inter-costal tube drainage is instituted

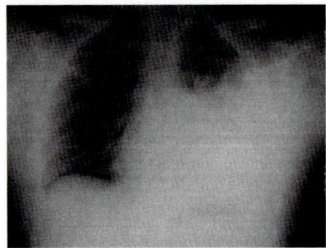

Fig. 39.1: X-ray of a case of empyema thoracis

- If pus is thick and fibrinous → either rib resection or decortications is carried out

Principle of Management

- Control of the infection
- Drainage of pus from the pleura
- Obliteration of the space and complete re-expansion of the lung

Drainage of Empyema

Various options available are:
- Intercostal tube thoracostomy
- Intrapleural instillation of streptokinase followed by tube drainage
- Video Assisted Thoracic Surgery (VATS) debridement of parietal pleura
- Decortication (Fowler-Delrome procedure). Thickened fibrosed visceral pleura which is not allowing the lung to expand, is removed from apex, diaphragmatic surface and lateral aspect of lung
- Rib resection drainage

Tube Thoracostomy

Indications of Chest Tube Insertion (General Indications)

- Pneumothorax
  - In any ventilated patient
  - Tension pneumothorax after initial needle relief
  - Recurrent pneumothorax
  - Large secondary spontaneous pneumothorax
- Malignant pleural effusion
- Empyema and complicated parapneumonic pleural effusion
- Traumatic hemopneumothorax
- Postoperative—for example, thoracotomy, esophagectomy, cardiac surgery

Position of Patient

- Supine with the arm on the side behind the patient's head to expose the axillary area

- An alternative is for the patient to sit upright leaning over an adjacent table with a pillow in the lateral decubitus position
- Insertion should be in the "safe triangle"
  - Anterior axillary line
  - Mid axillary line
  - Upper border of fifth rib

Size of Drain

- Pneumothorax   10–14 F drain
- Empyema   16–24 F drain
- Hemothorax   28–30 F drain

Intrapleural Streptokinase

Indications

- Acute or fibrinopurulent stage
- Presence of loculations
- Incomplete drainage after tube insertion

Contraindications

- Chronic stage
- Post-operative empyema
- Empyema with BPF (Broncho pleural fistula)

Technique

- Streptokinase 25000 IU in 50 cc of 0.9% saline solution
- Clamp the tube for 6 hours
- Open the clamp and connect tube to suction

Video Assisted Thoracoscopy

- Evacuation of necrotic material from pleural cavity essentially from parietal wall. Also known as debridement
- *Limitations:* Not effective in stage III empyema
- Complications, e.g. bleeding

Re-expansion of the Lung and Obliteration of the Space

- Decortication
- Muscle transposition
- Thoracoplasty

Thoracoplasty

- Described by Alexander et al.
- Principal is to remove the rigidity of chest wall and to restore contact between new flexible chest wall and residual lung.
- Posterior segments of 3, 4, 5th ribs between erector spinae muscle and serratus anterior muscle are removed.

Thoracic trauma is responsible for 70% of all deaths following road traffic accidents. Blunt chest trauma is fatal in as many as 10% of cases in isolation. In presence of other injuries, the mortality approaches 30%. Thoracic injury can be iatrogenic resulting from CVP line insertion or during upper GI endoscopy.

Penetrating thoracic trauma bears a mortality of 3% in cases of simple stabbing to as high as 15% in gunshot wounds. Less than 10 percent of blunt chest injuries and around 20 percent of penetrating chest injuries require thoracotomy.

Causes of Mortality Following Thoracic Trauma

- Hypoxemia leading to hypercarbia which in turn leads to acidosis. Metabolic acidosis is caused by hypo-perfusion of the tissues
- Hypovolemic shock
- Cardiac tamponade

Causes of Hypoxia During Chest Injury are Multiple but Few Important Factors are

1. Hypovolemic state due to blood loss
2. Ventilation perfusion mismatches resulting from contusion, alveolar collapse or hematoma
3. Changes in intra-thoracic pressure profile resulting from open or tension pneumothorax

Life Threatening Chest Trauma

It can be in the form of:
- Tension pneumothorax
- Open pneumothorax with sucking chest wound
- Flail chest
- Massive hemothorax
- Cardiac tamponade

Initial Management of a Case of Chest Trauma

- Airway, breathing and circulation need to be restored first (ABC should take first priorities as per ATLS guidelines)
- Inspection
  - Frequency and pattern of breathing
  - Look for foreign in the oropharynx
  - External evidence of trauma
  - Structural defects of thorax
  - Inspection for retraction of intercostal and supraclavicular muscles
- Palpation
  - Surgical emphysema
  - Paradoxical movement
  - Rib tenderness
  - Palpate for defects in the region of supra-clavicular joint which might result from posterior dislocation of clavicle head and can lead to airway obstruction. This type of injury usually manifest as stridor or change in voice quality if patient is conscious and able to speak. This type of injury can be managed by extending the shoulders or by pulling the dislocated clavicle head forward by holding it by towel clip. Once this type of dislocation is reduced it remains stable

- Auscultation and percussion
  - For pneumothorax resonant note on affected side
  - There may be reduced breath sounds in the axilla and shift of trachea to the opposite side.
- Once the patient is stabilised a radiograph of the chest is mandatory to decide the further treatment.

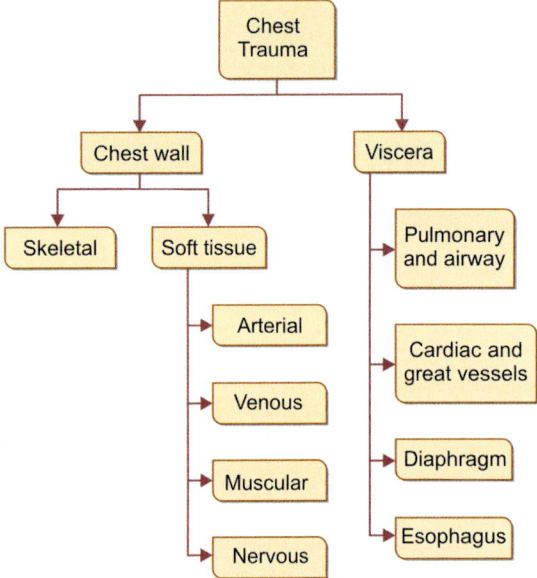

Fig. 40.1: Chest trauma anatomical classification

Fracture of the Ribs

Incidence

- Less common in children
- 1st and 2nd ribs are seldom fractured as they are protected by the clavicle
- Fracture is also less common in the 11th and 12th ribs as they are floating

Uncomplicated Rib Fracture

Presenting Features

- Local pain which increases on deep inspiration, coughing and sneezing
- Shallow and painful respiration
- Tenderness at the fracture site
  AP view of X-ray chest is done to demonstrate the fracture.

Treatment

- Treatment is aimed at relief of pain, the fracture heals by itself
- Systemic analgesics in the form of NSAIDs

- Injection of 2% xylocaine at either the fracture site or as an intercostal nerve block
- Immobilisation of the fracture by strapping the chest wall with an adhesive plaster although commonly done but is not effective
- To be effective the plaster must cross the midline both anteriorly and posteriorly and must include few ribs above and below the fractured rib

Drawbacks of Strapping

- Diminishes respiratory reserve
- May force broken rib ends inwards, causing damage to the lung parenchyma

Complications of Rib Fracture

- Shock
- Surgical emphysema
- Pneumothorax
- Hemothorax
- Flail chest
- Stove in chest
- Contusion and lung laceration
- Cardiac tamponed
- Injury to the diaphragm
- Injury to abdominal viscera, e.g. liver, spleen

Flail Chest

Flail chest results from double fracture of three or more ribs, causing instability of the chest wall. The flail segment shows paradoxical movement and compromises pulmonary and cardiac functions.

Types

- Lateral (Most common)
- *Anterior:* Result from a frontal impact. Sternum is separated from the ribs resulting in a direct compression of the heart during inspiration leading to decreased venous return and poor cardiac output
- *Posterior:* Strong muscle support prevents major paradoxical movements

Treatment

- If flail segment is small and not causing respiratory compromise, the patient must be managed in a high dependency unit and followed with regular blood gas analysis. Patient should receive good analgesic support till the flail segment stabilises.
- In severe cases endotracheal intubation must be done and positive pressure ventilation given for 3 weeks till the fracture becomes less mobile.

Traumatic Hemothorax

Traumatic hemothorax can arise due to bleeding from:
- Intercostal vessels
- Injured lung
- Large vessels
- Heart

Treatment

- Management of shock and blood transfusion
- Draining of hemothorax:
  - Causes re-expansion of the lung and compresses the torn vessel reducing further loss
  - Allows mediastinal structures to return to the midline thus relieving pressure on the contralateral lung
- Thoracotomy:
  - Continued brisk bleeding (more than 100 ml/15 minutes)
  - Continued bleed for more than 200 ml per hour for more than 3 hours
  - Initial drainage of more than 1 litre of blood at the time of insertion of the tube
  - Rupture of the aorta, bronchus or esophagus
  - Cardiac tamponade if needle aspiration is unsuccessful

Traumatic Pneumothorax

Traumatic pneumothorax is defined as presence of free air in the pleural cavity following trauma. Traumatic pneumothorax can be:
- *Simple:* Occurs due to air leak from the lung due to damage from fractured rib ends.
- *Tension:* Results from the communication of the major airway with the pleural cavity such that the air can only enter the pleural cavity on inspiration without any escape. This causes rapid collapse of the lung with shift of the mediastinum to the opposite side.
- Open pneumothorax with a sucking wound.

Tension Pneumothorax

Tension pneumothorax occurs when air is forced in thoracic cavity without any route of escape leading to complete collapse of lung on affected side, shifting of mediastinum to opposite side with decrease venous return and compression of opposite lung. Tension pneumothorax occurs by air leak through one way valve resulting from injury to lung or chest wall.

Aetiology of Traumatic Tension Pneumothorax

a. Positive pressure mechanical ventilation in a trauma patient with undiagnosed or unsuspected visceral pleural injury.
b. Simple pneumothorax after blunt or penetrating trauma may get converted in to tension pneumothorax if lung parenchymal injury fails to heal.
c. Open traumatic wounds in chest wall may result in tension pneumothorax if occlusive dressing is applied inappropriately or if traumatic defect create a flap valve like mechanism.
d. Tension pneumothorax can be as a result of displaced thoracic spine.

Tension pneumothorax is a clinical diagnosis and treatment should not be delayed for radiological confirmation.

Clinical Signs and Symptoms of Tension Pneumothorax

a. Respiratory distress, chest pain and air hunger
b. Tachycardia, hypotension, marked tracheal deviation, decreased or absent breath sounds on one side with hyper-resonant chest on affected side
c. Distended neck veins and central cyanosis
d. Muffled heart sounds

Treatment of Tension Pneumothorax

a. Immediate decompression of affected hemi thorax
b. By inserting a large bore needle 16–18 G in to the second intercostal space in the mid clavicular line
c. Once patient is stabilised intercostal tube is inserted in to fifth intercostal space in triangle of safety

Treatment of Simple Pneumothorax

- *Simple:*
  - Observation is done when there is less than 10% of lung collapse without any symptoms
  - If patient is symptomatic or there is more than 10% of lung collapse intercostal drainage must be done

Open Pneumothorax

This occurs if there is a large open defect of chest wall or if there is a sucking wound of the chest wall. There is a rapid equilibrium between intra-thoracic pressure and outside pressure. If the diameter of the open wound of the chest wall is about 2/3 rd of diameter of trachea, the air will take a path of least resistance and will enter thorax through wound rather than through trachea.

Treatment of Open Pneumothorax

Defect in the chest wall should be closed promptly by sterile occlusive dressing. Large dressing should be used so that it covers and overlaps the wound margin. Only three margins of dressing should be secured with tape and one margin of dressing should be kept free to provide flutter type of valve effect so that when patient breathes in the dressing occludes the wound, but during expiration unfixed margin of the dressing allows the air to escape from pleural cavity. If all margins of dressings are secured with tape before chest tube insertion, the air may accumulate inside chest wall cavity resulting in tension pneumothorax. Temporary Occlusive dressing can be of paraffin or petroleum gauze or of plastic material. A chest tube remote from the area of wound is placed as soon as possible. Definite surgical closure is carried out later on.

Indications of Inserting a Chest Tube in Chest Trauma

- Blunt trauma with more than 10% lung collapse
- Symptomatic pneumothorax
- Penetrating trauma with pneumothorax
- Radiologically appreciable hemi thorax
- Suspected severe lung injury and patient being transported by air or road
- Suspected significant lung injury in a patient undergoing general anaesthesia for management of other injuries

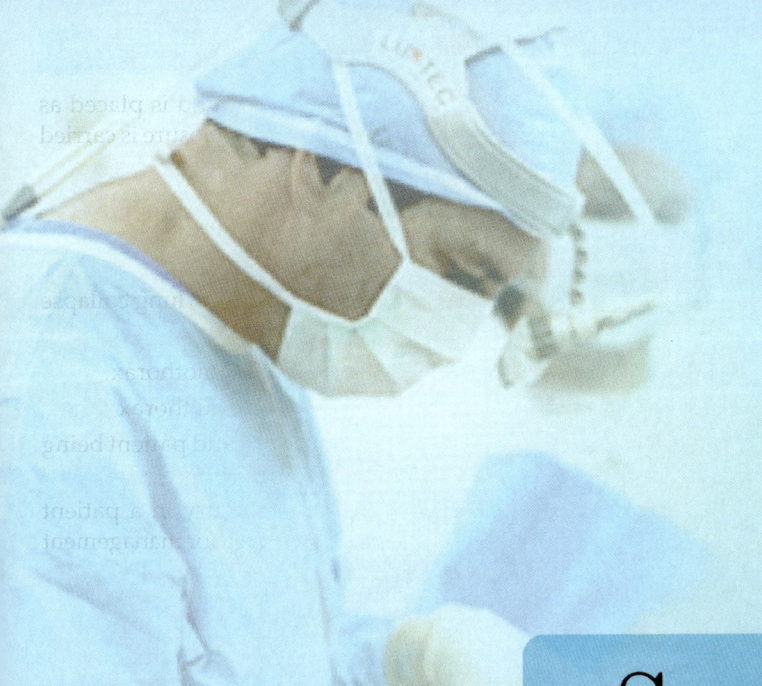

Section IV

41 | The Adrenal Gland

HISTORY

Table 41.1: Historical landmarks with regards to the adrenal gland

1563	Bartolomeo Eustachi	First described adrenal gland
	Albert von Kolliker	Identified cortex and medulla
1855	Thomas Edison	Identified adrenal failure and described its features
Around 1900		Adrenaline (or epinephrine) was isolated
1936	Hans Selye	Identified stress response and made contribution to understanding of hypothalamic-pituitary-adrenal (HPA) axis
1950	Edward Kendall, Tadeus Reichstein, Philip Hench	Received Nobel prize for physiology and medicine for ground breaking work on adrenal cortical hormones
1977	Roger Guillemin, Andrew Schally, Rosalyn Yalow	Received Nobel prize for describing peptide hormones in brain responsible for HPA axis

ANATOMY

- Paired structures in retroperitoneum lying above the kidneys
- Right adrenal is pyramidal-shaped and left one is crescent-shaped.
- They weigh about 4 ounce each.
- They are the among the most well perfused organs of the body ~2000 ml/kg/min

Relationships

Right Adrenal

- Abuts the posterolateral surface of the retro-hepatic vena cava.
- This gland has the right kidney inferolaterally, the diaphragm posteriorly, and the bare area of the liver anterosuperiorly.

Left Adrenal

- It lies between the left kidney and aorta.
- Related to the diaphragm posteriorly and the tail of the pancreas and splenic hilum anteriorly.
- Each adrenal gland is enveloped by its proper capsule, in addition to sharing Gerota's fascia with the kidneys. The adrenal capsules are immediately associated with the perirenal fat.

Histology

Adrenal Cortex

- Three layers
  - *Zona glomerulosa*: Outer layer of relatively small cells with moderately eosinophilic, lipid-poor cytoplasm. It has an undulating inner border and normally does not form a complete circumferential layer.

– *Zona fasciculata*: Thickest middle layer composed of long radial columns of large, clear, lipid-laden cells.
– *Zona reticularis*: Inner layer made up of small nests of compact, eosinophilic cells.

Adrenal Medulla

- It consists of clusters and short cords of chromaffin cells, which are large, polyhedral, and packed with basophilic secretory granules. Catecholamines within these granules yield a brown-colored reaction when treated with chromium salts, thus giving the cells their name.
- In contrast to the cortex, the adrenal medulla is richly endowed with autonomic nerve fibers and ganglion cells. Sympathetic fibers synapse directly with the chromaffin cells and constitute an interface between the nervous and endocrine systems.

Blood Supply

- Although the arterial supply is diffuse, the venous drainage of each gland is usually solitary.
- The arterial supply arises from three distinct vessels:
  - The superior adrenal arteries from the inferior phrenic arteries
  - The small middle adrenal arteries from the juxtaceliac aorta
  - The inferior adrenal arteries from the renal arteries.
- Of these, the inferior is the most prominent and is commonly a single identifiable vessel.
- The left adrenal vein is approximately 2 cm long and drains into the left renal vein after joining the inferior phrenic vein.
- The right adrenal vein is typically as short as it is wide (0.5 cm) and drains directly into the vena cava. In up to 20% of individuals, the right adrenal vein may drain into an accessory right hepatic vein or into the vena cava at or near the confluence of such a vein.

Embryology

- Adrenal cortex and medulla have different origins.

Adrenal Cortex

- The primordial cortex arises from the celomic mesodermal tissue near the cephalic end of the mesonephros during the fourth to fifth week of gestation.

- Biosynthetic activity can be detected as early as the seventh week. The cortical cell mass dominates the fetal adrenal at 4 months of development, and steroidogenesis reaches its maximum during the third trimester.

Adrenal Medulla

- The adrenal medulla arises from ectodermal tissues of the embryonic neural crest.
- It develops in parallel with the sympathetic nervous system, beginning in the fifth to sixth week of gestation. From their original position adjacent to the neural tube, neural crest cells migrate ventrally to assume a para-aortic position near the developing adrenal cortex. There, they differentiate into the chromaffin cells that make up the adrenal medulla.
- Both the cortical and medullary tissue can be found at extra-adrenal sites. When extra-adrenal, pheochromocytomas are also called paragangliomas.

ADRENAL HORMONES

Steroid Hormones

Synthesis

Cholesterol is transported into the mitochondria by Steroidogenic acute regulatory protein (StAR). This cholesterol undergoes a series of oxidative reactions catalyzed by membrane associated enzymes of P-450 (CYP) family to produce various steroid hormones in the adrenal gland. DHEA, androstenedione and cortisol are produced in zone fasciculata and reticularis, while aldosterone is produced in zona glomerulosa (Fig. 41.1).

Metabolism

- The steroid hormones are protein bound and their levels are affected by serum protein levels, e.g. in pregnancy, nephrotic syndrome and cirrhosis.
- The hormones have intracellular receptors and act by alteration in gene expression.
- They are metabolized by hydroxylation, sulfonation or conjugation to glucoronic acid in liver that is excreted in urine.

Glucocorticoids

Regulation

- ACTH binds to a G protein-coupled receptor on the adrenocortical cell surface and stimulates

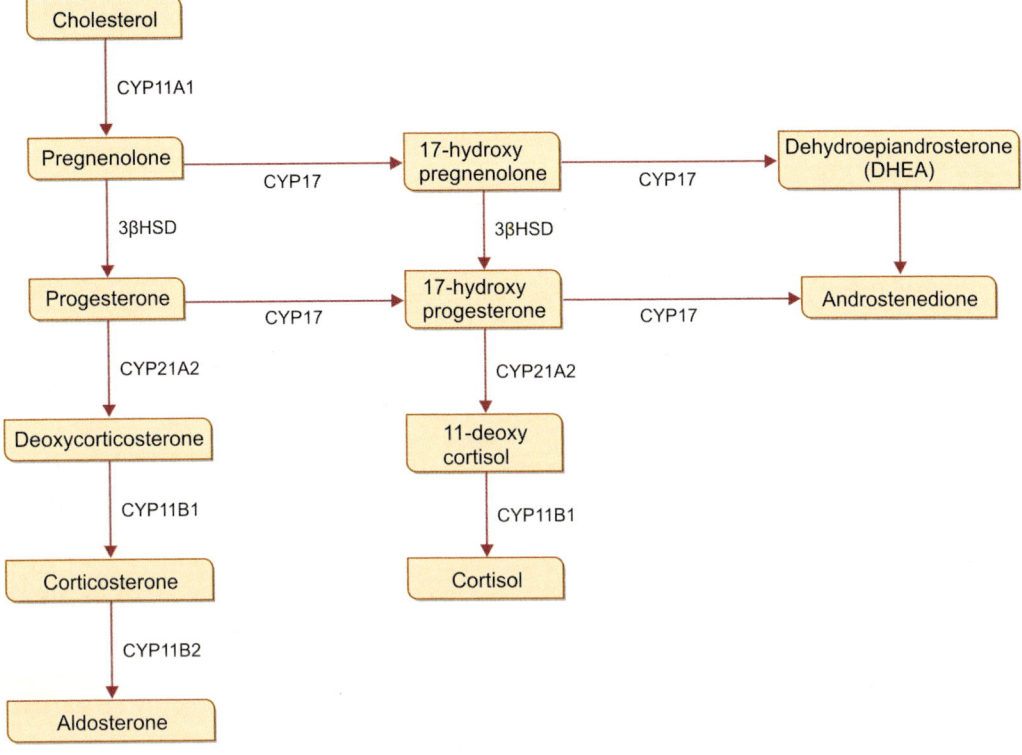

Fig. 41.1: Flowchart showing various steps in the synthesis of aldosterone and cortisol

glucocorticoid secretion, among other effects. (*see* Fig. 41.2)

- Steroidogenesis is acutely up-regulated via increased StAR-mediated cholesterol transport and pregnenolone synthesis by CYP11A1 (cholesterol side chain cleavage enzyme). Chronically, ACTH increases transcription of all steroidogenic enzymes and supports maintenance of normal adrenal cell mass.
- ACTH is released in a pulsatile fashion that normally displays a circadian rhythm. The highest levels of ACTH, and thus cortisol, are generally detected on waking, with levels gradually declining through the day to reach a nadir in the early evening.

Functions
- As a response to stress, the gluococorticoids generate catabolic state in the body.
- Net glycogen deposition in liver
  - Increased gluconeogenesis
  - Inhibition of peripheral glucose uptake
- Increased lipolysis
- Insulin resistance – protein breakdown

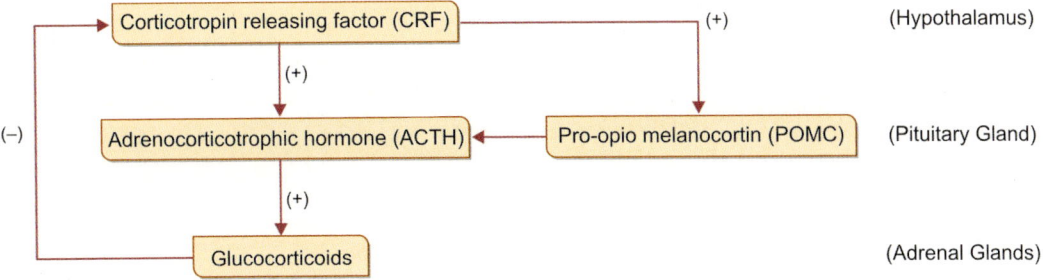

Fig. 41.2: Flowchart showing hypothalamo pituitory adrenal axis (HDA axis)

- Glucocorticoids exert a permissive and enhancing effect on catecholamine signaling by sensitizing arterial smooth muscle cells to β-adrenergic stimulation and increasing catecholamine concentrations in neuromuscular junctions. Cardiac contractility and peripheral vascular tone are thus maintained.
- They are potent, anti-inflammatory and immuno-suppressive agents
  - Reduce circulating lymphocyte and eosinophil counts while increasing neutrophil counts.
  - Cytokine and immunoglobulin production is decreased, and histamine release is suppressed.
  - Glucocorticoids also reduce prostaglandin synthesis via inhibition of phospholipase A2.

Mineralocorticoids

Regulation

- Regulated by the angiotensin level and potassium content of the body.
- Low sodium in distal convoluted tubule (in hypovolemia, shock, renal artery vasoconstriction, and hyponatremia) stimulates renin production from juxta-glomerular apparatus. Angiotensinogen, produced by liver, is converted to angiotensin I by this renin. The angiotensin I in turn is converted to angiotensin II in the lung.

This angiotensin II causes release of aldosterone by adrenal glomerulosa cells in addition to causing vasoconstriction.
- Hypokalemia reduces aldosterone secretion by decreasing renin secretion and by its direct effect.

Functions

- Aldosterone is responsible for maintaining water and electrolyte balance in the blood.
- Promotes sodium and chloride retention in the distal tubules. It causes increased secretion of potassium and hydrogen ions in the urine.
- Increased sodium delivery to distal tubules, in turn, negatively regulates aldosterone secretion.

Adrenal Sex Steroids

- Androstenedione, DHEA and DHEAS are produced in adrenal cortex and liver.
- DHEA and DHEAS are converted to more potent androgens responsible for normal pubic and axillary hair growth and maintain libido and a sense of well-being.
- The regulation of these hormones is poorly understood.

Catecholamines

Synthesis and Metabolism (see Fig. 41.3)

- Catecholamines are secreted by adrenal medulla
- Hydroxylation of tyrosine by tyrosine hydroxylase is the rate limiting step.

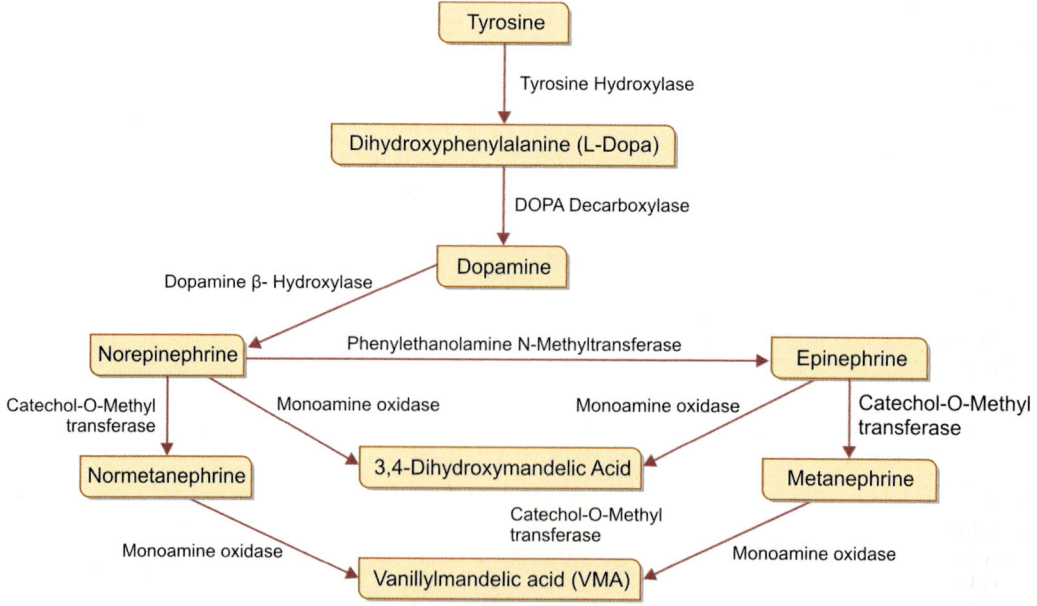

Fig. 41.3: Flowchart showing synthesis and breakdown of epinephrine and norepinephrine

- Phenylethanolamine N-methyltransferase is localized to chromaffin cells in adrenal medulla and organs of Zuckerkandl.
- Basal level of secretion of these hormones is low, with up to 50-fold increase due to sympathetic stimulation of adrenal medulla in response to physiological and psychological stress.
- Plasma half-life of epinephrine and norepinephrine is only 1 minute.
- Their concentration in synapses and blood is regulated through reuptake and degradation.
- Their metabolites, metanephrine and normetanephrine are stable and their values can be measured in blood in disease conditions like pheochromocytoma.
- They finally metabolize to VMA, which is excreted in urine after sulfonation or conjugation to glucoronic acid. It can be measured in urine as screening test for pheochromocytoma.

Functions
- The hormones act through α and β-receptors in the target organs.
- The β-receptors have more affinity for norepinephrine while α-receptors have more affinity for epinephrine.
- Overall, they mediate the "fight or flight" response of the body in response to stress. This is achieved by increasing the blood flow and delivery of oxygen to brain, heart and skeletal muscle at the expense of other organs.

Congenital Adrenal Hyperplasia
- This condition occurs due to defective glucocorticoids synthesis.
- This may occur because of deficiency of any of the six enzymes involved in steroid hormone biosynthesis, but deficiency of 21-hydroxylase (CYP21A2) is most common (90%).

Manifestations
- Deficiency of aldosterone
  - Due to deficient hydroxylation of progesterone

  - Manifests with salt wasting – hypovolemia, hyperkalemia and hyperreninemia
- Deficiency of cortisol
  - Due to deficiency in 21-hydroxylation of 17-hydroxyprogesterone
- Excess of adrenal androgens
  - Due to reduced negative feedback resulting in excess ACTH secretion and accumulation of precursors to 21-hydroxylation, which are diverted to oxidation at 17th carbon
  - May present in simple virilizing form or as ambiguous genitalia in newborn girls.

Management
- Diagnosis is made by serum estimation of 17-hydroxyprogesterone
- Confirmed by genetic and provocative biochemical testing
- Treatment includes glucocorticoid and mineralocorticoid replacement
- Surgery is required for correcting female phenotype — female genitoplasty.

Adrenal Insufficiency
Clinical Features
- Weakness and fatigue
- Anorexia
- Nausea or vomiting
- Weight loss
- Hyperpigmentation — caused by ACTH induced melanogenesis.
- Hypotension
- Electrolyte disturbances (hyponatremia and hyperkalemia).

Types
Primary Adrenal Insufficiency (Addison's Disease)
- Hormonal deficiency arises due to internal adrenal disease
- Mechanisms
  - Congenital adrenal hypoplasia/dysgenesis
  - Defective steroidogenesis

Table 41.2: Actions and locations of various sympathetic receptors

Receptor	Location	Actions
β_1-receptor	Myocardium	Increased heart rate and contractility
β_2-receptor	Uterus, bronchi, skeletal muscle arterioles	Smooth muscle relaxation
α_1-receptor	Skin, GIT	Vasoconstriction
α_2-receptor	Presynaptic locations in CNS	Mediate attenuation of sympathetic outflow

- Adrenal destruction
  ◊ Autoimmune
  ◊ Infectious adrenalitis (tubercular, fungal, viral)
  ◊ Metastasis to adrenal gland
  ◊ Adrenal hemorrhage (waterhouse-Friderichsen syndrome) – common in meningococcus septicemia with pediatric and asplenic patients being more prone.

Secondary Adrenal Insufficiency
- Due to reduction in ACTH levels
- Causes
  - Steroid withdrawal
    ◊ After more than 5 days of high dose steroid (more than 20 mg equivalent of prednisolone per day)
    ◊ After more than 3 weeks of low dose steroid
    ◊ After surgical correction of Cushing's syndrome
  - Panhypopituitarism
    ◊ Neoplastic or infiltrative replacement
    ◊ Granulomatous disease
    ◊ Pituitary hemorrhage/infarction — Pituitary infarction associated with severe postpartum hemorrhage is called Sheehan's syndrome.

Adrenal Insufficiency in Acutely Ill
- Caused by reversible suppression of HPA axis
- Proposed mechanisms
  - ACTH resistance
  - Decreased responsiveness to glucocorticoids
- Management
  - Glucocorticoids in physiologic doses, i.e. 400 mg/d of hydrocortisone or lower or equivalent for 5 to 7 days
  - High doses may actually harm the patient.

Adrenal Crisis
- Due to sudden complete loss of adrenal function like waterhouse-Friderichsen syndrome and certain hypercoagulable states.
- Also occurs in patients with marginal adrenal function when exposed to significant acute physiological stress.
- Manifests with shock, abdominal pain, fever, nausea and vomiting, electrolyte disturbances, and occasionally, hypoglycemia.

- Mechanisms
  - Mineralocorticoid deficiency — inability to retain sodium and water resulting in loss of intravascular fluid volume
  - Glucocorticoid deficiency — diminished cardiovascular response to catecholamines.
- Management
  - Resuscitation with large volume of crystalloid infusion (>2 L of isotonic saline)
  - Glucocorticoid administration – Hydrocortisone 100 mg 6–8 hourly or Dexamethasone 4 mg q24 hourly
  - Exogenous mineralocorticoid may not be given as they take several days to be effective.

Diagnosis
- Depends on clinical suspicion in intensive care setting
- Confirmed by hormone estimation — basal and provocative.

Steroid Replacement Therapy
Normal Maintenance
- Glucocorticoids – Prednisolone 5 mg/d
- Mineralocorticoids – Fludrocortisone 0.1 mg/d.

For Surgical Stress
- Increased doses may be needed in patients with adrenal insufficiency.
- Patients undergoing adrenalectomy for Cushing's disease may need perioperative corticosteroid administration to prevent adrenal crisis.

Primary Hyperaldosteronism (Conn's Syndrome)
- Excess secretion of aldosterone from one or both adrenal glands
- 1–7% of patients with hypertension have hyperaldosteronism
- Mean age 50 years
- Male predilection
- Present with resistant hypertension and hypokalemia
- Patients are at increased risk of stroke, myocardial infarction, atrial fibrillation, and left ventricular hypertrophy
- Causes
  - Unilateral aldosterone-producing adenoma (Aldosteronoma)

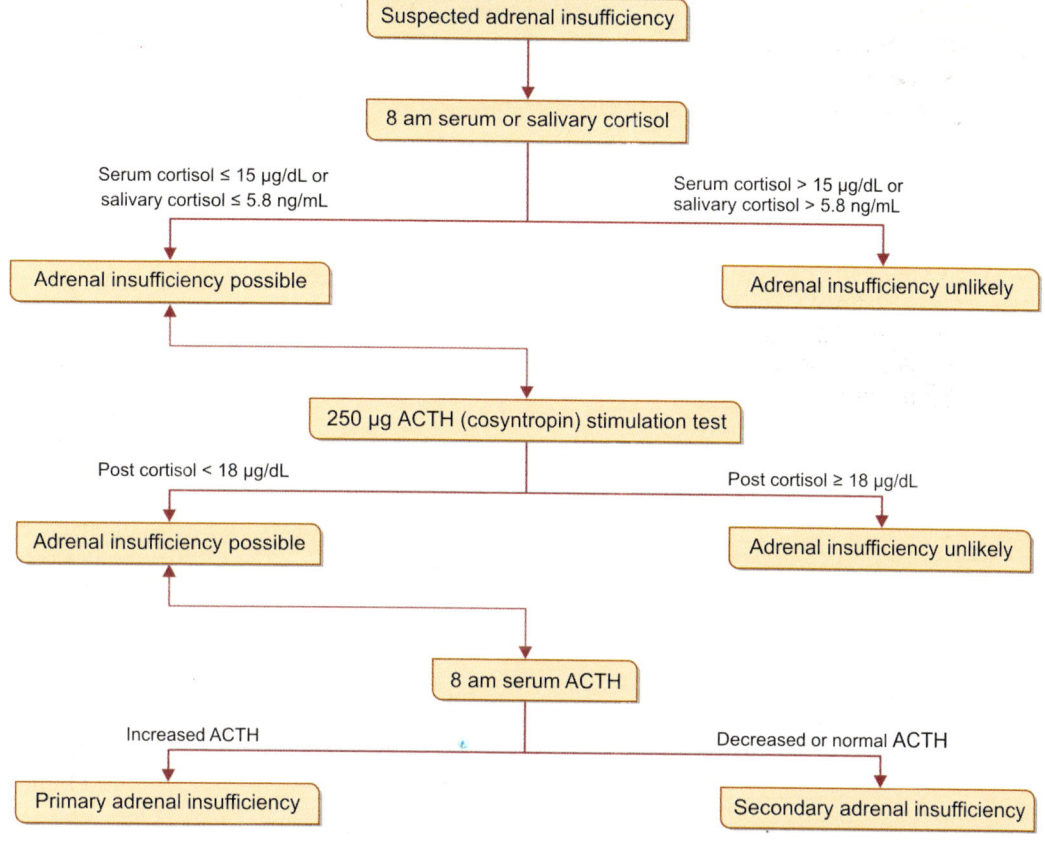

Fig. 41.4: Flowchart showing various steps in investigations of adrenal insufficiency

- Bilateral adrenal hyperplasia (Idiopathic Hyperaldosteronism)
- Aldosterone-producing adrenocortical carcinoma
- Familial hyperaldosteronism
  ◊ Type 1 (glucocorticoid-remediable aldosteronism)
  ◊ Type 2 (non–glucocorticoid-remediable aldosteronism).

Diagnosis

- Ratio of plasma aldosterone concentration to plasma renin activity
  - After discontinuation of interfering medications such as spironolactone, angiotensin-converting enzyme inhibitors, diuretics, and β-adrenergic blockers.
  - Ratio >30 is suggestive of primary hyperaldosteronism (sensitivity 90%)
  - Addition of absolute aldosterone concentration >15 mg/dL improves specificity

- Patients positive for the disease and less than 30 years should be genetically screened for autosomal dominant familial hyperaldosteronism type-1
- Confirmed by suppression test
  - A state of hypovolemia/sodium excess is created by IV saline loading (2–3 L of isotonic saline given over a 4–6 hour period, followed by measurement of plasma aldosterone) or oral salt loading (200 mEq = 5000 mg sodium daily over a 3-day period, followed by measurement of 24-hour urine aldosterone excretion)
  - Non-suppression of aldosterone is confirmatory
- Thin cut (3 mm) CT scan helps to localize tumor if unilateral enlarged gland is seen
- Selective venous sampling
  - Indicated in patients where thin slice CT scan is normal, or when hypertension persists even after unilateral adrenalectomy of tumor bearing adrenal (the tumor in such cases may

Table 41.3: Steroidal supplementation based on degree of surgical stress		
Degree of surgical stress	*Surgeries*	*Dosage*
Minor	OPD procedures, minor procedures like hernia	Hydrocortisone 25mg/d
Moderate	Routine abdominal, peripheral, vascular or orthopedic surgery	Hydrocortisone 50–75mg/d
Severe	Major resections, cardiopulmonary bypass	Hydrocortisone 100–150mg/d

be non-functional adenoma and the hypertension may be due to contralateral microadenoma or bilateral hyperplasia)

- Serum aldosterone and cortisol levels are estimated in bilateral adrenal veins and peripheral blood simultaneously
- Greater than five-fold elevation of the cortisol level as compared to peripheral blood suggests successful cannulation, failure of test is usually due to failure to cannulate right adrenal vein successfully diagnosed by normal cortisol levels in the selective sample
- Functional scanning with radiolabeled 131I-6-β-iodomethylnorcholesterol (NP-59) may be used to lateralize the tumor, but is ineffective in small tumors.

Surgery
- Laparoscopic adrenalectomy is the procedure of choice.

Outcome
- 75 to 95% success rates have been reported
- Criteria
  - Reduction in blood pressure and antihypertensive medications (all medications can be stopped after 1 day of surgery except β-blockers, which need to be tapered lest rebound should happen)
  - Normalization of blood or urinary aldosterone levels
- Patients who are less likely to respond to surgery: male, age older than 45 years, family history of hypertension, long-standing hypertension, and no response to spironolactone
  - Due to essential hypertension
  - Due to irreversible cardiovascular alterations resulting from chronic disease.

Cushing's Syndrome
- Described by Harvey Cushing in 1912.

Clinical Features
- Obesity
- Easy bruising
- Muscle weakness
- Hypertension
- Plethora (a red facial appearance caused by thinning of the skin)
- Hirsuitism
- Physiologic derangements resulting from glucocorticoid excess
  - Hypertension (present in >70% of cases)
  - Hyperglycemia
  - Truncal obesity
  - Cardiovascular complications may lead to early mortality.

Causes
- Exogenous corticosteroid use for treatment of various inflammatory disorders.
- *Cushing's disease:* Due to ACTH secreting pituitary adenoma
- Increase secretion by adrenal gland
- Ectopic ACTH producing tumors – Neuroendocrine tumors, bronchogenic tumors.

Diagnosis
- Increased cortisol secretion can be tested by
  - 24 hour urinary cortisol excretion — do the test twice in case of normal; for moderately raised urine cortisol late evening salivary cortisol estimation may give the diagnosis
  - Late evening salivary cortisol level – cutoff value of 550 mg/ml has 93% sensitivity and 100% specificity
- Localization of the cause of Cushing's disease
  - Serum ACTH estimation
    ◊ Non-detectable levels (< 5 mg/ml) are seen in primary adrenal Cushing's syndrome (ACTH-independent Cushing's syndrome) – Solitary adrenal adenoma, adrenocortical carcinoma, bilateral micronodular or macronodular hyperplasia.

◊ Normal or raised ACTH levels are seen in ACTH-dependent Cushing's syndrome
- CT scan abdomen/chest – detects adrenal adenoma and adrenocortical carcinoma. May help to detect peripheral source of ACTH.
- MRI pituitary fossa–detects pituitary microadenomas that are more than 6 mm.
- High-dose dexamathasone suppression test – 2 mg dexamathasone q6 hourly given for 48 hours and then urinary or serum cortisol is measured. Suppression by high dose dexamethasone suggests pituitary microadenoma, non-suppression suggests peripheral source of ACTH (like bronchogenic tumor). Dexamethasone is chosen because it does not cross-react with present biochemical assays for cortisol.
- Bilateral inferior petrosal sinus ACTH sampling with CRF stimulation – study done if in case of ACTH-dependent Cushing's syndrome, the MRI fails to detect microadenoma.

Management

- Perioperative glucocorticoid administration is necessary to prevent the adrenal crisis.
- For patients undergoing adrenalectomy for adrenal adenoma or adrenocortical carcinoma,
  - Hydrocortisone 100 mg q8 hourly for 24 hours post-operatively is given. The steroid is then tapered slowly over weeks.
  - Perioperative antibiotics for 24 hours are given as these patients are prone to surgical site infection.
- For patients undergoing pituitary surgery (through transnasal transsphenoidal approach)
  - Steroids are withheld for first 48 hours. Subnormal serum cortisol estimation on post-op day 1 or 2 is suggestive of cure. The glucocorticoid supplementation is then started for usually 6 months, to give time to HPA axis to recover.
  - If the post-op cortisol levels remain high, repeat pituitary surgery, radiation to pituitary fossa or bilateral laparoscopic adrenalectomy remain options.

Subclinical Cushing's Syndrome

- It is characterized by
  - Incidentaloma
  - Biochemical evidence of hypercortisolism
  - No typical clinical evidence of Cushing's syndrome
- Natural history is not known
- The patients are at risk of hypertension, dyslipidemia, and impaired glucose tolerance
- Surgical therapy does not show consistent improvement
- Therapy is primarily medical.

Adrenocortical Carcinoma

- Rare – incidence 1:1,000,000
- No gender predilection
- Mostly 40 to 50 years old, minor peak at 5 years age
- Presentation
  - More than half of them are functional tumors and present with Cushing's syndrome or virilization
  - Mean tumor size at presentation is 9–12 cm
- Diagnosis
  - CT scan shows a heterogeneous mass with irregular/indistinct borders, central necrosis, and invasion of adjacent structures.
  - Large tumors, esp. right sided, may have intravascular extension into inferior vena cava or right heart
  - Metastases to the lymph nodes, liver, and lungs may be found.
- Treatment
  - Radical open surgery — En-bloc resection of the tumor with adjacent organs and lymph nodes. Patients with vascular tumor thrombus may need cardiopulmonary bypass to prevent tumor thromboembolism.
  - Chemotherapy — It is a relatively chemoresistant tumor. Only mitotane (o,p-DDD, or 1,1-dichloro-2-[o-chlorophenyl]-2-[p-chlorophenyl] ethane), a derivative of the insecticide DDT, has shown some efficacy in adjuvant/neoadjuvant settings.
- Prognosis
  - Overall adrenocortical carcinoma is associated with poor survival with 5 years survival reported between 15–20% range.
  - Patients who undergo incomplete resection of adrenocortical carcinomas have extremely limited life expectancy (median survival, < 1 year).

- Even those who undergo successful surgery are prone to the development of local recurrence and metastases, which typically occur within 2 years.

Sex Steroid Secreting Tumors

- Extremely rare
- May be feminizing, but mostly are virilizing
- Almost all feminizing tumors are malignant while one-third of virilizing tumors are malignant
- Diagnosis of virilizing tumors is made by 24-hour urinary estimation of testosterone, DHEA and DHEAS
- Management is by laparoscopic adrenalectomy for benign and open surgery for malignant tumors as they may invade local structures.

Pheochromocytoma

- First described by Felix Frankel in 1886. It derives its name's meaning "dusky-colored tumor" from the Greek *phaios* due to its characteristic color when stained with chromium salts.
- Successful management was first reported in 1926 by both Cesar Roux and Charles Mayo.
- Affects 0.2% of hypertensive patients
- Most in age group 40–50 years
- No gender predilection.

Clinical Features

- Classic triad – headache, diaphoresis, and palpitations. All patients have at least one of the symptoms.
- Hypertension – either sustained or episodic – is present in 90% of patients.
- Also called "Biologic Time Bomb" because of potentially lethal effects of bioactive compounds.
- Was also called "10% Tumor" because 10% are bilateral, 10% malignant, 10% extra-adrenal, and 10% familial.
- Differential diagnoses include hyperthyroidism, hypoglycemia, coronary artery disease, heart failure, stroke, drug-related effects, and panic disorder.

Diagnosis

- 24-hour urinary level of catecholamines and their metabolites viz. metanephrines
- Serum level of metanephrines – high sensitivity (99%) but low specificity (<85%). This test can be used to rule out pheochromocytoma as the cause of hypertension.
- Factors that may cause false results
  - Sympathomimetics (present in many cold remedies)
  - Phenoxybenzamine (frequently initiated when suspicion of pheochromocytoma is raised)
  - Acetaminophen (which interferes with the plasma free metanephrine assay)
  - Many psychotropic drugs (notably tricyclic antidepressants)
  - Major physical or psychological stressors
  - Episodes of acute pain
  - Critical illness
- Anatomic localization can be done by CT scan or MRI.
- Scinitigraphy
  - ^{131}I- or ^{123}I-labeled metaiodobenzylguanidine (MIBG) – highly specific but with low sensitivity (77–90%) – can be used to detect multifocal/extra-adrenal disease.
  - Positron emission tomography (PET) using ^{18}F-labelled catecholamine can also be used.

Molecular Genetics

- Associated syndromes
  - MEN type II
  - Von hippel-lindau syndrome
  - Neurofibromatosis type I
- Mutation recognized
  - Germline mutations in the B and D subunits of succinate dehydrogenase gene family, which is responsible for oxidative phosphorylation in mitochondria, are identified in 10% of familial cases. The mutations are inherited in autosomal dominant fashion with 75% penetrance.
  - Succinate dehydrogenase B mutation carriers have high rates of extra-adrenal (abdominal or thoracic) pheochromocytomas and malignant disease, whereas succinate dehydrogenase D carriers tend to have multiple tumors and hormonally inactive paragangliomas of the head and neck.
  - Genetic counseling and testing is encouraged for patients in whom pheochromocytoma is diagnosed before the age of 50.

Table 41.4: Normal values of various adrenal metabolites

Test	Cutoff value (in mols/μmol)	Cutoff value (in mg/μg)
Plasma free metanephrine	0.3 nmol/L	59 μg/L
Plasma free normetanephrine	0.6 nmol/L	110 μg/L
Urinary total metanephrines	6.6 μmol/day	1.3 mg/day
Urinary epinephrine	191 nmol/day	35 μg/day
Urinary norepinephrine	1005 nmol/day	170 μg/day
Urinary dopamine	4571 nmol/day	700 μg/day
Urinary vanillylmandelic acid	40 μmol/day	7.9 mg/day
Plasma free normetanephrine	0.61 nmol/L	112 μg/L
Clonidine suppression test	Elevated levels of plasma free normetanephrines, and reduction of more than 40% after administration of oral clonidine 0.3 mg	

Perioperative Care

- Perioperative mortality has decreased to 2% from 26–50% (about 50 years earlier).
- Causes
  - Intraoperative hypertension – due to excess catecholamine release in response to anesthetic induction agents or handling of the tumor.
  - Postoperative hypotension – due to withdrawal of catecholamines. In preoperative period, excess catecholamines induce a state of relative hypovolemia. As the catecholamine source is removed, it results in peripheral arterial vasodilation and increase in venous capacitance, thus causing profound hypotension.
- Preoperative control
  - α-blocker – Nonselective α-blocker is the drug of choice for preoperative control of hypertension and tachycardia. Phenoxybenzamine is started in dose 10 mg q12 hourly and gradually increased till maximum of 40 mg q8hourly. The period of preoperative conditioning lasts at least 2 weeks to allow adequate reversal of α-adrenergic receptor down-regulation. This restores sensitivity to vasopressor agents, which can then be used to treat the patient postoperatively.
  - β-blocker may be given to patients with persistent tachycardia. β-blockers are never the first agent administered because a decrease in peripheral vasodilatory β-receptor stimulation results in unopposed α-adrenergic tone, which may exacerbate hypertension.
  - Volume expansion by giving preoperative crystalloids may be needed.

Surgery

- Close communication between surgeon and anesthetist is required.
- Invasive monitoring including arterial BP monitoring and CVP recording is mandatory.
- Anesthetist should be ready with fluids, IV α- and β-blockers and vasopressors, if they are needed.
- Surgeon should observe the principle of minimal handling of the tumor.
- Adrenalectomy, either open or laparoscopic, results in over 90% success rate.
- Laparoscopic resection is contraindicated when preoperative imaging demonstrates local invasion.

Malignant Pheochromocytoma

- Defined by the presence of metastasis.
- It includes presence of tumor implants in distant sites where neuroectodermal tissue is not normally found. It excludes multifocal primary tumors.
- Incidence varies from 2.5–40%.
- The pheochromocytoma may metastasize to axial skeleton, lymph nodes, liver, lung, and kidney.
- Management rests on surgical excision of all tumors, which may have a palliative role even if cure is not possible.
- High dose ^{131}I-MIBG may be used, which has shown moderate early response. But no long term effect has been seen.
- Medical management includes control of hypertension using selective α_1-blockers.
- Prognosis is poor with overall 5-year survival between 20% and 45%.

Incidentaloma

- They are "Incidentally discovered adrenal masses" through imaging performed for unrelated disease.
- Incidentalomas are found in 2.1% of autopsies and 1–4% of abdominal imaging studies. The prevalence rises to greater than 4% in patients older than 60 years.

Differential Diagnosis — Causes

- Nonfunctioning adenoma (60%)
- Pheochromocytoma (10%)
- Cortisol producing adenoma (5%)
- Aldosteronoma (1%)
- Adrenocortical carcinoma (5%)
- Adrenal cyst (5%)
- Ganglioneuroma (5%)
- Myelolipoma (9%)

Evaluation

- History – guided towards previous malignancy, hypertension, and symptoms of glucocorticoid or sex steroid excess
- Hormone estimation, as suggested by history and general examination
- CT-guided fine-needle aspiration is rarely helpful in the evaluation of adrenal masses and may be hazardous. It is reserved for patients with extra-adrenal tumors which may be associated with adrenal metastasis.

Management

- Surgery is indicated in all patients with hormone secreting incidentaloma
- Other indication is malignant potential
  - <4cm – 2% will turn malignant
  - 4–6cm – 6% are adrenocortical carcinomas
  - Tumors larger than 6 cm carry a greater than 25% risk for malignancy
- Suspicious imaging characteristics – heterogeneity, high attenuation, or irregular margins
- Most adrenal incidentalomas can be removed laparoscopically, except for those displaying obvious malignant features on imaging
- If patient chooses observation repeat imaging in 6 to 12 months should be done, given the fact that 5–25% of adrenal masses may increase in size.

Metastasis to Adrenal Gland

- Common site for distant metastasis due to rich blood supply

- As many as 25% of cancers ultimately metastasize to adrenals
  - Half of them are bilateral
- Common primary tumors that metastasize to adrenals are cancer of lung, gastrointestinal tract, breast, kidney, pancreas, and skin (melanoma)
- Although exclusive metastasis to adrenal gland is rare, excision of such tumor may provide survival benefit to the patient
- Thus evaluation of such a tumor includes detailed radiological investigations (like CT/MRI of head in breast or melanoma; triphasic CT evaluation of liver plus thin 3 mm slice CT scan of lungs in gastrointestinal malignancies). PET scan may be done when appropriate
- Patients with isolated bilateral adrenal metastasis should be investigated for adrenal insufficiency by serum cortisol and ACTH estimation before surgery, so as to correct hormonal levels before surgery lest adrenal crisis should occur.

Adrenalectomy – Technique

Open Anterior Transabdominal Adrenalectomy

- After induction of general anesthesia, the regional block (like epidural catheter) is inserted for management of postoperative pain
- Patient is then positioned supine with a bolster elevating the ipsilateral side slightly
- Urinary and nasogastric catheters are placed
- Incisions – subcostal or chevron

Left Adrenal

- Incise the left 'while line of Toldt', mobilize splenic flexure, spleen and tail of pancreas to expose left adrenal gland
- Alternatively, the adrenal gland can be exposed through lesser sac and incising peritoneum just below tail of pancreas
- Left adrenal vein is divided between ligatures
- Arteries are divided as the adrenal gland is mobilized.

Right Adrenal

- Mobilize liver by dividing triangular and falciform ligaments
- Right adrenal gland and inferior vena cava are exposed by performing Kocher's maneuver

- Plane between adrenal and inferior vena cava is developed first. There may be many vessels including the right adrenal vein which are ligated and divided before mobilization of adrenal gland.

Laparoscopic Lateral Transabdominal Adrenalectomy

- After induction, the patient is placed in 80 degree lateral decubitus position with the involved side upwards
- The table bridge is elevated to widen the gap between costal margin and iliac crest
- Gastric decompression is done.

Left Adrenal

- Four subcostal 11 mm ports are used with intervening distance about 5 cm each
- Dissection is started by mobilizing spleen medially till greater curvature of stomach is visible
- Splenic flexure of colon is then mobilized and retracted medially
- Along left crus of diaphragm, the inferior phrenic vein courses medial to left adrenal gland and drains into left adrenal vein. The left adrenal vein is encountered at the infero-medial border of the gland near renal hilum, where it is divided between clips. Small adrenal arteries can be coagulated and divided
- The glans is then mobilized from the kidney and posterior abdominal wall. The specimen is placed in catchment device, morcellated and removed.

Right Adrenal

- Ports same as that on left side
- Right triangular ligament is divided
- Hepatic flexure is mobilized and retracted inferiorly
- Dissection is done between adrenal gland and inferior vena cava
- The right adrenal vein is a potentially perilous structure to manage because it is short, wide, variable, and confluent with thin-walled, large capacitance vessels (the inferior vena cava in >80% of cases, followed by the renal vein and uncommonly the right hepatic vein) that can bleed briskly if directly injured (e.g. by cautery), lacerated by undue traction on adjacent structures, or sheared by clips
- An accessory adrenal vein may be found in 10% patients
- Rest of the procedure is same as that for left side.

Complications

- Venous hemorrhage and bleeding from solid organ capsular injuries
- Hollow viscus injuries
- Pancreatic injuries and fistulas
- Port site hernias and port site metastases
- Surgical site infections
- Subphrenic abscesses.

Bladder Outflow Obstruction (BOO)

BOO is a urodynamic concept and the diagnosis is based upon:

- *Low flow rate:* Peak urinary flow<10 ml/second for a voided volume >200 ml at least on two occasions (Fig. 42.1)
- High voiding pressure > 80 cm of water (normally it is < 60 cm of water).

Pathogenesis

BOO can result from:

- Detrusor instability
- Neurological dysfunction
- Weak bladder contractions

The common disease entities resulting in bladder outlet obstructions are:

- Benign hyperplasia of the prostate
- Bladder neck stenosis
- Bladder neck hypertrophy
- Prostate cancer
- Urethral stricture
- Neuropathic bladder with sphincter dys-synergia.

Complications

- Acute retention
- Chronic retention with upper tract damage
- Impaired emptying resulting in stasis and infections
- Bladder calculi

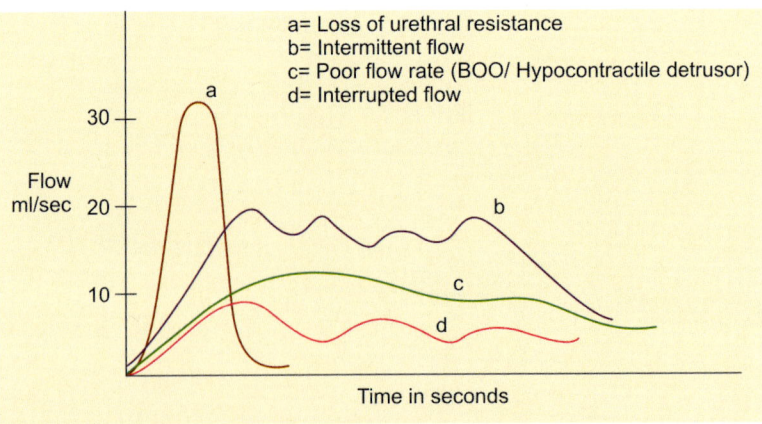

Fig. 42.1: Uroflowmetry patterns

- Bladder diverticulum
- Hematuria.

Clinical Features

1. Patient usually presents with symptoms of LVTS, e.g. narrowing of stream, hesitancy, sense of incomplete evacuation of bladder.
2. Recurrent urinary tract infection.

Work up of Patient with BOO

1. Blood urea and serum creatnine estimation as patient can have chronic renal failure

2. Urine culture sensitivity examination to rule out UTI.
3. Ultrasound examination of KUB, prostate size and post void residual urine. BOO can lead to back pressure changes.
4. Urethroscopy and cystoscopy to rule out any obstructive pathology in the lower urinary tract.

Treatment

Treatment is directed towards cause.

43 Benign Prostatic Hyperplasia (BPH)

ANATOMY (Fig. 43.1)

- Anterior Fibro-muscular zone (30%)
  - 1/3rd of prostate , no glandular tissue
- Glandular epithelial cells (70%)
  - Peripheral zone (most cancers)

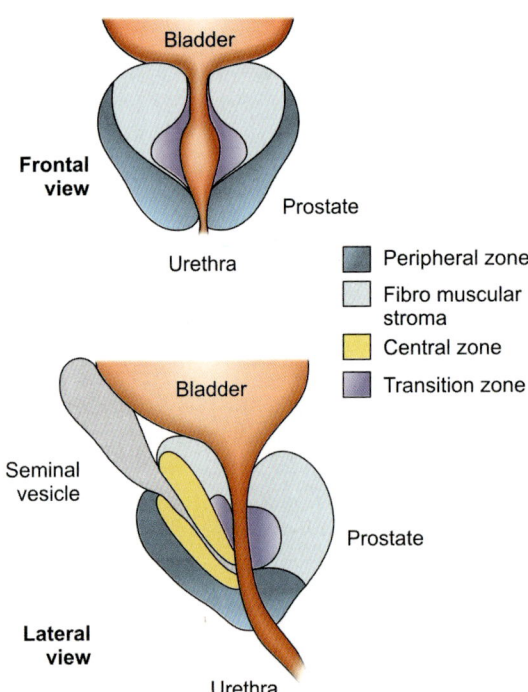

Fig. 43.1: Anatomy of prostate

- Central zone
- Transition zone (BPH, low grade cancer).

Incidence

- Moderate to severe Lower Urinary Tract Symptoms (LUTS) occur in 25% of men over 50 years, and the incidence rises with age
- 27–35 % of men age 60–79 will need some form of treatment
- Approximately 90% of men will develop histological evidence of BPH by 80 years of age
- Incidence is increasing because
  - Men are living longer with relative increase in proportion of Men over 50 years.
  - Men are better informed about health matters.

Etiology

- There may be reawakening of the urogenital sinus to proliferate leading to hyperplasia
- Change in hormonal milieu with alterations in the testosterone/estrogen balance
- Induction of growth by prostate growth factors
- Increased stem cells activity and decreased stroma cell death (apoptosis)
- Significant percentage of LUTS is due to age related detrusor instability and other systematic medical conditions like Polyuria, diabetes and geriatric sleep disorders. These are unrelated to prostate enlargement but often attributed to prostate enlargement.

- There is increased number of epithelial and Stroma cells in the peri-urethral area of the prostate thus known as hyperplasia of the prostate. The increased no. of cells may be due to proliferation or due to impaired programmed cell death leading to cellular accumulation.
- Smooth muscle tone in the prostatic capsule is increased due to increased activity of alpha 1 A receptors.

Anatomical Changes

- Urethra gets elongated, compressed, and becomes slit like with exaggerated curvature. There is distortion of urethra if only one lobe is enlarged
- Detrusor hypertrophy, trabeculations and diverticulum formation
- Dilated veins at base of bladder (Bladder piles).

Pathophysiology

- Slow and insidious changes over time
- Complex interactions between
  - Prostate urethral resistance, and intravesical pressure, which depends upon
    - ◇ Detrusor function
    - ◇ Neurological integrity
- Initial hypertrophy of detrusor → detrusor decompensation → poor tone → diverticula formation → increasing urine volume → Hydronephrosis due to back pressure changes → upper tract dysfunction.

Understanding Lower Urinary Tract Symptoms

Storage symptoms or irritative symptoms
- Frequency
- Nocturia
- Urgency
- Urge incontinence
  (Due to hyperactivity of alpha receptors at bladder neck)
  Voiding symptoms or obstructive symptoms
- Slow stream, or narrowing of stream
- Intermittent flow
- Loss of stream formation
- *Hesitancy:* The patient has to wait for a while before he can start act of micturation.
- Straining
- Terminal dribbling
- Sense of incomplete evacuation of bladder.

Patho-physiology of Symptoms

Frequency

- Reduced functional bladder capacity due to
  - Unstable detrusor contractions or
  - Due to reduced bladder compliance.

Nocturia

- Loss of circadian rhythm in sodium and water excretion.

Hesitancy

- Detrusor bladder neck dyssynergia

Other late presenting signs/symptoms
- Abdominal/flank pain with voiding
- Uremia - fatigue, anorexia, somnolence
- Hernias, hemorrhoids, bowel habit change
- Recurrent UTI
- Bladder calculi
- Haematuria due to rupture of dilated veins at base.

Other relevant points on history
- GU History (STD, trauma, surgery)
- Other disorders (e.g. neurological, diabetes)
- Medications (anti-cholinergic)
- Functional Status AUA Score for severity of symptoms ranges from 0–35
  - 0–7: mild
  - 8–19: moderate
  - 20–35: severe.

Physical Signs

- May be few
- Look for obvious signs of uremia or CRF (Anemia, HTN, irritability)
- Palpate for full bladder, palpable kidneys
- Examine urethral meatus for phimosis and palpate urethra for stricture
- Digital rectal examination (DRE) is the most important clinical examination: a smooth enlargement, "non-palpable" nodularity with a loss of distinction between the lobes. A soft/firm consistency, underestimates enlargement, can't feel seminal vesicles.
- Signs on DRE indicating malignancy:
  - Firm to hard nodules
  - Irregularities, unequal lobes
  - Indurations
  - Stony hard prostate
  - Any palpable nodular abnormality suggests cancer and warrants investigation.

Investigations for BPH

- Blood urea, Serum creatinine and electrolytes if clinically indicated
- Prostate specific antigen (PSA) (total and free)
- Ultrasound of prostate bladder, kidneys with post void residual urine and size of prostate with any suspicious area of malignancy. Post void residual urine of more than 100 ml is significant.
- Peak urinary flow rate (uroflometry). Normal is more than 15 ml per second. In between 10–15 ml per second is border line and less than 10 ml per second is highly suggestive of obstruction. Peak flow should be measured for a voided volume at least 150 to 200 ml on two occasions. If the voided volume is less than 150 ml, estimation is not reliable.
- International prostate symptom score (IPSS) should be done for every patient
- Preoperative cystoscopy is not routinely indicated however it is performed to rule associated pathology in bladder if patient presents with Haematuria. Bleeding per urethra cannot be attributed to BHP unless carcinoma urinary bladder has been ruled out. Pre-operative cystoscopy is also indicated to evaluate bladder if the patient is planned for retropubic prostatectomy. However at the time of performing TURP cystoscopic evaluation of bladder is mandatory before actually starting the procedure to rule out any unexpected pathology in the bladder.
- Urine culture.

Differential Diagnosis

- Urethral stricture
- Bladder neck contracture
- Carcinoma of the prostate
- Carcinoma of the bladder
- Bladder calculi
- Urinary tract infection and prostatitis
- Neurogenic bladder

Difficulties in Diagnosis and Management

- The symptoms of BPH are the same as those of early prostate cancer
- Confirmation of the presence of prostate cancer may be difficult
- The need to treat (proven) cancer may not always be clear cut.

Prostate Cancer

- No symptoms specific for early prostate cancer
- Presenting symptoms are therefore those of BPH
- Biopsy of the prostate should be performed in those with abnormal DRE, or PSA above age-specific reference range.

Prostate Specific Antigen

- Single-chain glycoprotein of 240 amino acid residues and 4 carbohydrate side chains
- Physiological role in liquefaction of seminal coagulum
- Prostate specific, but not cancer specific
- In addition to prostate cancer, an elevated level may be found in
  - Increasing age
  - Acute urinary retention/Catheterization
  - After TURP/prostate biopsy
  - Prostatitis
  - BPH
- A reduced level may be found in patients treated with Finasteride
- Fallacies
  - Men with prostate cancer may have a normal PSA
  - Men with BPH or other benign conditions may have a raised PSA
  - May not even be prostate-specific
- Refinements in the use of PSA
  - PSA density—levels of PSA are standardised in relation to size of prostate. It is the ratio of PSA and size of prostate (PSA density) >0.15 that indicates malignancy.
  - PSA velocity (rate of change of PSA) (>0.75 ng/mL/yr).
  - Age-specific PSA
    - ◊ 40–49 years old   <2.5 ng/ml
    - ◊ 50–59 years old   <3.5 ng/ml
    - ◊ 60–69 years old   <4.5 ng/ml
    - ◊ 70–79 years old   <6.5 ng/ml
  - *Free: Total PSA ratio* <0.18 strongly suggests possibility of carcinoma prostate)
  - Delay performing test 48 hours after recent ejaculation or local trauma and wait at least 6 weeks after biopsy or TURP.
  - If PSA elevated wait 2–4 weeks and repeat to confirm. Some experts recommend anti-biotics before repeating the test.

Goals of Treatment for BPH

a. Relieving LUTS
b. Decreasing bladder outlet obstruction
c. Improving bladder emptying
d. Ameliorating detrusor instability
e. Reversing renal insufficiency
f. Preventing disease progression.

Treatment Modalities for BPH

Medical Therapy

- α-blocker therapy, i.e. Tamsulosin, Prazosin, Alfuzosin
  - Selective α-1a receptor blockers *may* have fewer side effects
- 5-α-reductase inhibitors, i.e. Finasteride or Dutasteride. The rational for androgen suppression is based on observation that the embryonic development of the prostate is dependent on the dihydrotestosterone (DHT). The testosterone is converted to DHT by an enzyme 5 alpha reductase and the genetic deficiency of this enzyme leads to rudimentary prostate and feminized external genetilia. Maximum reduction of prostate volume after initiation of androgen suppression is obtained within 6 months. Therefore androgen suppression therapy must be continued at least for 6 months. 5 alpha reductase enzyme occurs in two forms, i.e. type 1 and type 2. Type 1 occurs in skin and liver. Type 2 occurs in prostate. Finasteride inhibits only type 2 isoenzyme. Dutasteride inhibits both type 1 and type 2 isoenzyme.
  - The men with large prostates (> 40cc), taking long-term Finasteride therapy are less likely to develop acute retention, or require surgical intervention
- Phytotherapy, i.e. saw palmetto or beta sitosterols

Surgery

Indications

- Chronic retention
- Acute retention (recurrent)

- Severe obstructive symptoms with objective evidence of obstruction (Indicated for AUA score >20; post void residual urine >100 ml or peak flow ratio <10 ml/sec).
- Complications of BPH:
  - Hematuria
  - Recurrent UTI
  - Back Pressure changes
  - Diverticulum/stone
- Surgical therapies
  - Transurethral resection of prostate (TURP) still the gold standard therapy, against which all other therapies are compared. It is performed endoscopically using a Resectoscope (Fig. 43.2).
  - Laser evaporisation of prostate by KTP laser.
    ◊ Expensive to set up
    ◊ Significantly reduced blood loss
    ◊ Catheter may be required for longer time post operatively
  - Open prostatectomy rarely required if TURP is contraindicated.
- Minimally invasive techniques (MITs)
  - Transurethral microwave thermotherapy (TUMT)
  - Transurethral needle ablation (TUNA)
  - Transrectal high-intensity focused ultrasound (HiFU)
    ◊ HiFU currently requires GA, is costly and time consuming, and appears unlikely to be popular at present
  - Transurethral electrovaporisation (TUVP)
  - The subjective response after MITs and TURP appear similar, but objective results are superior for TURP.

Transurethral Resection of Prostate

- TURP is the present Gold standard to which other therapies can be compared.
- Cited as the "benchmark for surgical therapies"

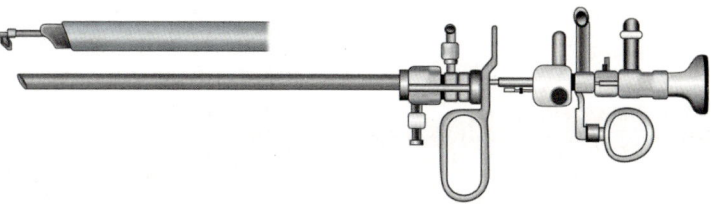

Fig. 43.2: Resectoscope used for performing TURP

- Treatment of choice for prostates sized 30 to 80 gm.
- TURP is efficient, cost-effective and dependable with low long-term complications and re-treatment rates
- 18% morbidity, <2% mortality, 5% require repeat TURP.

Indications

- Patients with mainly obstructive symptoms with definitive objective evidence of Obstruction as in Q_{max} less than 10 ml/sec for a voided volume of 200 ml or more on two occasions or a post void residual volume more than 100 ml
- Patients presenting with chronic retention of urine
- Obstructive uropathy due to BPH
- Recurrent UTI with BPH
- Recurrent hematuria in whom other causes have been ruled out
- Acute urinary retention (recurrent episodes ≥ 2)
- Complications of BOO like diverticulae or calculi
- Moderate to severe AUA score not responding to medical management.

Contraindications

- Huge prostate size more than 80 gm
- Associated cardiac conditions like CHF in a setting of fluid overload
- Pathology of hip joint precluding Lithotomy position
- Large size diverticulum that cannot be managed endoscopically
- Large Bladder stones that cannot be managed endoscopically
- Associated urethral conditions like complicated stricture or previous hypospadias repair
- Patients requiring simultaneous ureteric reimplantation
- Associated inguinal hernia along with BPH
- Patients with known coagulopathy

Pre-operative Preparation

- A preoperative sterile urine culture is preferable before conducting the procedure
- Prophylactic cover is given in the form of a second generation cephalosporin with or without an aminoglycoside before the initiation of surgery.

- Spinal anesthesia or general anesthesia
- The patient is positioned in a lithotomy position
- While positioning the patient the thighs should not make an angle of more than 45 degrees with the horizontal plane.

Procedure

- Parts are cleaned and draped
- Urethra is calibrated
- Resectoscope sheath is inserted per urethra with an obturator sheath. If distal urethra is inadequate to accommodate 28 Fr sheath, a smaller sheath may be used.
- A Dorsal internal Urethrotomy and ventral meatotomy can also be performed
- Surgical landmarks are identified and resection is performed in three stages as described by Nesbitt
- Bladder is filled with upto 150 ml of the irrigation solution
- Resection is done from 12 to 9 'o' clock starting near the bladder neck. The gland near the neck is resected in the form of small chips till the circular fibres of the neck are visible
- The complete anterior quadrant near the neck from 12 to 3 'o'clock is now resected. The posterior quadrants near the neck are then individually resected upto 6 'o' clock
- In the Second stage of the surgery the rest of the gland is removed leaving the part closest to the external sphincter
- The resection begins from 12 'o' clock position going towards 3 and 9'o' clock on either sides such that the lateral lobes fall down and are easily removed in the later part of this stage
- In the last stage the part lying in close vicinity to the verumontanum is chipped off, preserving the extrinsic sphincter especially at 12'o' clock which is the most common site for sphincteric injury
- Irrigation rate is slowed and all bleeders are coagulated using the loop
- The chips are evacuated using an Ellik's evacuator though the resectoscope channel

Post-operative Care

- Once the procedure is completed a three way 24 Fr Foley's catheter is introduced and inflated with 20 ml of distilled water
- Return fluid post TURP must be light pink or rosy pink. Venous bleed if present is controlled by instilling 100 ml fluid and applying traction for upto 7 minutes

- Long periods of traction can lead to ischemia of the bladder neck and stricture
- Patient is given post operative oral antibiotic cover till the catheter has been removed.
- Once the urine is clear the urethral catheter can be removed and patient discharged after ensuring normal passage of urine

Complications

- Bleeding:
  - Mostly occurs due to lack of adequate hemostasis during surgery
  - Heavy postoperative bleed must be managed by review Cystoscopy and removal of the clots
  - Any visible bleeders should be coagulated
  - In case the bleeding continues the bladder may be opened up as an emergency surgery and prostatic fossa packed
- *Clot retention (3.5%):* Cystoscopy and clot evacuation should be done
- Capsular perforation (2%)
  - It is characterized by extravasation of fluid
  - Manifested by restlessness, nausea, vomiting and abdominal pain despite anesthesia
  - Once detected hemostasis must be secured and procedure terminated
  - A supra pubic cystostomy may be done if significant extravasation is suspected.
- TUR Syndrome (2%)
  - Patient becomes symptomatic usually when serum sodium falls below 125 meq/l
  - Usually occurs if resection time exceeds more than 90 min usually in gland volume of more than 75 mg.
  - TUR syndrome is manifested by confusion vomiting, hypertension with bradycardia.
  - 20 ml per minute fluid is absorbed by patient amounting up to a total of 1000 ml during the complete procedure

- Incontinence
- Retrograde ejaculation
- Urethral stricture
- Bladder neck contracture

Open Prostatectomy

- Offers more complete removal of the gland under vision
- No incidence of TUR syndrome and lower rates of recurrence and reoperation
- It employs a lower midline incision with disadvantage of more blood loss and longer post operative stay
- Associated with more morbidity with regards to the incision line and prolonged hospitalization, but it results in better IPSS, PFR improvement, less re-operation rate, and less dysuria.
- Following methods are used for open prostatectomy:
  - Suprapubic (Frayer's procedure)
  - Retropubic (Millin's procedure)
  - Trans-perineal (Young's procedure)

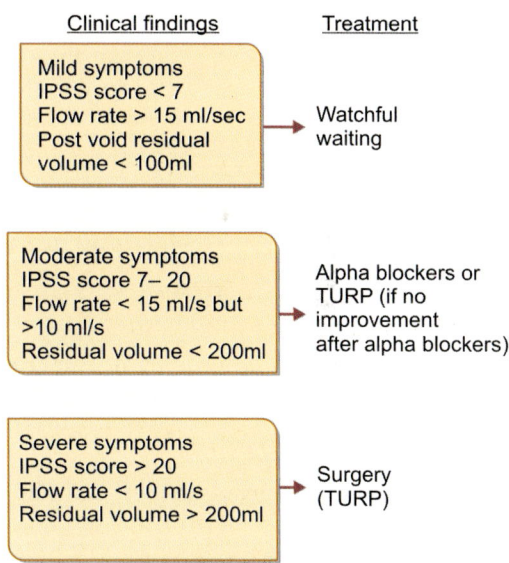

Fig. 43.3: Algorithm for management of BPH

44 | Prostatitis

Prostatitis is the inflammation of the prostate which can be acute or chronic. Infection and inflammation of the prostate usually involves the seminal vesicle and the posterior urethra also.

Acute Prostatitis

- It is an acute inflammation of the prostate gland caused by organisms like *E. coli* (Most common), *S. aureus, S. albus, Streptococcus faecalis, Neisseria gonorrheae* etc.
- The route of these infections may be hematogenous (descending) or secondary to urinary tract infection (ascending).

Clinical Features

- General features like shivering, malaise, backache, fever
- Local features like
  - Pain during micturation
  - Urine containing threads in the initial voided sample
  - Perineal heaviness
  - Rectal irritation
  - Rarely urethral discharge may be seen
- On per rectal examination the prostate is tender.

Treatment

- Prolonged administration of Trimethoprim or ciprofloxacin. Trimethoprim and ciprofloxacin has high concentration in prostate.

Chronic Prostatitis

Chronic prostatitis was classically considered the sequel of untreated acute prostatitis. The responsible organism is difficult to find and it has been suggested that Chlamydia may be a potential etiological agent. It is characterised by recurrent, relapsing UTI caused by persistence of pathogen in the prostatic fluid despite of antibiotic therapy.

· Clinical Features

- Posterior urethritis with symptoms of dysuria, urgency, frequency, nocturia and low back pain.
- Chronic perineal and prostatic pain
- Perigenital pain with intermittent fever
- Chronic backache

Diagnosis

- On per rectal examination the prostate is normal or soft boggy and tender
- Prostatic fluid obtained by prostatic message shows pus cells with or without bacteria
- On urethroscopy the posterior urethra may appear to be inflamed and pus may be seen exuding from the prostatic urethra. The verumontanum is likely to be enlarged and edematous

Treatment

- Antibiotics must be administered according to bacterial sensitivity test or based on etiology.

45 Prostate Cancer

- Most common non-cutaneous cancer in men.
- Accounts for 21% of all cancers.
- There is increased risk with age with 30% presenting between age 70–79 and 67% between age of 80–89.
- Estimated life time risk of disease is 17 % with a life time risk of death being 2.57%.
- It is the fifth most common malignancy worldwide and second most common in men.
- Only in 2 % of men it is diagnosed in men less than 50 years of age.
- Median age of diagnosis is 68 years with 63% being diagnosed after 65.
- Slowly progressive (as a rule): low grade - good prognosis, high grade - poor prognosis, and moderate grade - variable prognosis.

Risk Factors

- Advance age is the most important risk factor.
- *Diet risk:* High animal fat consumption, high zinc, low vegetable and low fish (omega-3 fatty acids) intake, low selenium intake, low fruit, low vegetable intake.
- Hormonal risk: high levels of testosterone, high insulin level, and high insulin-like growth factor.
- Low UV light exposure, high pesticide exposure.
- No increase in risk with BPH or after vasectomy.

Screening

- Digital rectal examination (DRE) can detect tumors in the posterior and lateral aspects of the gland. Can detect extension. Accuracy depends on experience of examiner.
- **PSA:** Must be interpreted in clinical context, higher sensitivity and lower specificity than DRE.
- Referral for TRUS and/or sextant biopsy if DRE or PSA abnormal.
- PPV for PSA >4 or DRE is ~30%.
- Screening is controversial. No consensus as morbidity and mortality data inconclusive.
- If decision to screen: yearly DRE/PSA until co-morbidities/age (75) limit life expectancy to 10 yrs
- Refer if abnormal DRE or PSA>4.
- If PSA <4, refer men who experience a PSA rise of more than .75 ng/mL/year (based on last three measurements obtained over 12 to 24 months).

Signs

- Stony hard prostate.
- Hematuria, Blood in the semen
- Irregular, firm, hard nodule on DRE.
- Signs of obstructive uropathy/Rising AUA Score.
- Neurologic cord compression signs.
- Pathologic fractures/bone pain.
- Sudden onset of erectile dysfunction, painful ejaculation.

Diagnosis

- Prostate biopsy by FNA or Biopsy.
- 33–50% chance of biopsy being malignant.
- *Differential diagnosis*: BPH, chronic prostatitis, prostatic TB, old biopsy fibrosis, prostatic cysts, prostatic calculi.

Clinical Staging

- **DRE:** Size, location, volume, local extension
- TRUS/Endorectal coil MR to determine local extension
- *CT abdomen and pelvis:* Pre-op pelvic node assessment
- *PSA:* Highest in transition zone tumors and well differentiated tumors. Its greatest value is in detecting recurrence
- *Bone scan:* For ruling out metastasis

Staging

TNM Staging

- T1 are microscopic and non-palpable
- T2 are palpable but confined to gland
- T3 protrude beyond the gland capsule
- T4 are fixed and extend well beyond the gland

Gleason Scale

- Based on tumor histology
- Grade 1 Gleason is the most well-differentiated
- Grade 5 is the most poorly differentiated
- Combined scores are reported (primary + secondary) (2–10)

Treatment

Clinically Localized Disease

- Radical prostatectomy (Open, laparoscopic or robotic assisted). Robotic assisted radical prostatectomy is gaining popularity
- Radiation therapy (external beam or interstitial implantation)

- Watchful waiting
  - 70 to 80% of prostate carcinoma are hormone dependent and 70–80% of men respond to hormonal therapy.
  - LHRH agonist causes induction of androgen deprivation without orchidectomy.
  - Commonly used LHRH agonist are Goserelin acetate and Leuprolide acetate. They are used in injectable form.
  - Orchidectomy is another commonly used method of hormonal manipulation.
  - Suppression of both testicular and adrenal testosterone (complete androgen suppression) produces longer lasting response.
  - Complete androgen suppression can be obtained by combination of antiandrogen agent + orchidectomy or LHRH agonist
  - Commonly used antiandrogen is either bicalutamide or flutamide.

Most Important Treatment Issues in Deciding Radical Prostatectomy

- Patient's medical condition/age
- Gleason grade and PSA
- Is it organ confined
- Estimation of outcome for individual patient
- Potential side effects of treatment
- Greatest treatment benefit-> "moderate to poor grade cancers in younger, healthier age group."
- Least treatment benefit-> "lower grade cancers in older, sicker age group".

Non Localized Disease/Metastatic

- Hormonal therapy
- *Chemotherapy:* Docetanel incised
- *Lymphomatic management:* Bone health, voiding symptoms

46 Voiding Dysfunction

Includes Problems of

- Bladder emptying
  - Obstructive conditions, e.g. benign prostatic hyperplasia (BPH)
- Bladder storage
  - Overactive bladder
  - Stress incontinence
  - Mixed incontinence
  - Overflow incontinence

Overactive Bladder

Present with

- Frequency
- Urgency
- Urge incontinence

Pathophysiology of urinary incentinence:

- Due to pelvic floor weakness with normal sphincteric mechanism (Stress incontinence)
- Due to detrusor instability with normal anatomy of pelvis floor and normal sphincter (True incontinence)
- Neuropathic incontinence due to nerve lesions
- Congenital incontinence due to ectopic ureter, duplicate or single system, with epispadias or exstrophy.
- False incontinence as a result of obstructive lesions (overflow incontinence).
- Traumatic

Urinary Incontinence

- *Definition:* Urinary incontinence is uncontrolled leakage of urine causing hygienic and social problems.
- Occurs mostly in older adults, more common in females.

Stress Incontinence

- Stress incontinence occurs when a small amount of urine escapes while the person coughs, sneezes, laughs, jumps or lifts something heavy.
- Occurs due to weakness in external urethra sphincter, mostly in women. Main pathology is hypermobility of vesicourethral segment, pelvic floor weakness and intrinsic sphincter deficiency.

Urge Incontinence

- Associated with sudden strong disease to pass urine
- Often results from detrusor overactivity.

Overflow Incontinence

- Overflow incontinence happens when urine leaks from an overfilled bladder.
- Occurs due to detrusor failure.

Mixed Incontinence

- Mixed incontinence occurs when a person has both the symptoms of urge incontinence and stress incontinence.

- Associated factors are
  - Sudden increase in intra-abdominal contractions
  - Uninhibited detrusor contractions
  - Weak external sphincter

Factors Associated with Bladder Control Problems

- Age
- Childbirth
- Gender
- Menopausal status
- Surgery
- Prostate enlargement
- Lifestyle
- Medications
- Concomitant illnesses

10 Warning Signs of Bladder Control Problems

- Any leakage of urine
- Leakage of urine, regardless of amount, on coughing, sneezing, laughing or standing.
- Leaking urine on the way to the toilet.
- Bed wetting at any age over six years.
- An urgent need to pass urine, being unable to hold on.
- Passing urine more frequently than 8 times a day and only passing small amounts.

- Blood in the urine.
- Inability to urinate (retention of urine).
- Pain when passing urine.
- Progressive weakness of the urinary stream or a stream that stops and starts instead of flowing out smoothly.

Investigation

  - Stress incontinence is usually diagnosed by urodynamic characteristics. They have a low urethral pressure profile with reduced closing pressure. Functional urethral length is shortened. This functional urethral shortening is in the proximal segment. Net urethral closure pressure is reduced in response to stress, e.g. coughing or sneezing.
  - Cystography for demonstration of anatomical abnormality may be done.
  - Urge incontinence is associated with detrusor overactivity on urodynamics.

Treatment

  - For stress incontinence the treatment of choice is proper suspension and support of the vesicourethral segment in a normal position through various approaches.
  - The treatment of urge incontinence is behavioral therapy for bladder training and anticholenergic pharmacotherapy.

47 Evaluation for Hematuria

- *Macroscopic hematuria:* Gross blood in urine.
- *Microscopic hematuria:* More than 3 RBCs/HPF (2–3 properly collected samples).

Macroscopic Hematuria

- As little as 1 ml/litre of blood can stain urine red
- Needs thorough evaluation
- Presenting symptom of 85% cases of bladder cancer and 40% cases of renal cell carcinoma.

Microscopic Hematuria

- Can be transient or continuous
- Blood can originate from anywhere along the urinary tract
- Some patients have no identifiable etiology
- Aim is to identify patients with significant disease
- Minimize the cost and morbidity of unnecessary tests.

Causes of Red Colored Urine

- Blood
- Hemoglobinuria
- Anthrocyanin in beets and blackberries
- Drugs
  - Pyridium
  - Phenothiazines
  - Rifampin
  - Phenolpthalien
  - Cyclophosphamide
- Myoglobinuria
- Chronic lead and mercury poisoning.

Microscopic Hematuria

- Timed urine collection and counting chambers
  - Detected in 9–18% of healthy individuals
  - Upper limit of normal is 500,000 to 600,000/12 hr with a urine volume of 300 ml
  - Technique is time consuming.

Urine Dipstick Test

- Chemical reagent strip
- Peroxidase like activity of hemoglobin catalyses the activity of chromogen indicator
- A green color indicates Hematuria
- Degree of color change proportional to amount of Hematuria.
- 91–100% sensitive
- 65–99% specific
- Should be confirmed by microscopic evaluation of urinary sediment.
- False positive in myoglobinuria/hemoglobinuria/acidic urine/antiseptic solutions: povidone iodine.

Urine Microscopy

- Centrifuge 10 ml of urine at 2000 rpm for 10 minutes

- Resuspend sediment and examine under high power field X400
- 2 RBC/HPF is equivalent to upper threshold limit of 500,000 RBC/12 hours.

Specimen Collection

- Mid stream clean catch format
- Without instrumentation
- In a wide mouthed sterile container
- Evaluated within one hour
- If delay expected refrigerate at 4–5 degrees.

Glomerular Hematuria

- Erythrophagocytes (renal tubule cells with ingested RBCs)
- Red cell casts
- Dysmorphic RBC >80%
- Protienuria > 1 gm/day
- Elevated S. creatinine levels
- Pallor
- Causes
  - IgA Nephropathy (Berger's disease)
  - Thin glomerular basement membrane disease.

Non-malignant Cause Suspected on Examination

- Menstruation
- Vigorous exercise
- Sexual activity
- Viral illness
- Repeat urinalysis within 48 hours

In hematuria associated with urinary tract infection (microscopy showing pus cells, repeat microscopy 6 weeks after antibiotic therapy).

Urinary Cytology

- Depends upon exfoliative cells
- Sensitivity increases with grade of tumor
- Lower grade and low stage tumor have negative cytology – intracellular attachment better preserved.
- Improved sensitivity by early morning voiding sample or barbotaged sample during cystoscopy
- False negative rate for low grade cancer 10–50%
- 95% accuracy for high grade tumor
- Results depend upon expertise of cytologist
- Positive urine cytology is diagnostic of urothelial malignancy

- Negative cytology do not exclude urothelial cancer
- Bladder wash cytology yields more tumor cells
- High false positive rates
- Chromosomal markers for bladder malignancy
  - Homozygous loss of chromosome band 9p 21
  - Polysomy of chromosome 3, 7, 11
  - Threshold of more than 5 cells with polysomy 84% sensitive and 92% specific.

FISH – Urovysion

- Flouroscence in situ hybridisation assay is known as Urovysion
- Approved by USFDA
- Probes for centromeres of chromosome 3, 7, 11 and locus specific probe for 9p21
- Useful for recurrent bladder cancer
- High sensitivity for new cases of carcinoma urinary bladder
- Detected 95% cases of high grade carcinoma in comparison to 41% on cytology
- More sensitive but slightly less specific than urine cytology
- Useful initial diagnostic test for both new and recurrent bladder cancer.

Nuclear Matrix Protein 22 (NMP22)

- First described in 1974
- NMP22 is a non chromatin structure that supports nuclear shape and organizes DNA
- Takes part in DNA replication, transcription and RNA processing
- Helps in proper distribution of chromatin to daughter cells
- Found in nuclear matrix of all cells
- Released in urine from nuclei of tumor cells
- Can be up to 25 times higher in malignancy in comparisons to healthy persons
- Assay can be done in urine with high sensitivity and specificity.
- Grossman et al compared NMP22, cystoscopy and voided urine cytology and found that
  - Cystoscopy alone detected 91% of the cases
  - NMP22 and Cystoscopy had nearly 99% sensitivity
  - NMP22 was found to be more sensitive than cytology
- Advantages
  - Does not require expert analysis
  - Does not depend upon intact cells

- Cost less than half of cytology
- No definitive cut off point.

Cystoscopy

- Indications
  - Gross hematuria
  - Microscopic non glomerular hematuria if:
    - ◊ More than 40 years
    - ◊ Cigarette smoking
    - ◊ Family history of carcinoma urinary bladder
    - ◊ Occupational hazard
    - ◊ Previous history of urothelial malignancy
    - ◊ Suspicious cells on cytology
    - ◊ H/O urological disorder/disease
    - ◊ H/O Pelvic irradiation
    - ◊ H/O irritative voiding symptoms
- Types
  - *Flexible:* Difficult procedure to learn but can be done out on patient basis
  - *Rigid:* Therapeutic procedure can also be carried out.
- Fluorescence cystoscopy
  - Filtered blue light is used 375-440 nm
  - Intravesical instillation of a photosensitiser usually (5-ALA) or hexaminolaevulinate (HAL) is performed
  - Malignant lesion selectively absorbs light and is visualised on scopy.
    CT urography: If the cystoscopy is normal, and cause of hematuria cannot be ascertained then CT urography is indicated.

Bladder Carcinoma Management: Current Trends

INCIDENCE

- 4th common malignancy in males and 8th most common cancer in females
- 2.9% of all cancers deaths in men and 1.5% in women
- Urothelial cancer is related to environmental factors and age. Its incidence increases with age with peak incidence in 8th decade of life.
- Bladder cancer is the 9th most common malignancy globally and 13th most common cause of death.
- Bladder cancer in many cases is associated with slow N-acetyl transferase -2 gene polymorphism which leads to less activity of N Acetyl Transferase (NAT). NAT is responsible for detoxification of Nitrosamines a known bladder carcinogen.

Predisposing Factors

- Beta-naphthylamines in cigarette smoke
- Occupational exposure to dyes in petroleum, dye and aniline industries (aromatic compounds) is seen in 15–35% of cases in men.
- Epithelial trauma
- Family history
- Aromatic amines which bind to DNA are main environmental risk factors leading to mutation.
- There is a mutation in p53 tumour suppressor gene.
- There are 2–4 times more chances of developing bladder cancer in smokers and risk is related

linearly to duration and quantity of smoking. It accounts for 50% of cases in men and 30% of cases in females.
- Chronic urinary tract infection is associated with high risk of developing urinary bladder cancer.
- Cyclophosphamide has been proven to cause bladder cancer and the risk is directly related to duration and dose of cyclophosphamide. Phosphoramide mustard is the primary metabolite which is found to be mutagenic.
- Loss of genetic material on chromosome 9 appears to be consistent finding.

Pathology

- 92% are transitional cell carcinoma, 6% as squamous cell carcinoma and 2% are adenocarcinoma. On histological examination angiolymphatic invasion and pagetoid spread, i.e. growth of cancer cells underneath the layer of normal appearing urothelium are two bad prognostic signs.

Pathological Staging (Fig. 48.1)

Ta	Papillary tumor confined to urothelium
Tis	(CIS) Flat high grade lesion which is confined to urothelium
T1	Tumor which invades lamina propria
T2	Tumor which invades detrusor muscle
T2a	Tumor invades inner half of detrusor muscle or mucularis propria

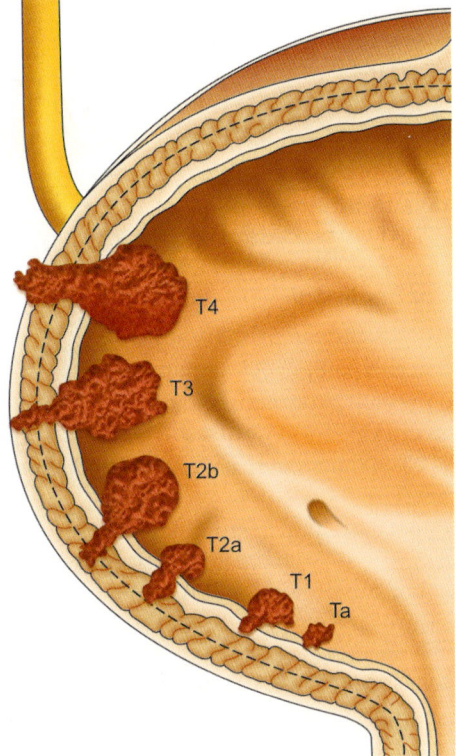

Fig. 48.1: T-staging of carcinoma bladder

T2b	Tumor invades outer half of detrusor muscle or muscularis propria
T3	Tumor which invades extravesical fat.
T3a	Microscopic invasion
T3b	Macroscopic invasion presenting as extravesical mass
T4	Tumor invades prostate, seminal vesicle, uterus, vagina, pelvic wall and abdominal wall.

T staging is determined by a combination of transurethral resection and bimanual examination under anesthesia. Bimanual examination under anesthesia is carried before and after TURBT.

Grading

- *Grade 0* (**Papillary lesion):**
  - Fine fibro- vascular core,
  - Covered by normal bladder mucosa and
  - Never recurs after endoscopic resection
- *Grade 1:* (**Well differentiated tumors):**
  - Thin fibro- vascular core, thickened uro-thelium
  - More than seven cell layers,

- Slight anaplasia, pleomorphism with rare mitotic figures.
- Often recur after endoscopic resection
- *Grade 2* (**Moderately differentiated tumors):**
  - Wide fibro- vascular core with disturbance of base to surface cell maturation
  - Loss of cell polarity
  - Nuclear pleomorphism and frequent mitotic figures
- *Grade III* (**Poorly differentiated):**
  - No differentiation of cells
  - Marked nuclear pleomorphism, higher N:C ratio and frequent mitotic figures

Prognostic Indicators Predicting to Muscle Invasion

- Grade and presence of carcinoma in situ
- Presence of tumor associated antigen 138 (TAA 138)
- Hyauloronidase activity.
- Increased urinary excretion of fibronectin
- Amplification of the C-erb B2 oncogene
- Deletion of chromosome 9
- p53 mutation
- Epidermal growth factor receptor
- Multiple aneuploid cell lines.
- Presence of expression of Lewis X blood group

Diagnosis

Cytology

- Microscopic cytology of urinary sediment or saline bladder to detect malignant cells. (Saline bladder washes more accurate)
- Microscopic cytology is more sensitive in high grade tumours or carcinoma in situ but can be falsely negative in 20% of cases.

Newer Tests for Screening of Bladder Cancer

- Hyaluronic acid (Hyaluronidase activity)
- Nuclear Matrix protein (NMP) 21
- Telomerase activity in urine

Cystoscopy

- Standard procedure for diagnosis and staging-cystoscopy and bimanual examination under anesthesia (EUA) before and after resection.
- Tumor mapping done first
- All visible tumors removed and muscle under it resected plus multiple biopsies taken of suspicious sites.

- Random biopsies from normal areas of bladder to detect field change are controversial
  - Except in patients with positive urine cytology with no obvious tumor.
- *Tumor encroaching the ureteric orifice:* resection without fulguration with D-J stent.
- *Tumor in diverticulum:* Do biopsy only because of high risk of perforation.

Radiology

CT Scans: To determine tumor extent, nodal metastasis and distant spread (Accuracy in nodal metastasis is 40–70%). It will also give information about kidneys and back pressure changes.

MRI: Same resolution, better sensitivity. There is no difference between CT and MRI. MRI is indicated if there is uremia or allergic to dye.

Chest X-Ray: done in all cases.

Bone scan: In symptomatic patients.

STAGING

TNM Staging

T definitions: Defined above

N definitions

Nx: Regional lymph nodes can not be assessed

N0: No regional lymph node metastasis.

N1: Metastasis in a single lymph node 2 cm or less in greatest dimension.

N2: Metastasis in a single lymph node 2 cm to 5 cm or multiple lymph nodes not more than 5 cm

N3: Metastasis in a lymph node more than 5 cm in greatest dimension.

Distant Metastasis (M staging)

Mx: Distant metastasis can not be assessed

Mo: No distant metastasis

M1: Distant metastasis.

AJCC stage subgroups

Stage 0: Ta, or Tis, N0, Mo

Stage I: T1, N0, M0

Stage II: T2a or T2b, N0, M0

Stage III: T3a or T3ba or T4a, N0, MO

Stage IV: T4b, N0, M0 or Any T with N1 to N3 with M0 or Any T, any N, with M1.

Treatment

For the purpose of treatment, bladder cancer can be grouped in to three major groups:

- Superficial
- Muscle Invasive
- Metastatic.

Superficial Bladder Cancer

- 80% of all bladder cancers
- Transurethral Resection of Bladder Tumour (TURBT) is procedure of choice.

Aims of Treatment

- To eradicate the primary lesion
- To prevent superficial relapse
- To prevent progression to muscle invasive and less curable form of disease
- Initial management is complete transurethral resection
- Depending upon cystoscopic and pathological findings, superficial bladder cancers can be further sub divided in low risk group and high risk group. (*see* table top on next page)

Further Management of Low Risk

- Periodic cystoscopic examination and urine cytology every 6 month for 2 years and yearly for at least 5 years
- Recurrence and progression are managed by transurethral resection
- Bladder tumour antigen (BTA) and nuclear matrix protein (NM22) in voided urine as supplement to cystoscopic and cytological evaluation

Further Management of High-risk

- Intravesical chemotherapy
- CIS and recurrence after BCG: BCG agent of choice.
- Combination of intravesical BCG and subcutaneous BCG is better.
- Cystectomy for patients after 2nd failure
- Immediate single mitomycin-C instilation: prolongs recurrence free survival.

Follow up for High Risk Group

- Cystoscopy and cytology 3 monthly for 2 years, 6 monthly for next 5 years and yearly after.

Muscle Invasive Bladder Cancer

- 15% of all bladder cancers
- Stage II and III of AJCC staging

Table 48.1: Classification of bladder carcinoma

S. No.		Low risk	High risk
1.	Appearance	Papillary fine stalk	Papillary thick stalk or sessile
2.	Size	up to 3cm	> 3cm
3.	Number of lesions	up to 3	> 3
4	Transurethral resection	Complete	Incomplete
5.	Stage	T_a	T_1, T_{cis}
6.	Grade	I-II	III
7.	Molecular markers		
	Immunostaining for mutated p53 antigen	Absent	Present
	Aneuploidy	Absent	Present
8.	Multiple, frequent recurrence	No	Yes

Table 48.2: Some common agents used for intravesical therapy

Drug	Dose	Induction scheme	Toxicity
Mitomycin C	20 – 60 mg	Weekly × 6–8 weeks	Chemical cystitis, Skin reactions
BCG	80 mg	Weekly × 6 weeks	Cystitis, Hematuria
Interferon Alpha	10–100 Million Units	Weekly × 6 weeks	Flu like symptoms
Valrubicin	80 mg	Weekly × 6 weeks	Bladder irritation

- Aim of treatment for muscle invasive disease is to cure the patient and to determine which modality of treatment is best for a particular patient
- Divided into bladder sparing and non bladder sparing modalities.

Bladder Sparing Modalities

- Transurethral resection alone in superficial solitary muscle invasive disease (T2a)
- Partial cystectomy in muscle invasive tumour without CIS or dysplasia if tumour located at dome or posterior wall and at least 2 cm available surgical margin for resection.
- Radiotherapy as definitive treatment: Total dose 5000–7000 Gy. Complete response in 40% to 50%. 5 year survival rate: 30–40%. Local recurrence major problem (25% of deaths). Not favoured these days as primary treatment.
- Bladder preservation using concurrent or sequential chemo radiotherapy:
  - TURBT and chemotherapy provides durable local control in less than 20% of patients
  - Radiation alone is not sufficient
  - Rationale:
    ◊ Cisplatin and 5FU are capable of radiosensitization of tumour tissue
    ◊ 50% of muscle invasive disease harbor occult metastasis

Non-Bladder Sparing Modalities

- Radical cystectomy standard treatment (Fig. 48.2)
- Local control rates at 5 and 10 years are >90% and 88%
- 5 year survival rate: 40- to 60%
- Preoperative radiotherapy 4000 Gy followed by surgery has shown benefit in prolonging survival
- No survival benefit from post cystectomy single agent or multidrug agent adjuvant chemotherapy
- Indications:
  - Muscle-invading tumours unsuitable for segmental resection
  - Low stage tumour unsuitable for conservative management due to multicentricity and frequent recurrences resistant to intravesical instillation
  - High grade tumours (T_1G_3) associated with T_{is}
  - Bladder symptoms, such as frequency or haemorrhage - "bladder cripple"

Metastatic Bladder Cancer

- Choosing the most effective palliation. Systemic chemotherapy is the only option for metastatic bladder cancer.
- Despite good response, disease continues to recur and long term survival is poor.

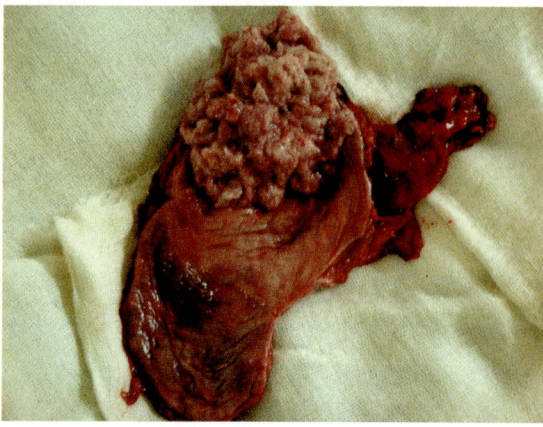

Fig. 48.2: Radical cystectomy specimen

- *Single agent chemotherapy:* Complete response is uncommon. Responses last for about 3 to 4 months. Cisplatin administered every 3 to 4 weeks and methotrexate in the weekly or biweekly schedule has given pooled response rate of 30 and 29% respectively.

Response to Single Agent Chemotherapy

Agent	Response rate (%)
Cisplatin	30
Methotrexate	29
Iforosamide	28
Gallium nitrate	17
Doxorubicin	10
Vinblastine	16
Carboplatin	13
5 FU	15
Epirubicin	15
Paclitaxel	40

Combination Chemotherapy

- Most accepted modality for metastatic bladder cancer
- *MVAC regimen:* Most popular regimen MVAC comprises of methotrexate, viblastine, doxorubicin and cisplatin (response rate: 40–70% and 25–30% complete response.
- Long term follow up 5 year survival of 32% (nodal disease) and 17% (advanced metastatic diseases)
- *Toxic effects:* myelosuppression, sepsis, mucositis, nephrotoxicity and neuropathy
- *To reduce toxicity:* eliminating vinblastine and methotrexate on days 15 and 22, and replacing doxorubicin with epirubicin and cisplatin with carboplatin
- Current front line chemotherapy for metastatic bladder cancer remains MVAC and CMV. MVAC regimens has produced better response rates and survival than single agent cisplatin or CISCA.

Summary of Treatment Options for Bladder Cancer

Stage	Treatment option
Tis	Complete TURBT with intravesical BCG
Ta	Complete TUR
T_1	Complete TUR followed by intravesical chemo or immunotherapy
T_2–T_4	Radical cystectomy neoadjuvant chemo followed by radical cystectomy Radical cystectomy followed by adjuvant chemotherapy
Any TN + M+	Systemic chemotherapy followed by surgery

49 Surgical Anatomy of the Kidney and Ureter Kidney

- 150–130 gm. Paired reddish brown organs Each measures 10–12 × 5 × 7 × 3 cm
- Fetal lobulations persist till 1st year of life
- *Dromedary hump* is a normal focal renal parenchymal bulge caused by downward pressure by liver/spleen
- Right kidney is shorter and wider due to compression by the liver.

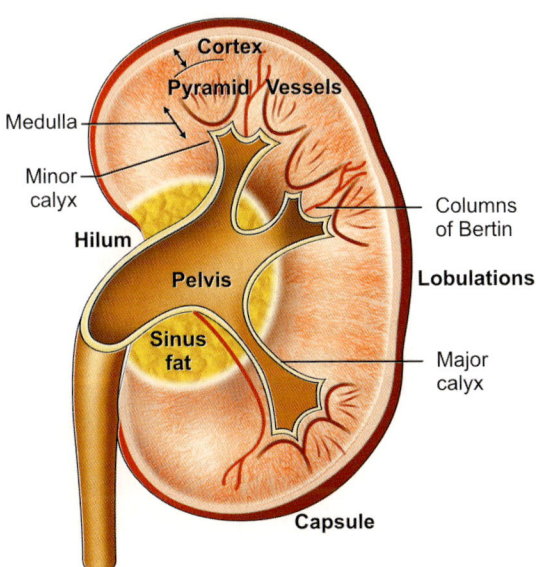

Fig. 49.1: Gross anatomy of the kidney

- Vascular structures and collecting ducts unite to form the renal sinus
- Surrounded by sinus fat which is a landmark for surgical procedures
- Sinus narrows to form the renal hilum medially.
- Kidney is divided grossly and microscopically into cortex and medulla.
- Vessels run above the sinus fat. Dissection should therefore be done below the sinus fat to avoid injury to the retropelvic vein.

Renal Medulla

- Made up of separate, distinct, conical areas called pyramids.
- Darker than cortex.
- Apex of the pyramid is a renal papilla.
- Each papilla is cupped by individual minor calyx.

Renal Cortex

- Covers the pyramids and extends between them.
- Extensions of the cortex run between the renal pyramids called *Columns of Bertini*
- Lighter in color than the medulla.
- Renal vessels traverse to periphery through Columns of Bertini.

Anatomical Relations

- Right kidney resides between top of 1st and bottom of 3rd lumbar vertebrae.
- Left kidney resides 1 to 2 cm higher, between 12th thoracic and 3rd lumbar vertebrae.

- It may be required to go through the bed of 11th and 12th rib for complete mobilization of left kidney
- Lower pole lies laterally and anteriorly in relation to the upper pole.
- Medial aspect of both kidneys is rotated anteriorly at an angle of 30 degrees.

Anterior Relations

- Right kidney
  - Right adrenal gland
  - Liver
  - 2nd part of duodenum
  - Hepatic flexure
  - Small Intestine
- Left kidney
  - Left adrenal gland
  - Stomach
  - Spleen
  - Pancreas
  - Splenic flexure
  - Descending colon
  - Jejunum
- During a transperitoneal approach to the kidneys, it may be required to kocherize the duodenum anteriorly along with mobilization of the hepatic flexure on the right side and mobilization of the splenic flexure of colon on left side.
- Colon is particularly susceptible to injury as it may be retrorenal in 16%

Posterior Relations

- Right kidney
  - 11th and 12th rib
  - Quadratus lumborum
  - Psoas muscle
- Left kidney
  - 12th rib
  - Quadratus lumborum
  - Psoas muscle

Perirenal Structures – Gerota's Fascia

- Anatomic barrier to the spread of malignancy as well as a means of containing perinephric fluid collections.
- Covers kidney on 3 sides
- Medially it extends across the midline
- Inferiorly it remains as an open potential space.

- Perinephric fluid tracks inferiorly and can lead to psoas abscess
- Kidney is removed along with Gerota's fascia in radical nephrectomy

Renal Artery

- Renal artery is a branch of the abdominal aorta
- Splits usually into five segmental branches
- Segmental arteries are end arteries
- During partial nephrectomy one must be very careful with regards to the arterial supply of the segment to be preserved

Renal artery → Segmental artery → Lobar artery → Interlobar artery → Arcuate artery → Interlobular artery → Afferent arteriole

- Segmental arteries are end arteries supplying discrete areas of the kidney with no collaterals
- Any occlusion causes infarction
- First and most constant branch is the posterior segmental branch
- Uretropelvic junction obstruction occurs when it crosses anterior to the ureter.
- An avascular plane lies longitudinally just posterior to the lateral aspect of the kidney.
- Posterior segmental artery is the most commonly injured during endourological procedures (retropelvic in 50%)

Brodel's Line

- Anterior and posterior artery divisions meet posteriorly just lateral to renal pelvis.
- This forms an avascular plane marked by Brodel's line
- It is the preferred site of incision during nephrolithotomy

Renal Vein

- Venous drainage communicates freely through venous collars around the infundibula forming collateral circulation.
- Occlusion of a venous segment has little effect on the outflow
- Interlobular veins drain the post glomerular capillaries.

Efferent vein → Arcuate vein → Interlobar vein → Lobar vein → Segmental vein → Renal vein

- In the renal pelvis the vein is the most anterior structure followed posteriorly by the artery and pelvis

- Right renal vein is 2–4 cm in length
- Left renal vein is 6–10 cm in length
- Right renal vein is shorter than the left and has more chances of avulsion.

Renal Vein Tributaries

- Right renal vein
  - Right lumbar artery
- Left renal vein
  - Left lumbar artery
  - Left adrenal artery
  - Left gonadal artery

Lymphatics

- Lymphatics mainly follow the blood vessels through columns of Bertin
- Form large trunks within the renal sinus
- Right side drainage is to the right interaortocaval and right paracaval nodes
- Occasional drainage to retrocrural or left lateral para aortic nodes.
- Lymphatics on left drain mainly into the left lateral para aortic nodes including nodes anterior and posterior to the aorta
- Additional drainage is to retrocrural nodes or directly into the thoracic duct above diaphragm.
- Lymphadenectomy was done in renal cell carcinoma from diaphragm to bifurcation of aorta, but now only selected involved and pedicle nodes are removed.

Collecting System

- Tip of the medullary pyramid are known as renal papillae
- Usually 7–9 per kidney
- Papillae can be 4–18 in number
- Each papilla is cupped by the minor calyx
- Minor calyx narrows into the infundibulum and then into major calyx.

Calyceal System

- Calyces in direct apposition to renal papilla are defined as minor (5–14)
- May be simple or compound (draining 2–3 papillae)
- Three calyceal groups: superior/midzone (arranged in two parallel rows)/inferior
- Midzone calyceal configuration can be Brodel type or Hodson type.

Renal Innervation

- Sympathetic preganglionic nerves originate through T8 to L1
- Postganglionic fibers travel to the kidney via autonomic plexus surrounding the renal artery
- Parasympathetic fibers originate form the vagus
- Autonomic fibers have a vasomotor function.

Ureter

- 22 to 30 cm in length
- Divided into 3 parts (Fig. 49.2)
  - Upper ureter extends from renal pelvis to upper sacrum
  - Middle ureter extends from upper to lower sacrum
  - Lower ureter extends from lower sacrum to the bladder.
- Also divided as abdominal and pelvic ureter.

Histology

- Inner layer of transitional epithelium
- Covered by lamina propria
- Together for the mucosal lining
- Inner longitudinal and outer circular smooth muscle layer
- Muscle layer is continuous with that of pelvis and calyces.
- Outermost layer is the adventitia

Blood Supply

- Abdominal arteries approach medially while pelvic branches approach laterally.
- Upper ureter supplied by
  - Renal
  - Gonadal,
  - Common Illiac artery and
  - Abdominal aorta
- Lower ureter supplied by the branches of internal Illiac like
  - Superior vesical,
  - Middle rectal, and
  - Vaginal arteries
- Ureteric mobilization
  - Ureteric blood supply is segmental
  - Mobilization is done lateral to medially as the blood supply is from medial to lateral side in abdominal part of ureter.

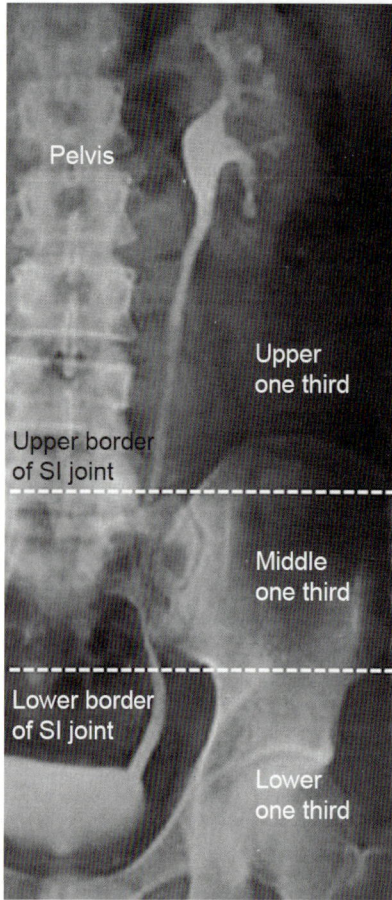

Fig. 49.2: Parts of the ureter

– Periadventitial tissue must not be removed.
– Extreme care is required during use of energy sources or negotiating during ureteroscopy at the level of pelvic brim because of close relation of ureter with illiac vessels.

Lymphatics

- In pelvis drainage is to internal, external and common Illiac nodes
- Left abdominal ureter drains in to the left para aortic lymph nodes
- Right ureter is drained primarily to the right paracaval and inter-aortocaval lymph nodes.

Nerve Supply

- Controversial role of autonomic innervation
- Intrinsic activity regulates peristalsis
- Cells in minor calyx of the renal collecting system act as intrinsic smooth muscle pacemaker sites
- Preganglionic sympathetic output from T10 to L2
- Postganglionic SMA, Aortic and hypo gastric plexus
- Parasympathetic output from S2–S4

Normal Constrictions

- Common site of lodging of stone
- First at uretero-pelvic junction where pelvis tapers into proximal ureter
- Second at site of extrinsic compression by illiac vessels when they cross
- Third and true physical restriction is during intramural passage through the bladder.

Anatomical Relations

- Right ureter related to ascending colon, cecum, colonic mesentry and appendix
- Left ureter related to descending and sigmoid colon
- Crossed anteriorly by gonadal vessels in lower one third and uterine artery in pelvis.
- Crosses anterior to Illiac vessels on entry into the pelvis.

50 Hydronephrosis

- Hydronephrosis is defined as the aseptic dilatation of the pevicalyceal system most commonly due to partial or complete obstruction to the outflow of urine. However it can be due non obstructive pathology like severe vesico-ureteric reflux or in Prune Belly syndrome (Fig. 50.1)
- Hydronephrosis can be unilateral or bilateral.

Adverse Effects of Hydronephrosis are

- Loss of renal cortical function due to cortical atrophy

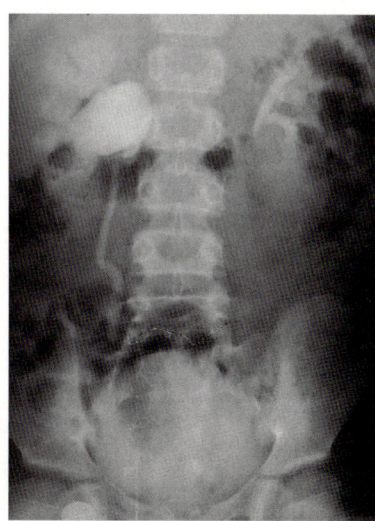

Fig. 50.1: Intravenous pyelogram showing hydronephrosis of the right kidney

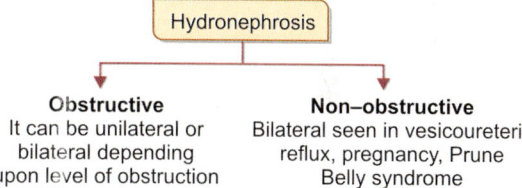

Fig. 50.2: Types of hydronephrosis

- Pyonephrosis and septicaemia if infection supervenes
- Stone formation
- Haematuria

Causes

Unilateral Obstruction

- Extramural obstruction
  - Neoplasm of adjacent structures, e.g. Carcinoma cervix, carcinoma Colon involving ureter
  - Retroperitoneal fibrosis
    ◊ Idiopathic
    ◊ Drugs like methysergide
    ◊ Chronic ambulatory peritoneal dialysis
  - Retro-caval ureter
- Obstruction in the wall
  - Congenital narrowing: PUJ obstruction
  - Ureterocele
  - Congenital small ureteric orifice
  - Inflammatory stricture

- Following
  - ◊ Removal of impacted ureteric calculus
  - ◊ Repair of damaged ureter
  - ◊ Tuberculous infection
- Ureteric neoplasm
- Intraluminal causes
  - Calculus
  - Blood clot
  - Sloughed papilla in papillary necrosis
    - ◊ Diabetes
    - ◊ Analgesic abusers
    - ◊ Sickle cell disease

Bilateral Obstruction

- Congenital
  - Stricture of external urethral meatus
  - Phimosis
  - Posterior urethral valve
  - Congenital bladder neck stenosis (Marion's disease)
- Acquired
  - Benign hypertrophy of prostate
  - Prostatic carcinoma
  - Benign hypertrophy of prostate
  - Post-operative bladder neck scarring
  - Urethral stricture
  - Phimosis
  - Urethral obstruction can lead to detrusor muscle hypertrophy and obstruction of intramural part of ureter.

Pelvic Ureteric Junction (PUJ) Obstruction (Fig. 50.3)

- It is defined as functional or anatomic impediment to urine flow from the renal pelvis to the proximal ureter leading to back pressure changes in kidney and loss of function if obstruction remains unattended.
- Primary pathology is poor drainage of the renal collecting system resulting in progressive renal damage.

Pathophysiology

- Primary UPJ obstruction is thought to be due to developmental anomalies
- Secondary UPJ obstruction is secondary some other pathology which can be due to
  - Previous renal surgery
  - After recurrent stone passage

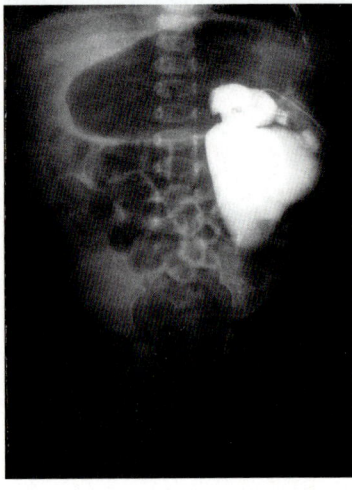

Fig. 50.3: Nephrostogram showing pelvi-ureteric junction obstruction

- Recurrent urinary tract infection
- Associated with vesicoureteric reflux.

Primary PUJ Obstruction

- Insertion anomalies
  - Non dependent insertion of ureter into pelvis
- Functional abnormalities
  - Presence of a non-peristaltic segment in the ureter because spiral musculature is replaced by abnormal longitudinal muscle bundles or fibrous tissue.
  - Abnormal collagen architecture within the narrowed ureteric pelvic junction
- Intrinsic obstruction
  - Tissue valves forming mucosal folds and ureteric polyps which develop due to anatomical abnormalities
- Extrinsic obstruction
  - Aberrant or accessory blood vessels.
  - Kinks
  - Bands

Symptoms

- Unilateral hydronephrosis is more common
- Female: male = 2:1
- Right side is more commonly affected
- Symptoms
  - Mild dull ache in the loin (77%), feeling of fullness associated with nausea or vomiting
  - Sensation of dragging or heaviness
  - Acute renal colic

- Hematuria (9%), which can be spontaneous or associated with trivial trauma
- Reno vascular hypertension
- Recurrent urinary tract infections, calculi formation (20%).
- Symptoms of chronic renal failure like malaise, weakness and loss of appetite
- Vague gastrointestinal complaints (5%).
- Patient may present with the episodes of flank pain, nausea, and vomiting followed by periods of rapid diuresis with large volumes of liquid intake (**Dietl's crisis**). It occurs after drinking fluids which promotes diuresis like coffee or beer.
- Signs
  - Renal angle tenderness
  - Palpable kidney mass/palpable bladder
- Fluid present in the hydronephrotic kidney is not stagnant. It undergoes constant absorption and secretion due to pyelo-lymphatic, pyelo-venous and pyelo-tubular flow.

Investigations

- Blood urea, serum creatinine
- Urine microscopy, routine and culture

Ultrasound

- It is the initial diagnostic study
- The findings of moderate-to-severe hydro-nephrosis of the renal pelvis and calyces without concomitant hydro-ureter are indicative of UPJ obstruction.
- If the UPJ obstruction has existed untreated for some time, a thin renal parenchyma may also be apparent.
- Presence of hydronephrosis along with increased renal resistive index (RRI) more than 0.7 is highly suggestive of UPJ.

Intravenous Urography

- This used to be the investigation of choice in the past but it has been replaced by CT Urography these days.
- The initial finding on IVU is a delayed nephro-gram which may persist for 24 hours or longer
- Delayed gradual filling of the collecting system up to the level of obstruction of the ureter
- Severity of hydronephrosis correlates to the degree and duration of the UPJ obstruction
- Pyelo-sinus extravasations and pyelo-venous backflow may be demonstrated

CT scan

- In UPJ obstruction there is marked delay of the passage of contrast from a markedly dilated renal pelvis proximally to a non-dilated distal ureter
- In severe UPJ obstruction there is no enhance-ment of the affected kidney during the time of the CT scan
- The presence of aberrant crossing renal vessels, an extrinsic cause of UPJ obstruction can be easily demonstrated during 3-D reconstruction of images

Diuretic Renogram

- The gold standard investigation
- The patient should be well hydrated before renogram and bladder should be catheterized for continuous drainage throughout the study
- The MAG-3 diuretic renogram is the gold standard test because the agent is filtered as well as secreted by the renal tubules
- DTPA Scan
  - The DTPA does not measure tubular function as it is only filtered at the glomerulus
  - In an obstructed urinary tract, such as in UPJ obstruction, the excretion and passage of the tracer is delayed
  - At 20 minutes, the furosemide is administered and further images are obtained
  - If the tracer clears with the induced diuresis, obstruction can be excluded
  - If the tracer does not clear and if there is continued accumulation of the tracer and if t1/2 is greater than 20 minutes diagnosis of PUJ obstruction is confirmed
  - The normal t1/2s has been determined to be either 10 or 15 minutes
  - Patients with t1/2s between 10 and 20 minutes are labeled as indeterminate

Whitaker's Test

- This test is used to establish the diagnosis of UPJ obstruction in those cases which are indeterminate
- The Whitaker test requires am intra-pelvic catheter or nephrostomy tube placed by percutaneous puncture and simultaneously measure intra-pelvic and cystometric pressures. Cystometric pressure is measured by bladder catheter

- The fluid is infused via the nephrostomy tube at a flow rate of 10 mL/s, and the resulting pressure gradient between the renal pelvis and the bladder is measured
- Whitaker proposed ranges of normal pressure differential as high as 12 cm water and obstructive pressure differentials greater than 20 cm water

Retrograde Pyelogram

- Useful in detecting the site of obstruction

Treatment

Surgery is aimed at preservation of renal tissue

Indications

- Recurrent renal pain
- Increasing hydronephrosis
- Infection
- Deteriorating renal function

The Pre-operative Drainage of the System

It can be done by placement of an internal ureteric stent or a percutaneous nephrostomy tube

Indications

- Presence of symptoms associated with the obstruction
- Impairment of renal function which can be over all function or unilateral function
- Recurrent urinary tract infections, pyelonephritis
- Development of ipsilateral nephrolithiasis
- Development of hypertension
- If infection is associated with the obstruction
- Azotemia resulting from obstruction in a solitary kidney or bilateral disease
- Patients suffering from severe, unrelenting pain requiring emergent relief of obstruction

Goals of Treatment

- Relief of symptoms
- Preservation or improvement in renal function
- The ultimate goal is to provide a drainage system with unobstructed urinary flow

Approach

- Classified into following categories
  - Open surgical procedures – Pyeloplasty
  - Endoscopic procedures
  - Laparoscopic pyeloplasty
  - Robot assisted pyeloplasty

Endoscopic Procedures

- Involve fullness thickness incision of mucosa of obstructing proximal ureter
- Can be performed by ante-grade or retrograde approach and incision is given up to peri-pelvic and periureteric fat
- Incised ureter is stented to help maintaining patency, helping in healing and preventing extravasation
- A percutaneous approach is indicated in patients having PUJ obstruction associated with pelvicalyceal stones, which can be managed simultaneously
- Contraindications to a percutaneous endopyelotomy include
  - Long segment (>2 cm) of obstruction
  - Active infection
  - Untreated coagulopathy
  - Obstruction of PUJ by crossing vessels.

Open Pyeloplasty

- If PUJ obstruction is associated with involvement of long segment of proximal ureter.
- In patients in whom previous less invasive procedures have failed.
- In situations when less invasive procedure are contraindicated.
- In patients where most important consideration is successful outcome and improvement in renal function like patients with single functioning kidney or in patients who have impaired renal function due to bilateral UPJ.
- Patient with secondary UPJ obstruction.
- UPJ obstruction with crossing aberrant lower polar vessels

Requisites of Successful Pyeloplasty

- Resulting anastomosis should be water tight, tension free and widely patent.
- Resultant anastomosis should result in dependent drainage.
- After reconstruction there should be funnel shaped transition between pelvis and ureter.
- One should avoid loss of functional renal parenchyma and ligation of renal vessels.

Approaches

- Extra peritoneal flank approach: It is the most popular approach to the UPJ. Incision is through the bed of the twelfth rib and provides excellent exposure of the UPJ.

- Anterior extra peritoneal approach: This approach is useful in patients with horseshoe kidneys, or where there is anterior malrotation of the kidney.
- The posterior lumbotomy approach might have role in cases with a significant extra peritoneal component of the UPJ.

Anderson-Hyne's Dismembered Pyeloplasty

- Used regardless of position of insertion ureter in to pelvis i.e. both in high insertion and dependent insertion
- Allows reduction of a redundant pelvis and correction of a tortuous proximal ureter.
- If the obstruction is due to accessory or aberrant lower pole vessels anterior or posterior transposition of the UPJ can be carried out.
- Complete excision of abnormal UPJ itself is only possible in dismembered Pyeloplasty

Foley's Y-V Pyeloplasty

- Described for repair of a UPJ obstruction due to a high ureteric insertion.
- Foley YV-plasty is contraindicated if there are aberrant renal vessels at lower pole which needs transposition.
- If simultaneous reduction of redundant renal pelvis is required then, this technique is not useful.

Culp De Weerd's Spiral Flap Pyeloplasty

- The Culp-DeWeerd's spiral flap Pyeloplasty is indicated in cases of accessible extra-renal pelvis with insertion of ureter in a dependent, oblique position.
- The spiral flap is of significant value if UPJ obstruction is associated with a relatively long segment of proximal ureteric stricture.

Scardino Prince Vertical Flap Pyeloplasty

- Limited clinical application, because it can only be employed only when a dependent UPJ is situated at the medial margin of a large, square ("box-shaped") extra renal pelvis.
- The vertical flap is preferable for relatively long areas of proximal ureteric narrowing

Davis Intubated Ureterostomy

- Described for surgical repair of very long or multiple ureteral strictures.
- May be combined with any of the standard pyeloplasty procedure but preferably with a spiral flap procedure because the spiral flap can be made longer.

Ureterocalycostomy

- When UPJ obstruction or proximal ureteral stricture is associated with a relatively small intra-renal pelvis.
- When the UPJ is associated with rotational anomalies such as horseshoe kidney in order to provide completely dependent drainage.
- Ureterocalycostomy is used as a salvage technique for the failed pyeloplasty.

Post-operative Care

- External drains are removed 24 to 48 hours after urinary drainage has ceased.
- Internal stents if inserted remain in situ for 4 to 6 weeks.
- If a nephrostomy tube is present, a nephrostogram is obtained on 7 to 10 days post-operatively.
- The tube is clamped for 12 to 24 hours and removed if there is no flank pain, fever, or leakage around the tube.

Laparoscopic Pyeloplasty

- First reported in 1993 by Schuessler and associates
- Resembles the steps of the open approach with adherence to identical surgical principles.
- Performed though either a trans-peritoneal or retroperitoneal route.
- The transperitoneal allows a larger working space and the retroperitoneal approach provides more direct access to the UPJ.

Nephrectomy

- If the function of obstructed kidney is less than 10% of total function
- Only done if opposite kidney is normal.

51 Management of Renal Calculi

- Diclofenac sodium is the drug of choice
- Alternate drugs used only if pain persists
- Opioids are associated with increased risk of vomiting
- Prevention of recurrent Colic
  - Diclofenac sodium 50 mg 8 hrly X 7 Days
  - Reduces Inflammation
  - Reduces risk of recurrent pain

Facilitation of Stone Passage (for Lower Ureter)

- Alpha blocking agents, e.g. Tamsulosin (29%)
- Calcium channel blockers (9%)
- Alpha blockers inhibit ureteral basal tone and peristaltic activity
- Dilates ureteric lumen
- Calcium channel blocker reduces ureteric spasm and inhibits fast peristaltic activity

Active Stone Removal

Indications for Active stone removal

- Stone diameter > 7–10 mm
- Adequate pain relief cannot be achieved
- Stone obstruction causing infection
- Pyonephrosis or signs of Urosepsis
- Single kidney with obstruction
- Bilateral obstruction

Modalities for Active Stone Removal

- Extra corporeal shock wave lithotripsy (ESWL)
- Percutaneous Nephrolithotomy (PCNL)
- Open Pyelolithotomy
- Open Nephrolithotomy
- Laparoscopic Pyelolithotomy

Extra Corporeal Shock Wave Lithotripsy (ESWL)

- 1969 – Dornier started a study on effect of shock wave on tissue
- Feb 1980 – HM3 lithotripter introduced
- Many generations of lithotripters
- Modern Lithotripters are smaller and Cheaper
- >80% of simple renal calculi can be treated
- First experimental lithotripter in 1970
- Chaussay et al in 1980 did first successful case in Germany
- Can remove >90% stones
- Outcome depends upon size, number, location and hardness of stones and patient habitus
- Number of ESWL sessions
  - Should not exceed more than 5
- To avoid renal tissue damage and bleeding complications.

Contraindications

- Pregnancy
- Severe spine deformity
- Morbid obesity
- Aortic or renal artery Aneurysm
- Uncontrolled blood coagulation
- Uncontrolled urinary tract infection
- Distal obstruction

- Stone >2 cm or Staghorn calculus (Relative contraindication)

Types of Lithotripter

- Electrohydraulic (spark gap generator)
  - Shock wave produced by underwater spark discharge
  - Short electrode like
  - Produces focused shock wave from an ellipsoid
- Electromagnetic
  - Plain or cylindrical shock wave focused by an acoustic lens
  - Less painful more effective in stone breaking
  - Higher rate of sub capsular hematoma
- Piezolelectric
  - Focused accuracy
  - Longer service life
  - Less discomfort

Mechanism of Stone Breakage

- Spall fracture
- Squeezing- splitting or circumferential splitting
- Shear stress
- Cavitations
- Dynamic fractures

Changes in Kidney During ESWL

- Reversible
  - Mild tubular necrosis
  - Casts and RBC
  - Mild interstitial edema and hemorrhage
- Irreversible changes
  - Disruption of Nephrons
  - Large hematoma – cortex and medulla
  - Fracture of glomerular peritubular arteries
  - Rupture and occlusion of veins and arteries

Optimal shock wave frequency

- 1.0 to 1.5 Hz
- Increase in shock wave frequency causes more tissue damage
- No consensus on number of shock waves per session
- Depends upon the type of lithotripter

Interval between sessions

- Longer for electro hydraulic and electro-magnetic lithotripters
- Shorter for piezoelectric equipment

Stone location vs outcome

- Renal pelvic stones – 85–90% stone free rate
- Upper and middle calyx – 75–80% stone free rate
- Lower calyx – 60% stone free rate

Stone size vs outcome

- Stone < 20 mm – 66–99%
- >20 mm – 45–60 %

Complications

- More complications in stone size more than 20 mm
- Surface area > 300 mm^2
- Pain
- Hydronephrosis
- Fever
- Urosepsis

Double J Stents

- Reduce the obstructive and infective complications
- Especially useful if stone size > 20 mm
- Does not improve outcome in terms of stone free state
- Prevents obstruction and loss of ureteral contraction

Stone composition

- *Harder stones, e.g.:* Calcium oxalate monohydrate and cystiene needs increased number of shock waves at higher intensities
- *Softer stones, e.g.:* Struvite provide good results

Percutaneous Stone Extraction

Historical Aspects

- **1941-** Extracted renal calculus from an operatively established nephrostomy tract (Rubel and Brown).
- **1956 -** Used percutaneous nephrostomy drainage for obstruction and infection (Goodwin).
- **1976 -** Established percutaneous tract for stone removal (Fernstorm and Johansson).

Indications

- Body habitus precluding SWL, e.g. morbid obesity
- Obstruction distal to the stone
- Moderate to large size cysteine stone
- Stones with upper tract foreign body, e.g.- broken DJ dilating balloons

- Large stone with branched calculi.
- Failure of SWL.
- Presence of implanted cardiac defibrillator.
- Transplanted and pelvic kidney.

Preoperative Preparation

- Complete blood count
- Serum electrolytes
- Blood urea/S.creatinine estimation
- Aspirin/antiplatelet drugs to be stopped 7 days prior to surgery
- Urine culture and sensitivity
- CT Urogram or IVU to display stone burden
- Group and cross match blood
- Treat UTI
- First generation cephalosporin given just prior to percutaneous access and continued 24 hours later
- Urethral catheter inserted before puncture

Anesthesia

- General
  - Mandatory for upper pole puncture
  - Best means of protecting the airway when patient is prone
- Spinal
  - If patient is unfit for GA
  - High block needed to relieve all renal pain
  - Vasovagal reaction can occur by distension of pelvis
- Local Anesthesia

Technique-Four Sequential Steps

- Establish percutaneous access – opacification of collecting system is necessary
- Dilate tract
- Stone manipulation with fragmentation and extraction
- Post extraction drainage and tamponade of tract

Opacification of collecting system is necessary

- Necessary for proper location of calcyx
- Preoperativety catheter is inserted to opacify calyceal system
- Also prevents passage of fragments in to ureter
- Allows retrograde irrigation

Patient position

- Prone or slightly oblique with ipsilateral site elevated to 20 degrees
- Patients with rotational anomalies of kidney
- Contralateral side is elevated to allow more medial rotation of anteriorly placed pelvis
- Posterior infundibula and calyces project more laterally
- Supine oblique (elevation of ipsilateral side)
- Patient not tolerating prone position
- For ultrasound guided access (avoids rib generated artifacts)
- CT guided access

Site selection

- Posterior calyx is selected because major vascular renal structures surrounding renal pelvis are avoided
- Transparenchymal route stabilized and nephrostomy catheter inserted
- Direct puncture of renal pelvis avoided to safeguard posterior branch of renal artery
- Medial punctures avoided
- Ideal Site for puncture
  - Site providing shortest tract to renal calyx from below the 12th rib
  - Sub coastal approach
  - Intercostals approach for upper pole of calyx
  - Two plane fluoroscopy to identify accurate size
  - 18 gauge translumbar angiography diamond tipped needle is used for puncture
  - Needle entry confirmed by return of urine from needle
- Guide wire (J wire) passed through the needle into the pelvis
- Tract dilated by dilators (Amplatz dilator) upto 30 F
- Rigid nephroscope used
- Puncture of inferior calyx associated with increased risk of colon injury
- Upper calyceal puncture done only if
  - The stone is predominantly in the upper calyx
  - Horse shoe kidney
  - Supracostal puncture needed

Postoperative Care

- Estimate of volume of irrigation and output should be kept
- Furosemide 10–20 mg i.v. Given at the end of procedure
- I.v. fluids administered for 24 hours to ensure diuresis

- Antibiotics continued for 48–72 hours
- 24–26 Fr nephrostomy tube left in situ.
- Role of nephrostomy tube:
  - Tamponade bleeding from track
  - Allows renal puncture to heal
  - Allows proper drainage of urine
  - Allows secondary PNL if required
- Nephrostogram done at day 1–2 to look for any residual calculus

Complications

- 1.1 to 7% major and 11–25% minor complications associated
- Include:
  - Bleeding
  - Intra/extraperitoneal extravasation of irrigation fluid
- Injury to liver or spleen
- Hydro/hemopneumothorax
- Duodenal/colonic injury
- Perforation of renal pelvis and ureter

Open Surgery

- With Advances in ESWL and PCNL open surgery is needed in only –5.4 % of cases

Indications

- Complex stone burden
- Treatment failure of ESWL and PCNL
- Morbid obesity
- Skeletal deformity, contractures and fixed deformities of hips and legs
- Comorbid medical disease
- Concomitant open surgery
- Non-functioning lower pole
- Non-functioning kidney
- Patient's choice
- Stone in ectopic kidney
- Intrarenal anatomical abnormalities
  - Infundibular stenosis
  - Stone in calyceal diverticulum
  - Obstruction of ureteropelvic junction

Operative Procedures

- Simple and extended pyelolithotomy
- Pyelolithotomy
- Nephrolithotomy
- Based on historical experience open surgery is thought to be superior in terms of stone free rate.

52 | Malignant Neoplasms of the Kidney

Renal Cell Carcinoma (RCC)

Incidence

- Affects 2–3% of all adult malignancies
- More common in Urban dwellers and males
- In patients with Von Hippel-Lindau disease there is high incidence of renal cell carcinoma
- More common in sixth to seventh decades
- Acquired cystic disease in CRF patient having long term dialysis, have high incidence.

Etiology

- Arises from proximal convoluted tubule
- Tobacco smokers
- Industrial contaminants of cadmium
- Colloidal thorium dioxide
- Diethylstilbestrol.

Cytogenetics

- Deletions and translocation involving the short arm of chromosome 3 (3p)
- Molecular activation of proto-oncogenes
- Overexpression of *c-myc* and epidermal growth factor receptor (EGRF) (*c-erb B-1*) mRNA and
- Under-expression of HER-2 (*erb B-2*) mRNA
- Both TGF alpha and EGRF are overexpressed in RCC.

Multidrug Resistance (MDR)

- RCC is a chemotherapy resistant tumour.

- MDR appears to be related P-glyco-protein, P 170 encoded by the MDR1 gene, which is an energy dependent drug efflux pump for hydrophobic compounds, e.g. chemotherapy drugs
- Glutathione detoxification mechanism seen in RCC.
- Reduced topoisomerase activity in RCC.

Histological Subtypes

- Conventional (70–80%) Clear cell, granular cell and mixed. Arise from PCT
- Chromophilic (10–15%) in acquired renal cystic disease from PCT
- Chromophobic (3–5%) from intercalated cells of collecting duct
- Collecting duct type (from collecting duct): may respond to chemotherapy
- Unclassified.

Pathology

- Varies in size
- Unilateral or bilateral
- Pseudocapsule
- Cut section
  - Variegated appearance
  - Areas of yellowish or brownish soft tumor interposed sclerotic bifrontal areas
  - Patches of necrosis and hemorrhage
- Clear cell, granular cell, tubulopapillary and sarcomatoid

- Tumor thrombus
- Calcification.

Clinical Presentation

- Asymptomatic
- Classic triad of
  - Flank pain
  - Gross hematuria
  - Abdominal mass (too late triad)
- Symptoms due to metastases
- Weight loss, fever, night sweats and sudden development of a varicocele
- Para-neoplastic syndrome
- Stauffer's syndrome. RCC with altered liver function test.

Prognostic Factors

- Pathologic stage, tumor size and nuclear grade
- Nuclear ploidy
- Renal vein involvement, extension to regional lymph nodes, extension through Gerota's fascia, involvement of contiguous organs and distant metastases.

Robson's Staging of RCC

I	Tumor within capsule
II	Tumor invasion of perinephric fat (confined to Gerota's fascia)
III	Tumor involvement of regional LN and/or Renal Vein or IVC
IV	Adjacent organs or distant metastases
TNM	Classification of RCC
Tx	Primary tumor cannot be assessed
T0	No evidence of primary tumor
T1	Tumor <7 cm in greatest dimension limited to the kidney
T2	Tumor >7 cm in greatest dimension limited to the kidney
T3a	Tumor invades adrenal gland or perinephric tissues but not beyond Gerota's fascia
T3b	Tumor extends into RV or IVC below diaphragm
T3c	Tumor extends into IVC above diaphragm or wall of IVC
T4	Tumor invades beyond Gerota's fascia
NX	Regional LN cannot be assessed
N0	No regional LN metastases
N1	Metastases in a single LN
N2	Metastases in multiple LN

MX	Presence of distant metastases cannot be assessed
M0	No distant metastases
M1	Distant metastases.

AJCC Stage Grouping

Stage 1	T1N0M0
Stage 2	T2N0M0
Stage 3	T1-2 N1M0
	T3N0-1 M0
Stage 4	T4 N0-1M0
	Any T N2,M0
	any T any N with M1.

5 Year Survival

Stage 1 – 75%
Stage 2 – 63%
Stage 3 – 38%
Stage 4 – 11%

Five year survival rates of 47% to 69% have been reported after complete surgical resection of renal tumors with IVC involvement in patients with no evidence of metastatic disease.

Investigations

- Renal biopsy/FNAC unnecessary due to
  - High false negative rate
  - Potential sampling error
  - Potential risk of tumor seeding
  - Difficulty in interpreting small biopsy sample/ FNAC.

Role of Biopsy

- With history of other primary malignances
- Patients with metastatic disease with unknown primary
- To find out if renal mass is primary or metastatic
- If there is suspicion of renal abscess, or lymphoma.

CT Scan

- Accurate staging (90% accuracy)
- Function of opposite kidney can be assessed
- Involvement of IVC and renal veins can be detected.
- Limitation of defining cephalic extension in IVC
- Supplemented with Doppler ultrasound
- Enhancement after IV contrast more than 15 Hounsefield unit is diagnostic of RCC.
- Helps in staging of RCC.

MRI

Indications

- Contrast allergy
- Renal function impairment
- Equivocal finding in CT
- More accurate in T3a and T4
  - Cannot assess function of opposite kidney.
- MRI is superior to CT is assessing IVC involvement.

Angiogram

No role except

- In pre-operative vascular mapping for nephron sparing surgery
- Before angiography infarction of large tumors.

Chest X-ray/CT Thorax

Plain X-ray chest in all cases

CT chest only if

- Patient with chest symptoms
- Single pulmonary nodule on X-ray and resection planned
- As a part of protocol for experimental immune or chemotherapy.

Treatment

Localized RCC - Surgical Treatment

- Radical nephrectomy
- Laparoscopic radical nephrectomy
- Renal-sparing surgery
- Laparoscopic partial nephrectomy
- Laparoscopic cryo ablation.

FDG PET Scan

- Useful in monitoring response to systemic therapy in patients with metastatic disease
- More accurate than CT in detecting recurrence or progression.
- No role in initial work up.

Radical Nephrectomy

- Standard treatment
- Trans peritoneal approach
- Early ligation of renal pedicle
- En block removal of kidney, peri-renal fat, Gerota's fascia and upper ureter (1/3rd)
- Adrenal only removed if
  - Pre operative CT shows involvement of adrenal
  - Involvement found on table

- Tumor in Upper pole
- Tumor more than 5 cm
- Extensive lymphadenectomy not indicated
  - Except in high tumor grade, sarcomatoid component, histological tumor necrosis, tumor size >10cm or T3 or T4 tumor if two or more of above factors are present.

Laparoscopic Radical Nephrectomy

Indications

- Less than 8–10 cm
- No local invasion
- No renal vein involvement
- No lymphadenopathy.

Partial Nephrectomy

- Bilateral renal tumors
- Malignancy in solitary functioning kidney
- Patients who have risk of renal failure in long term
- Hypertensive patients
- Recurrent renal stone disease
- Diabetics.

Laparoscopic Cryoablation

- Tumor less than 3 cm
- Kidney mobilized laparoscopically
- Cryo probe inserted in tumor
- Cryo ablation by liquid nitrogen or argon IVC Extension of RCC
- Radical nephrectomy with thrombectomy
- The 3 year survival rate was 64% with an operative mortality of 4.7% (Novick et al. 1990).
- Cardiopulmonary bypass for supra-diaphragmatic thrombus.

Locally Invasive RCC

- Surgical excision of the tumor including excision of the involved bowel, spleen or abdominal wall muscle
- Role of radiotherapy is controversial
- Immunotherapy for residual tumor
- Angioinfarction.

Metastatic RCC

- Chemotherapy - Combination of 5-FU with IL-2 and alpha interferon has a response rate of 46% with 15% complete response. Angiogenesis inhibitors have a potential role.
- Hormonal therapy - ineffective
- Immunotherapy - alpha interferon and IL-2

- Surgery
  - Adjunctive nephrectomy
    ◊ Excision of solitary metastases
    ◊ 24.3% responded to interferon after nephrectomy compared with 8.3% who did not have prior nephrectomy (UCLA data 1990)
  - Palliative nephrectomy
    ◊ Severe hemorrhage
    ◊ Severe pain
    ◊ Paraneoplasic syndrome
    ◊ Compression of adjacent viscera.

Gene therapy of RCC

- Genetically engineered tumor infiltrating lymphocytes (TIL)
- Tumor cell vaccine.

Chemotherapy

- No role in metastatic clear cell carcinoma
- May have some effect in non clear cell carcinoma or tumors with sarcomatoid change
- Gemcitabine and doxorubicin have some activity.

Urothelial Tumors

Epidemiology

- 10% of all renal tumors
- 5% of all urothelial tumors
- Associated with Balkan nephropathy
- Risk factors
  - Smoking
  - Coffee drinking
  - Analgesics - Phenacetin
  - Occupational factors - chemical, petro-chemical and plastic industries

  - Chronic infection
  - Cyclophosphamide.

Pathology

- Transitional cell carcinoma - 90%
- Squamous cell carcinoma - 0.7 to 7%. Frequently associated with infected staghorn calculi of long-term duration
- Adenocarcinoma - <1%. Associated with calculi, obstruction and inflammation.

Pattern of Spread

- Epithelial spread
- Lymphatic extension
- Hematogenous dissemination.

Diagnosis

Clinical presentation

- Hematuria
- Flank pain.

Imaging

- CT Urography
  - Filling defect in the renal pelvis with contrast enhancement
- Ultrasonography is imaging modality for initial evaluation
- Magnetic resonance imaging of CT contra-indicated
- Cytopathology by
  - Ureteroscopy and nephroscopy
- Metastatic evaluation:
  - Cystoscopy in all patients rule out transitional cell carcinoma of urinary bladder.

Treatment

- Total nephroureterectomy.

53 Congenital Anomalies of the Kidney

DEVELOPMENT OF KIDNEY

- Metanephric blastema develops into adult renal parenchyma, while the ureteric bud gives rise to the collecting system.
- The presence and orderly branching of a ureteric bud is needed for development of kidney.
- There is simultaneous medial rotation of the collecting system that occurs with renal migration.
- Kidney and renal pelvis normally rotate 90 degrees ventrally and medially during ascent of the kidney.

Classification

Anomalies of number

- Agenesis
  - Bilateral
  - Unilateral
- Supernumerary kidney

Anomalies of Volume and Structure

- Hypoplasia
- Multicystic kidney
- Polycystic kidney which can be of infantile and adult type.
- Other cystic disease
- Medullary cystic disease

Anomalies of Ascent

- Simple ectopia
- Cephalic ectopia
- Thoracic kidney
- Crossed ectopia

Anomalies of Rotation

- Incomplete
- Excessive
- Reverse

Anomalies of Form and Fusion

- Crossed ectopia with and without fusion
- Unilateral fused kidney (inferior ectopia)
- Sigmoid or S-shaped kidney
- L-shaped kidney
- Unilateral fused kidney (superior ectopia)
- Horse-shoe kidney

Anomalies of the Collecting System

- Calyceal diverticulum
- Hydrocalyx
- Megacalycosis
- Unipapillary kidney
- Extrarenal calyces
- Extrarenal pelvis
- Bifid pelvis

Anomalies of Renal Vasculature

- Aberrant, accessory or multiple vessels
- Renal artery aneurysm
- Arteriovenous fistula

Horse-shoe Kidney

- Most common of all renal fusion anomalies

- It consists of two distinct renal masses connected at their respective lower poles by a band which can be made of parenchyma or fibrous tissue which crosses the mid line of the body
- It was first described during an autopsy by Da Carpi in 1522
- In 1564 Botallo gave first extensive description of a horseshoe kidney
- Horseshoe shaped kidney is seen in 0.25% of population, i.e. about 1 in 400 people
- More common in males with male to female ratio more than 2:1
- In 95 percent of cases kidney are joined at their lower poles before their rotation on long axis. As a result pelvis and ureter are anteriorly placed and cross in front of the isthmus
- In small subset of cases kidneys are joined at upper poles
- Upward migration of horseshoe kidneys is generally incomplete and kidneys lie lower down in the abdomen. It is presumed that full ascend is prevented by obstruction of movement of isthmus by inferior mesenteric artery
- Parenchymatous isthmus has its own blood supply
- Isthmus is located near L3 or L4 just below the origin of inferior mesenteric artery
- Isthmus passes in front of aorta and vena cava but it can pass between aorta and inferior vena cava as well
- One third of all patients remain asymptomatic
- Symptoms if present are related to hydro-nephrosis, infection, or calculus formation
- There may be vague abdominal pain which may radiate to the lower lumbar region
- Rovsing's sign may be present which is elicited by appearance of abdominal pain, nausea, and vomiting on hyperextension of the spine
- Episodes of urinary tract infection occur in 30% of cases
- Five percent to 10% detected after palpation of an abdominal mass
- Most of the times horseshoe shaped kidney is discovered incidentally during the course of investigation for some other pathology.

Bilateral Renal Agenesis

- Bilateral renal agenesis (BRA) or complete absence of the kidneys is a common lethal malformation occurring in 1 in 5000 births
- It is twice as common in males as females
- BRA appears to have a predominantly genetic etiology and many cases represent the most severe manifestation of an autosomal dominant condition with incomplete penetrance and variable expressivity
- Leads to oligo-hydroamnios, pulmonary Hypoplasia and Potter's syndrome.

Hypoplasia

Hypoplasia means kidney has lesser number of nephrons or calyces but normally functioning and not dysplastic or embryonic. The kidneys are morphologically normal with either reduced number of nephrons or smaller size of nephrons but with normal nephron density. Hypoplasia may be unilateral or bilateral. In unilateral cases the other kidney shows compensatory hypertrophy. Hypo plastic kidneys have ectopic ureteric orifices.

Anomalies of Differentiation of Renal Tissue

- Dysplasia is defined as maldevelopment of the kidney that may affect the size, shape or structure. Basically dysplasia is a histo-pathological diagnosis characterized by presence of embryonic, immature, mesenchymal tissue and embryonic renal components
  - Total
  - Unilateral
  - Bilateral
  - Segmental
  - Focal
- Polycystic disease
  - Adult type (autosomal dominant)
  - Infantile type (autosomal recessive) is associated with hepatic cystic disease associated with congenital hepatic fibrosis
- Simple cysts
- Multilocular cysts
- Medullary cysts
  - Sponge kidney
  - Medullary cystic disease with uremia (Autosomal dominant)
- Other developmental cysts (acquired)

54 | Genitourinary Trauma

- Genitourinary (GU) trauma, because of its often non-life-threatening nature and subtle presentation, is often overlooked and poorly recognized in the emergency department. However, approximately 10–20% of all injured patients have some kind of GU involvement which can lead to very debilitating long term sequelae such as incontinence and impotence
- Although the more life-threatening injuries of the primary survey must be addressed first, however one should be alert to the clues pointing to the presence of GU injuries
- One should have a complete understanding of GU injuries, how to deal with it and how it can impact patient outcome.

Urethral trauma is described in chapter of urethral injuries.

Bladder Trauma

- Adult bladder is an extraperitoneal organ
- Bladder dome is the weakest point
- *Blunt* trauma is the most common cause seen in 60–85% of the cases
- *Motor vehicular accident* is the no. 1 cause of bladder trauma
- Important to recognize
- Undiagnosed bladder rupture can lead to
  - Pelvic/abdominal wall abscess/necrosis
  - Peritonitis
  - Intra-abdominal abscess
  - Sepsis/death

- Types of rupture
  - Extraperitoneal
  - Most commonly associated with pelvic fracture (80–100%)
  - Bladder rupture occurs in 5–10% of all pelvic fractures.
  - Intraperitoneal
  - Extravasation of urine in abdomen
  - Sudden force on full bladder
  - Associated injuries must be ruled out
  - Mortality (20%)

Iatrogenic injuries to bladder during pelvic operations or during endoscopic procedures can also occur.

- Investigations
  - *Cystography:* Gold standard
  - *CT Cystography*
- Treatment
  - *Penetrating injuries:* Operative repair
  - *Blunt:*
  - *Intraperitoneal:* Almost all cases need surgical repair
  - *Extraperitoneal:* Urethral catheter drainage kept for 7–10 days.

Kidney Injury

- Retroperitoneal organ
- Cushioned by perinephric fat
- Gerota's fascia
- Along T10 – L4 vertebral level

- Ribs 10–12 lie anteriorly
- Fixed only through pedicle
- 1.2L of blood/min
- *Blunt trauma:* 80–90%
- Rapid deceleration/direct blow
- MUST be suspected if
  - Trauma to back/flank/lower thorax/upper abdomen
  - Flank pain/low rib fracture
  - Hematuria/Ecchymosis over the flanks
  - Sudden deceleration/fall from height
  - Lumbar transverse process fracture.

Classification (Fig. 54.1)

- Organ injury scaling committee
- Grade I
  - Contusion
  - Hematuria
  - Urologic studies normal
  - Hematoma
  - Subcapsular
  - Non expanding
  - Parenchyma normal
- Grade II
  - Hematoma
  - Perirenal
  - Nonexpanding
  - Laceration
  - < 1.0 cm
  - Renal cortex only
  - No urinary extravasation
- Grade III
  - Laceration
  - > 1.0 cm
  - Renal cortex only
  - No urinary extravasation
  - Intact collecting system

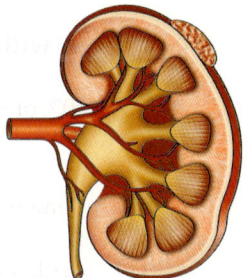

Grade I: Subcapsular, nonexpanding hematoma without parenchymal laceration

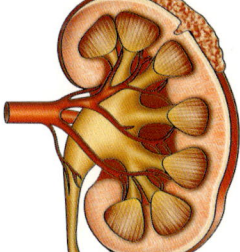

Grade II: Laceration of <1 cm parenchymal depth of renal cortex without urinary extravasation

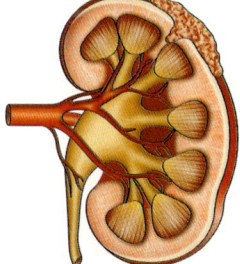

Grade III: Laceration of >1 cm parenchymal depth of renal cortex without collecting system rupture or urinary extravasation

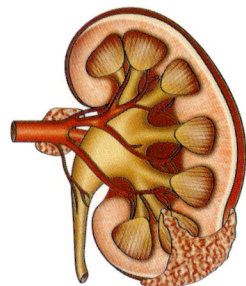

Grade IV: Parenchymal laceration extending through renal cortex, medulla, and collecting system or vascular main renal vessel injury with a contained hemorrhage

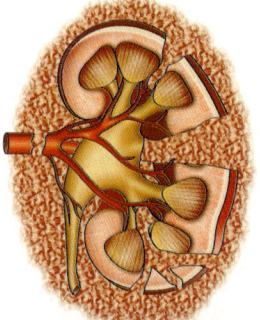

Grade V: Completely shattered kidney or vascular avulsion of renal hilum leading to devascularization of the kidney

Fig. 54.1: Grades of renal trauma

- Grade IV
  - Laceration
  - Renal cortex
  - Renal medulla
  - Collecting system
  - Vascular
  - Main renal artery/vein injury with contained hemorrhage
- Grade V
  - Completely shattered kidney.
  - Avulsion of renal hilum (pedicle) which devascularizes kidney
- Need for surgery; nephrectomy rates:
  - *Grade I:* 0; 0%
  - *Grade II:* 15; 0%
  - *Grade III:* 76; 3%
  - *Grade IV:* 78; 9%
  - *Grade V:* 93; 86%.

Investigations

- IVP
  - Used to be initial investigation of choice
  - Very poor sensitivity for penetrating injury
  - Limitation in staging renal injuries
  - Not the 1st choice anymore. Done only if patient unstable

- Contrast enhanced CT
  - Study of choice if stable
  - More sensitive and specific for staging
  - Detects other abdominal injuries.

Management

- Penetrating trauma:
  - Imaging for ALL (9% have NO hematuria)
- *Blunt trauma Imaging:*
  - Gross hematuria
  - Microscopic hematuria (>5 RBC/hpf) + shock (BP (systolic) < 90 mmHg)
  - Any child with > 50 RBC/hpf
- Absolute indication for surgery:
  - Uncontrollable renal hemorrhage
  - Multiply lacerated, shattered kidney
  - Main renal vessels avulsed
  - Penetrating injuries
- Grade I-II
  - Conservative
- Grade III-IV
  - Conservative if stable hemodynamically vs. surgery
- Grade V
  - Surgery.

55 | Urethral Injuries

- *Traumatic:* There is a history of blow to the perineum due to fall on projecting object. In modern days cycling accidents, falling in open manhole covers and gymnasium accidents due to fall from beam accounts for number of cases. It can occur in association with multisystem trauma like road traffic or industrial accidents. Fracture pelvis especially straddle fracture involving all four pubic rami are generally associated with urethral injuries. In about 10% of males and 6% of females sustaining fracture pelvis have associated urethral injuries.

  Posterior urethral in males is more commonly involved because it is densely adherent to pubis by urogenital diaphragm and pubo-prostatic ligaments. In children urethral injuries more commonly involve bladder neck because prostate is rudimentary in paediatric age group.
- Iatrogenic

Traumatic Strictures

- Blunt trauma
  - Pelvic fracture
  - Blow to the perineum
  - Falling astride
- Penetrating trauma

Iatrogenic Strictures

- Open surgery
- Traumatic catheterisation
- Insufflation of balloon in urethra
- Post endoscopy

Classification

- Urethral mucosal tear
- Partial rupture
- Complete rupture with
  - Minor distraction
  - Major distraction

  Clinical features: Patients usually present with
1. Retention of urine
2. Perineal haematoma
3. Bleeding from the external meatus
4. Classical finding of high riding prostate or a butter fly perineal haematoma may be frequently absent.

  Retrograde urethrogram (RGU): When blood at the urethral meatus is detected after trauma, immediate RG to rule out urethral injury can be done. To perform RGU small bore 16 F catheter is placed in to the fossa navicularis up to 1 cm after lubrication and balloon is inflated with 1 cc of water.

Management

In females with patients of urethral disruption due to pelvic fractures immediate primary repair or at least realignment of urethra over a catheter is indicated to avoid future urethra-vaginal fistula or urethral obliteration. Delayed reconstruction in female urethral injury should be avoided as female urethra is very short and likely to get embedded in scar if one waits for 6 weeks.

In male patients immediate supra-pubic tube placement is standard of care in men with posterior urethral injuries.

Associated pelvic ring fractures undergoes early surgical fixation.

Appropriate and adequate analgesics, e.g. NSAID are given and patient discouraged from passing urine if urethral injury is suspected. If the bladder is full and palpable percutaneous supra-pubic catheter is inserted to avoid extravasation of urine. A course of prophylactic antibiotics is started.

Injudicious urethral catheterization should be avoided as it converts a partial tear in to complete tear.

In presence of complete obstruction end to end urethroplasty can be performed 6 weeks post trauma and patient followed by regularly.

Complications

- Stricture formation (Fig. 55.1)
- *Erectile dysfunction:* Some degree of erectile is noted in 82% of cases with pelvic fractures and urethral injuries although average reported rate is 50%. Aetiology can be due to cavernous nerve injury, arterial insufficiency, venous leak or direct corporeal injury.
- Incontinence
  - Due to damage to external sphincter
  - Bladder neck injuries
- Fistula
  - Urethro-rectal
  - Urethro-cutaneous
- Peri-urethral complications
  - Urine extravasation
  - Periurethral abscess
  - Necrotising fasciitis of perineum
  - Pelvic abscess

Clinical Presentation

Urethral injuries should be suspected in any patient with blunt or penetrating trauma to:
- Lower abdomen
- Perineum
- External genitalia
- With pelvic fracture

The common presenting features are:
- Urethral bleeding
- Inability to void
- Scrotal hematoma in bulbar urethral injuries
- Acute urinary retention with palpable bladder
- Inability to palpate prostate on per rectal examination in major complete distraction injuries.

Investigations

- Retrograde urethrogram
- IVU
  - Excludes renal injuries
  - If bladder is present in pelvis and inverted tear drop in shape, it denotes partial injury or complete injury with minor distraction
  - If bladder is displaced out of pelvis and normal in shape it denotes complete urethral injury with major distraction.

Management

- Analgesics
- Prophylactic antibiotics
- Patient is discouraged from passing urine to prevent urinary extravasation

Bulbar Urethral Injuries

- Initially suprapubic cystostomy is performed
- Descending urethrogram is done at 14 days post injury

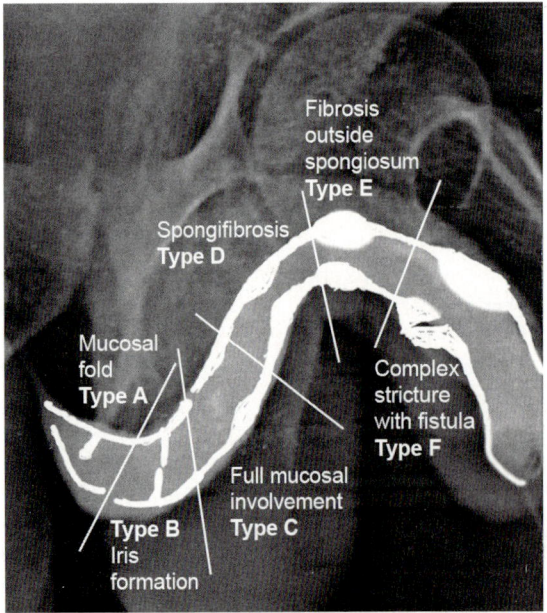

Fibrosis outside spongiosum
Type E

Spongifibrosis
Type D

Mucosal fold
Type A

Complex stricture with fistula
Type F

Full mucosal involvement
Type C

Type B
Iris formation

Fig. 55.1: RGU showing different types of urethral stricture

- If urethra is patent and there is not extravasation, SPC may be removed and patient followed up
- If the urethra is patent but extravasation is present the study is repeated after 2 weeks.

Drawbacks of Railroading

- Difficult surgery with bleeding from pelvic hematoma
- Increased incidence of erectile dysfunction and incontinence
- High stricture rate

Extravasation of Urine

- Superficial
  - Occurs in complete rupture of bulbar urethra or rupture of urethral abscess
  - Extravasation occurs in the deep layer of superficial fascia in the abdominal wall or in the scrotum and penis

- Extravasation is confined to
  - Mid perineal point by attachment of Colles' fascia to triangular ligament
  - To upper part of thigh by attachment of Scarpa's fascia just below the inguinal ligament
  - External spermatic fascia prevents it from entering into the inguinal canal
- Deep extravasation
  - Occurs in
    - Extraperitoneal rupture of bladder
    - Rupture of prostatic or membranous urethra
    - Perforation of prostatic capsule during transurethral resection of prostate
  - It occurs in the layers of pelvic fascia and retroperitoneal tissue
  - Treated by SPC drainage and drainage of retropubic space

56 Undescended Testis

A testis that halts in the path of normal descent.

Development of Testis and its Descent

- Bipotential gonad is present in gonadal ridge
- *Week 6–7:* SRY gene activates and differentiates the bipotential gonad into testis
- *Week 8–9:*
  - Sertoli cells produce Müllerian inhibitory factor (MIF) that cause regression of Müllerian structures
  - Leydig cells produce testosterone that guides the development of Wolffian structures
- *Third trimester:* Multifactorial descent of testis from near deep inguinal ring to scrotum
- Gubernaculum testis
  - Mucofibrous structure with base at scrotum and apex at testis and epididymis
  - *Outgrowth phase:*
    ◊ Mediated by insulin like factor-3
    ◊ The gubernaculum swells and in the process dilating the inguinal canal creating pathway for testicular descent
  - *Regression phase:*
    ◊ Gubernaculum undergoes cellular remodeling and becomes a fibrous structure rich in collagen and elastin fibers
    ◊ Gubernaculum provides pathway for the testicular descent, but it does not actively participate in testicular descent by pulling the testis as it is deficient in smooth or striated muscle fibers
- Mechanical and anatomic factors actively are involved in testicular descent:
  - Increased intra-abdominal pressure
  - Patent processus vaginalis
- Other factors contributing to testicular descent
  - Androgens contribute to testicular descent
  - Estrogens have an inhibitory role on testicular descent. Mothers exposed to diethylstilbestrol (DES) have increased incidence of cryptorchidism. The estrogens have such an effect through inhibition of insulin like factor-3
  - Epidermal growth factor induces placental gonadotropin release. This stimulates fetal testis to produce 'descendin' — an androgen independent growth factor
  - MIF causes regression of Mullerian structures which if present may cause mechanical obstruction in testicular descent
  - Calcitonin gene-related peptide (CGRP), secreted by genitofemoral nerve in rats under influence of androgens, causes contraction of cremasteric muscles and gubernaculum to aid in testicular descent. In humans, however, as gubernaculum is separate from cremaster, the role remains controversial
  - Role of epididymis in testicular descent is uncertain. Some researchers believe that gubernaculum is attached to epididymis,

which in turn takes testis with it. The incidence of epididymal anomalies associated with UDT is about 50%

Classification

See Fig. 56.1.

Differential Diagnosis

Ectopic Testis

A testis that has deviated from the path of normal descent. It may be present in inguinal region, femoral canal, perineum, penopubic area, or even contralateral hemiscrotum (called transverse testicular ectopia).

Retractile Testis

A normally descended testis that ascends by the action of cremasteric muscle. Such a testis can be pulled down into the scrotum and rests there without traction for sometime.

Acquired Undescended Testis

A testis that was once palpable in the scrotum (confirmed by palpation on an earlier occasion), that cannot be brought down into the scrotum without tension any longer is called ascended UDT. Such a condition may be due to retractile testis or secondary to inguinal surgery.

Vanishing Testis

An absent testis due to antenatal or perinatal torsion and resultant gangrene. When unilateral it results in monorchia, when bilateral it results in anorchia. Biopsy of the nubbin of tissue at the end of testicular vessels and vas will show hemosiderin and calicification.

Incidence

- At birth
  - *Premature boys:* 30%
  - *Full-term boys:* 3%
- At age 1 year: 1%
- Rate of secondary ascended testis among retractile testis has been reported between 2% and 45%
- *Palpable:* 2/3 to 3/4 of all UDT. Most of these lie either in inguinal canal or just distal to external inguinal ring
- *Associated anomalies:* Patent processus vaginalis, epididymal anomalies, and rarely, hypospadias, posterior urethral valves, prune belly syndrome and abnormalities of the upper tract
- Incidence of the UDT is reported to be on the rise due to environmental and lifestyle exposures to estrogens

Diagnosis

History

- Unilateral or bilateral absence of testis from scrotum
- Presence of swelling in inguinal region
- Pain in the inguinal region
- May present with trauma/torsion or tumor
- History of presence of testis on an earlier occasion suggests retractile testis as the cremasteric reflex is absent in first 2 years of life

Examination

- Examination to be done in warm environment as cold may stimulate cremasteric reflex and make testis impalpable
- Examine the boy in supine and cross-legged frog like position
- Look for the testis in the inguinal region. Gently run the fingers down the inguinal canal (may use jelly or powder for lubrication) to push subcutaneous tissue and feel for the testis. Slight pressure on mid-abdomen will increase intra-abdominal pressure and increase chances of palpation of testis

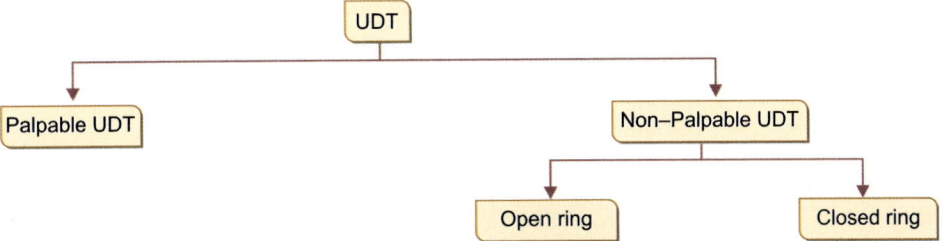

Fig. 56.1: Classification of UDT for the purpose of management

- In retractile/vanishing testis the scrotum will be normal while in UDT the hemiscrotum will be hypoplastic
- In monorchia, the contralateral testis will be hypertrophied

HCG Stimulation Test

- HCG stimulation test helps to differentiate bilateral UDT from anorchia
- Baseline testosterone, follicle-stimulating hormone (FSH), and luteinizing hormone (LH) levels are measured before administration of 2000 IU of hCG daily for 3 days, with a testosterone level determined on day 6
  - If the baseline FSH level is elevated (3 SD above the mean) in a boy younger than 9 years, anorchia is likely and no further evaluation is recommended
  - If baseline LH and FSH levels are normal and hCG stimulation results in an appropriate elevation of testosterone, testicular tissue is likely present and the patient should undergo exploration
  - If the testosterone level does not increase in response to hCG stimulation, testicular tissue may still be present and exploration should be performed
- The hCG stimulation test does not indicate whether testes or functioning testicular remnants are present

Radiological Investigations

- Ultrasound and MRI have been utilized in patients with impalpable testis, with varied accuracy. These investigations may have some role in obese patients in whom examination is difficult, but no definite advantage over clinical examination in other patients
- MR Angiography, with Gadolinium, has shown to be best radiological investigation for the purpose

Diagnostic Laparoscopy

- Diagnostic laparoscopy has >95% accuracy in defining the position of impalpable testis or confirming the absence of testis and is the investigation of choice for impalpable testis

Complications of UDT

- Infertility
  - A blunted normal testosterone surge at 60 to 90 days may result in a lack of Leydig cell proliferation and delay in transformation of gonocytes to adult dark spermatogonia. Histopathologic changes include a decrease in the ratio of spermatogonia per tubule and Leydig cell atrophy
  - Surgery at 9 months age has shown to preserve histological features of normal testis
  - Paternity rate in patients with unilateral UDT are similar to that in normal population
  - Patients with bilateral UDT, even on early surgery, result in only 50–65% paternity rate
- Malignancy
  - 50 to 60 times greater risk of developing testis
  - 1% of inguinal and 5% of intra-abdominal testis develop malignancy
  - 15–20% of testicular tumors develop in normally descended contralateral testis
  - Seminoma develops in uncorrected UDT while non-seminomatous germ cell tumors develop in UDT that have been corrected
  - Risk of developing malignancy is more if the corrective surgery is done after 10 years of age
  - Mechanism — two theories
    ◊ Raised intra-abdominal temperature acting as carcinogenic agent. This theory is supported by lesser incidence in testes in which orchiopexy is done at an early age
    ◊ Underlying genetic or hormonal defect causing cryptorchidism also causes malignancy. The support of this theory comes from the fact that even contralateral normally descended testis in patients with UDT is at higher risk of malignancy
- Other complications
  - Trauma
  - Torsion

Treatment

Indications

- Reduce the risk of malignancy
- Preserve fertility potential
- Reduce risk of torsion
- Allows easy examination of testis, if malignancy develops
- Improves endocrine function of testis
- For normal appearing scrotum

Timing

- Following factors guide timing of surgery
  - The chances of spontaneous descent after 1 year of age is negligible
  - The anesthetic risk for general anesthesia is reduced beyond 6 months of age
  - The chances of malignancy or infertility can be reduced by early surgery
  - The tissues are delicate in infancy, with testicular vessels at risk during dissection in spermatic cord
- Thus, the optimum time for orchiopexy is at or around 1 year of age
- Earlier surgery may be done if associated hernia is symptomatic

Hormonal Treatment

- HCG and Buserelin (a LHRH agonist) are used extensively in Europe for managing UDT
- These have shown success in treatment of low UDT (at or distal to external inguinal ring). The hormonal management is also successful in managing retractile testis
- Success rate of about 60% have been documented

Surgical Treatment

Palpable UDT

- Palpable unilateral or bilateral UDT are managed by orchiopexy

Steps of Orchiopexy

- The surgery is done under general anesthesia, often as a day care procedure
- A caudal block or ilio-inguinal block provides good post-operative analgesia
- The procedure is done through an inguinal incision over the internal ring along the Langer's line
- External oblique aponeurosis is opened in the line of fibers opening the external ring
- The spermatic cord dissection is done to perform high inguinal herniotomy. A 'high' herniotomy adequately mobilizes the testis so that it can be placed in scrotum without tension
- Retroperitoneal dissection may provide additional mobilization
- Prentiss' maneuver may be required for further reducing the tension. In this procedure, the spermatic cord is rerouted medial to the inferior epigastric vessels, thus medializing the internal ring

- Subcutaneous tunnel is created from inguinal region to scrotum. Space is created in the scrotum by blunt dissection
- A subdartos pouch is created in the dependent portion of the scrotum
- A clamp is then placed on the surgeon's finger in this scrotal incision, and its tip is guided into the inguinal canal by withdrawing the finger. The clamp is then used to grasp the adventitial tissue around the testis
- The clamp is then pulled back to guide the testis into the pouch. The mobilized testis is then fixed in the scrotal subdartos pouch by closing the neck of the sac or suture through the tunica vaginalis
- A suture through tunica albuginea is discouraged as it may induce testicular inflammation, damage intra-testicular blood supply and cause infertility risk. The testis remains in the scrotum by scarring with the everted tunica vaginalis which also reduces risk of torsion
- Biopsy of the testis for prognosticating about the risk of infertility/diagnosing carcinoma *in situ* may be done
- The wounds are closed in layers
- The procedure can also be done through a single high scrotal incision

Follow-up and Outcome

- The patient is seen 1 week later for wound healing and several months later for testicular examination
- The potential complications of this surgery are
  - Atrophy
  - Retraction
  - Hernia is a rare complication, more often seen in single high scrotal incision approach
- Orchiopexy has shown to have >95% success rate in several studies

Non-Palpable UDT

- About 18% of non-palpable UDT will become palpable when examined after induction
- Non-palpable UDT can be managed by open inguinal exploration or laparoscopy. We prefer diagnostic laparoscopy so that the blood supply to testis from cremaster can be reserved if staged orchiopexy is required

- Diagnostic laparoscopy may reveal
  - Vas and vessels entering the deep ring — this suggests that the testis is in inguinal canal. Inguinal exploration and orchiopexy should be done.
  - Atretic vessels and vas ending blindly — the testis had undergone torsion and is atrophic. The nubbin of tissue should be excised and sent for histopathology that will reveal hemosiderin deposit and calcification.
  - Atrophic testis—orchiectomy can be done through laparoscopic route.
  - Normal intra-abdominal testis
    - ◊ If the testis can be mobilized (as indicated by ability to take the testis to approach the contralateral deep ring easily), the orchiopexy can be accomplished in single stage. The advantages of laparoscopy in such a patient are magnification, adequate mobilization up to vessels origin, medializing the deep ring, thus resulting in tensionless orchiopexy.
    - ◊ If the testis cannot be mobilized, Fowler Stephen's Staged Orchiopexy can be done. The testicular vessels are clipped and divided. The collaterals from vasal vessels and cremasteric vessels grow to supply the testis. After 6 months of stage I, when the collaterals have grown, second stage procedure, i.e. orchiopexy is performed. The success rate of two staged Fowler Stephen's procedure is around 90%.
    - ◊ For high intra-abdominal UDT, autotransplantation (microvascular orchiopexy) can be done.

Bilateral Non-Palpable UDT

- Rule out intersex condition
- Management is otherwise same as that for unilateral non-palpable UDT

Secondary UDT

- Difficult surgery due to fibrosis from previous surgery.
- The dissection of cord is not tried. The spermatic cord is mobilized en bloc along with the external oblique aponeurosis, to preserve the blood supply of the testis. Dissection in the retroperitoneum and the Prentiss' maneuver gives length to the cord.

57 Testicular Cancer

- One of the potentially curable solid neoplasm accounts for 1% of all malignant tumor.
- 2–3 new cases per 100,000 US males per year are diagnosed.
- Affects young adults when testosterone fluctuations are maximum.
- Most common solid tumor in males ages 15–35 years.
- Marked variation in incidence among different countries/races.
- 99% of all testicular tumors are malignant.
- 90–95% are germ cell tumors.
- With advances in treatment techniques decrease in mortality from 50% before 1970 to less than 5% in 1997.

Risk Factors

- Cryptorchidism
  - 14 to 48 times the normal expected incidence
  - 7–10% of patients with testicular cancer have a history of cryptorchidism
  - Abnormal germ cell morphology
  - Elevated temperature
  - Interference with normal blood supply
  - 5–10% of patients with testicular cancer and a history of cryptorchidism develop cancer in the contralateral testis
  - Orchidopexy does not prevent development of cancer — just allows for early detection.
- Gonadal dysgenesis
  - 20–30% develop cancer (gonadoblastoma)
- Trauma
  - Prompts evaluation
- Atrophy (nonspecific vs. mumps orchitis)
  - Speculative
- Low and high birth weights
- Familial (early onset and bilateralism) in 8–14%
  - Majority sporadic
  - 2% of men with testicular cancer also have a relative with testicular cancer
  - 8–10 times more risk in brothers of patient with testicular tumor
  - 4–6 times more risk in sons of men with testicular tumor
  - The genes for familial testicular cancer have not yet been discovered
- Androgen insensitivity syndrome 5–10% risk
- Klinefelter's syndrome
  - 47, XXY karyotype
  - Characterized by
    ◊ Testicular atrophy
    ◊ Aspermatogenesis
    ◊ Eunuchoid habitus
    ◊ Gynecomastia
  - Increased risk for mediastinal GCT

Classification – Histological
Primary neoplasms of the testis

- Germinal Neoplasms (90–95 %)
  - Seminomas — 40%

◇ Classic typical seminoma
◇ Anaplastic seminoma
◇ Spermatocytic seminoma
– Embryonal carcinoma — 20–25%
– Teratoma — 25–35%
  ◇ Mature
  ◇ Immature
– Choriocarcinoma — 1%
– Yolk sac tumor
– Mixed (Embryonal commonly in mixed 20%)
• *Nongerminal neoplasms:* 5 to 10%
  – Specialized gonadal stromal tumor
    ◇ Leydig cell tumor
    ◇ Other gonadal stromal tumor
  – Gonadoblastoma
  – Miscellaneous neoplasms
    ◇ Adenocarcinoma of the rete testis
    ◇ Mesenchymal neoplasms
    ◇ Carcinoid
    ◇ Adrenal rest "tumor"

Secondary Neoplasm of the Testis

• Reticuloendothelial neoplasms
• Metastases

Paratesticular Neoplasm

• Adenomatoid
• Cystadenoma of epididymis
• Mesenchymal neoplasms
• Mesothelioma
• Metastases

Classification – Histological

• Pre pubertal group
  – Mainly teratoma or yolk sac tumor
  – Annual incidence — 0.12 per 10000
  – Deletion of 1p in the region of p36
  – Loss of 6q
  – Structural abnormalities of chromosome 2
  – Tumor cells in teratoma are mostly diploid
  – Yolk sac tumors are non-diploid
  – Develop during germ cell migration to the genital ridge
• Post pubertal group
  – Between 15–40 years
  – Incidence 6 per 10000
  – Mainly seminoma or non-seminoma

– In seminoma cells are hypertriploid
– If non-seminoma cells are hypotriploid
• Older groups
  – More than 40 years
  – Annual incidence 0.2 per 100000
  – Mainly spermatocytic seminoma
  – Cells are tetradiploid
  – Gain in chromosome 9

Testicular Tumor and Molecular Biology

• Proto-oncogenes in germ cell tumors

Seminoma and embryonal carcinoma	N-myc expression
Seminoma	c-K ras expression
Immature teratomas	c-erb B-1 expression

• Testicular germ cell tumor shows consistent expression of both:
  – Parental alleles of H19
  – IGF-2 genes

Presentation

• Painless swelling/mass with or without hydrocele (5–10%)
• 30–40% report dull/aching sensation
• 10% present with metastatic symptoms — cough, nausea, vomiting, CNS manifestations, lower extremity swelling secondary to iliac venous occlusive disease
• Gynecomastia
  – 5% germ cell tumors
  – 30–50% sertoli/leydig cell tumors
• More common on the right
  – 1–2% have bilateral disease at diagnosis. Of those with bilateral disease, 50% have a history of cryptorchidism

All patients with a solid, firm intratesticular mass that cannot be transilluminated should be regarded as malignant unless otherwise proved.

Differential Diagnosis

• Torsion
• Epididymitis
• Epididymo-orchitis
• Hydrocele
• Hernia
• Hematoma
• Spermatocele
• Syphilitic gumma

Natural History

- Epididymis or spermatic cord involved in 10% to 15%
- Increases risks of lymphatic or blood borne metastasis
- Involvement of the epididymis or cord may lead to pelvic and inguinal lymph node metastasis
- Tumors confined to the testis usually spread to retroperitoneal nodes
- Hematogenous spread occurs by direct vascular invasion or by way of thoracic duct and subclavian veins
- Lymphatic metastasis is common to all forms of germinal testis tumors
- Pure choriocarcinoma disseminates by means of vascular invasion
- Growth rate of GCTs is high except in seminoma
- Doubling times usually range from 10 to 30 days
- Due to short natural history of germinal tumors, 2-year survival taken as an endpoint for judging the effectiveness of therapy
- Longer follow-up after chemotherapy is mandatory, because relapse has been noted up to 10 years after treatment

Work-up

- Examination
  - Seminoma — painless, rubbery enlargement
  - Embryonal/teratocarcinoma — irregular mass
  - Delay in diagnosis of 4–6 months is frequent
- Ultrasound — Allows for evaluation of the mass, but also the contralateral testis
- CXR +/– Chest CT
  - In patients with a normal abdominal CT — Chest CT usually does not add much information
- Abdominal CT
  - Can identify small nodal deposits <2 cm
  - MRI and PET scan, no advantage over CT
- Markers
  - Elevation after orchiectomy generally represents metastatic disease
  - Conversely normalization does not rule out metastatic disease
  - Markers should undergo a predictable decline after orchiectomy. With XRT/chemo there is a "therapeutic lag" because there is no clear end of tumor destruction, therefore markers may make an unpredictable decline
  - In germ cell tumor — despite normalization of the markers after chemo, 10–20% are found to have viable tumor at RPLND
  - Elevation of tumor markers, multiple metastatic sites and bulk of disease are the major determinants of prognosis
  - Alpha-Fetoprotein (AFP)
    ◊ Expressed by the early embryo (also liver and GI tract)
    ◊ Single chain
    ◊ *Half-life:* 5–7 days
    ◊ Produced by pure embryonal, terato-carcinoma, yolk sac, mixed tumors (not pure choriocarcinoma or seminoma)
    ◊ Falsely elevated in liver dysfunction, viral hepatitis
  - Human chorionic gonadotrophin (hCG)
    ◊ Secretory product of the placenta
    ◊ Alpha unit (LDH, FSH, TSH) and beta unit
    ◊ *Half-life:* 24–36 hours
    ◊ Produced by syncytiotrophoblastic tissue
    ◊ All choriocarcinomas, 40–60% embryonal, 5–10% seminoma
    ◊ Falsely elevated in hypogonadism and marijuana use
  - Lactic acid dehydrogenase (LDH)
    ◊ Presents normally in smooth, cardiac and skeletal muscle, liver and brain
    ◊ Most useful in advanced seminoma or tumors where other markers are not elevated
    ◊ Many false positives
    ◊ DH correlates to tumor burden
  - Placental alkaline phosphatase (PLAP)
    ◊ Elevated by tobacco abuse and elevated in advanced disease (seminomas)
  - Gamma glutamine triphosphate (GGTP)—seminomas and sacrococcygeal teratomas
  - CD30 — embryonal carcinoma

Radical Orchiectomy

- Inguinal approach is used to avoid seeding the scrotum and disrupting lymphatics. Cord structures are ligated at the deep ring.
  - 65–75% of seminomas are confined to the testis at diagnosis
  - 60–70% of NSGCTs present with metastatic disease

- Trans-scrotal orchiectomy disrupts lymphatics, therefore changing metastatic pattern (more easily spreads to pelvic)
- If a trans-scrotal orchiectomy was done — will have to go back and excise the ipsilateral hemi-scrotum and spermatic cord, also biopsy inguinal nodes if palpable or enlarged on CT — if they are positive will need chemotherapy
• Wait 5 half-lives before rechecking markers

Staging

Staging system of the American joint committee on cancer and the international union against cancer

Primary Tumor (T)

pTX   Primary tumor cannot be assessed (if no radical orchiectomy has been performed, TX is used).

pT0   No evidence of primary tumor, (e.g. histologic scar in testis)

pTis   Intratubular germ cell neoplasia (Carcinoma *in situ*)

pT1   Tumor limited to the testis and epididymis and no vascular or lymphatic invasion

pT2   Tumor limited to the testis and epididymis with vascular/lymphatic invasion or tumor extending through tunica albuginea with involvement of tunica vaginalis

pT3   Tumor invades the spermatic cord with or without vascular/lymphatic invasion

pT4   Tumor invades the scrotum with or without vascular/lymphatic invasion

Regional Lymph Nodes (N)
Clinical

NX   Regional lymph nodes cannot be assessed

N0   No regional lymph node metastasis

N1   Lymph node mass 2 cm or less in greatest dimension or multiple lymph node masses, none more than 2 cm in greatest dimension

N2   Lymph node mass, more than 2 cm but not more than 5 cm in greatest dimension, or multiple lymph node masses, any one greater than 2 cm but not more than 5 cm in greatest dimension

N3   Lymph node mass more than 5 cm in greatest dimension

Pathologic

pN0   No evidence of tumor in lymph nodes

pN1   Lymph node mass, 2 cm or less in greatest dimension and ≤6 nodes positive, none >2 cm in greatest dimension

pN2   Lymph node mass, more than 2 cm but not more than 5 cm in greatest dimension; more than 5 nodes positive, none >5 cm; evidence of extranodal extension of tumor

pN3   Lymph node mass more than 5 cm in greatest dimension

Distant Metastasis (M)

M0   No evidence of distant metastasis

M1a   Nonregional nodal or pulmonary metastasis

M1b   Nonpulmonary visceral metastasis

Table 57.1: Serum tumor markers (S)

	LDH	hCG (mIU/ml)	AFP (ng/ml)
S0	≤ N	≤ N	≤ N
S1	<1.5 × N	<5000	<1000
S2	1.5–10 × N	5,000–50,000	1,000–10,000
S3	>10 × N	>50,000	>10,000

Table 57.2: Stage grouping according to the AJCC staging system

Stage grouping	T	N	M	S
Stage 0	pTis	N0	M0	S0
Stage I	T1–4	N0	M0	SX
Ia	T1	N0	M0	S0
Ib	T2	N0	M0	S0
	T3	N0	M0	S0
	T4	N0	M0	S0
Is	Any T	N0	M0	S1-S3
Stage II	Any T	Any N	M0	SX
IIa	Any T	N1	M0	S0
	Any T	N1	M0	S1
IIb	Any T	N2	M0	S0
	Any T	N2	M0	S1
IIc	Any T	N3	M0	S0
	Any T	N3	M0	S1
Stage III	Any T	Any N	M1	SX
IIIa	Any T	Any N	M1	S0
	Any T	Any N	M1	S1
IIIb	Any T	Any N	M0	S2
	Any T	Any N	M1	S2
IIIc	Any T	Any N	M0	S3
	Any T	Any N	M1a	S3
	Any T	Any N	M1b	Any S

Principles of Treatment

- Treatment should be aimed at one stage above the clinical stage
- Seminomas are radio-sensitive. Treat with radiotherapy
- Non-seminomas are radio-resistant and best treated by surgery
- Advanced disease or metastasis responds well to chemotherapy
- Radical inguinal orchidectomy is standard first line of therapy
- Lymphatic spread initially goes to retro-peritoneal nodes
- Early hematogenous spread rare
- Bulky retroperitoneal tumors or metastatic tumors initially "down-staged" with chemotherapy.

Seminoma

- Most common germ cell tumor
- Pure seminomas never secrete AFP
- 5–10% secrete hCG (usually classic)
- 90% stain positive for PLAP
- At diagnosis:
  - 65–75% confined to the testis
  - 10–15% with regional retroperitoneal nodes
  - 5–10% with advanced juxtarenal or visceral disease

Histology

- Classic variant 82–85% of cases
  - Age — fourth decade of life
  - Islands/sheets of cells with syncytio-trophoblasts (5–10%)
- Anaplastic 5–10% of cases
  - Stage for stage no different than classic
- Spermatocytic 2–12% of cases
  - Low metastatic potential — only one case of metastatic spermatocytic seminoma has ever been reported
  - Older population (>50)
  - 6% bilateral (as opposed to 2% of classic seminomas)
  - Confined to the testes
  - Stains negative for PLAP
  - Cured by orchidectomy

Stage I

- Radical inguinal ochidectomy followed by radiotherapy to ipsilateral retroperitonium and ipsilateral iliac group lymph nodes (2500–3500 rads)
- Approx. 80% with clinical stage I will also have pathologic stage I (XRT will treat those with clinical stage I and pathologic stage II)
- If tumor involved the tunica vaginalis or spermatic cord the scrotum should be involved in the field
- 5 year survival after XRT 95%
- Both need normal post-orchiectomy markers
- Radiotherapy (XRT)
  - 20% of clinical stage I have pathologic stage II
  - 2500 cGy to para-aortic nodes
  - Minimal acute morbidity
  - ***Long term concerns:*** Infertility, GI manifestations, secondary malignancies
  - ***Relapse rate 5% (rare after 5 years):*** Usually outside of retroperitoneum
  - Salvage chemotherapy after relapse
- Surveillance
  - Indicated only for compliant patients
  - Favorable tumors:
    ◊ Tumors <6 cm
    ◊ Absence of lymphatic or vascular invasion
    ◊ Normal post orchiectomy tumor markers
    ◊ Pure spermatocytic seminomas
  - Relapse rate 15% (90% in retroperitoneum)
  - After relapse treat with radiotherapy (XRT) or chemotherapy

Stage IIa, IIb

- XRT to the ipsilateral external iliac, bilateral common iliac, paracaval, para-aortic and cisterna chyli
- Bulky IIb disease or disease close to the kidney — chemotherapy first
- If history of herniorraphy or orchidopexy, should also do XRT to the inguinal region (shield contralateral testis).

Stage IIC, III

- Radical inguinal orchidectomy is followed by chemotherapy
- Cisplatin based chemo [4 cycles of EC (Etoposide, Cisplatin) or 3 cycles of BEP (Bleomycin, Etoposide, Cisplatin)]
- 90% will have a complete response
- If residual disease — surgery
- Residual retroperitoneal masses are usually fibrosis

– RPLND warranted if >3 cm and well circum-scribed

Non-Seminomatous Germ Cell Tumor (NSGCT)

Histological Variants

- Embryonal
  - Peak age 25–35 years
  - May secrete both AFP and β-hCG
  - 3% pure and 50% of mixed germ-cell tumors
  - PLAP positive, AFP and hCG-positive cells are present in 33% and 21%
  - Metastatic deposits usually contain teratoma (80%)
  - Epitheloid cells in glands or tubules with pale cytoplasm, 1+ nucleoli and giant cells
- Choriocarcinoma
  - Peak age 20–30 years
  - Worst prognosis of all testis tumors
  - Hematogenous spread (especially to lungs)
  - Always secrete β-hCG
  - <0.05% of pure lesions but present in about 4% of mixed germ-cell tumors
  - Central hemorrhage, syncytiotrophoblasts (eosinophilic cytoplasm) and cytotrophoblasts (closely packed, clear cytoplasm, single nuclei)
  - Highly aggressive
  - Bizarre spread to places like the spleen
- Yolk sac (Infantile embryonal)
  - Peak age: infants and children
  - Pure <2% and 40% of mixed germ-cell tumors
  - Also may spread hematogenously
  - Secretes AFB and β-hCG
  - Epithelial like cells arranged in glands with vacuolated cytoplasm
  - Embryoid bodies (Schiller-Duvall bodies) resemble 1–2 week old embryos surrounded by syncytiotrophoblasts and cytotrophoblasts
- Teratoma
  - Peak age 25–35 years
  - 5% pure and 50% of mixed germ-cell tumors
  - Poor response to chemotherapy and XRT
  - Pure forms should not secrete AFB or β-hCG
  - Can arise from malignant transformation after chemotherapy for NSGCT
  - Contains all 3 germ layers in the mature form and is undifferentiated in immature form

- Mixed germ cell tumors
  - 50% of germ cell tumors
  - Any of the above elements can be present in combination

Treatment

Stage I

- Radical orchidectomy followed by retroperitoneal lymph nodes dissection
- Retroperitoneal lymph node dissection (RPLND) (Fig. 57.1)

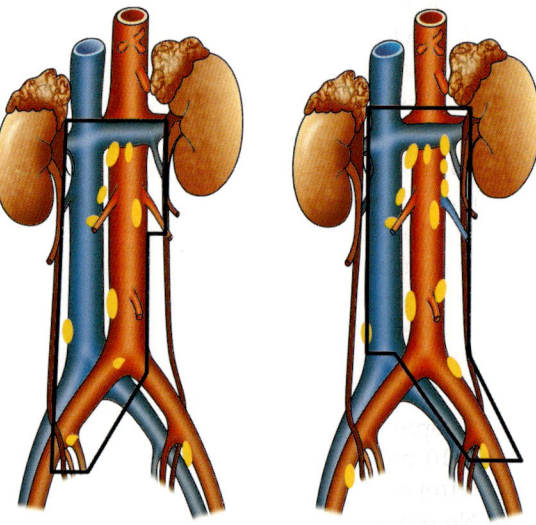

Fig. 57.1: Modified RPLND templates for right and left sides

- Allows for more accurate staging
- 30% clinical stage I is pathologic stage II
- Definitive treatment for N1 — cure rate post RPLND in stage I is 95%
- N2 will need post RPLND chemotherapy — N2 disease has a 50% relapse with RPLND therefore chemo is necessary
- Relapse rate 5–13% (5–10% outside of RPLND field: primarily in the lungs)
- Treat relapses with chemotherapy (BEP/EP)
- Major morbidity is ejaculatory dysfunction
  ◊ Modified nerve sparing RPLND preserves function in 90–99%
  ◊ Identify the sympathetic nerves
  ◊ Dissection is limited to below the level of the IMA on the ipsilateral side only
  ◊ Morbidity from disruption of the sympathetic nerves

◊ Morbidity is increased after XRT or chemo because of a desmoplastic reaction
  - Follow up after RPLND: Clinical examination, CXR and trauma markers every 2 months for 1 year, and every 4 months for 1 year and then annually (relapse beyond 2 years is rare).
- Surveillance
  - Appropriate for:
    ◊ Compliant patient
    ◊ Tumor confined to tunica albuginea
    ◊ No vascular/lymphatic invasion
    ◊ Normal markers after orchiectomy
    ◊ No further disease seen on radiographic imaging
    ◊ Absence of embryonal cell
    ◊ Presence of yolk sac elements
  - *Follow-up:* Physical examination, CXR, markers
    ◊ Monthly for 1 year
    ◊ Bimonthly for 1 year
    ◊ Every 3–6 months for 5–10 year (no precise end point)
    ◊ CT scan every 2–3 months for first 2 years then every 6 months
  - Relapse rate 25% and usually occurs in first 8–10 months (commonly outside of the retroperitoneum)
  - No economic difference between modified RPLND, chemotherapy or surveillance
- Chemotherapy
  - Traditionally not used for lower stages
  - 2 cycles of BEP
  - Added advantage of treating metastatic disease that RPLND misses
  - Initial data promising but long term unconfirmed

Stage IIA-IIB

- RPLND with possible adjuvant chemotherapy
- RPLND
  - Advocated for lower volume disease
  - Cures 50–70% of stage IIa/b without further intervention
- Chemotherapy
  - BEP X 3, EP X 4
  - Favored for patients with nodes >3 cm
  - 2 cycles of chemo decreases the relapse rate from 50% to 2% in stage IIa and IIb

- If markers normalize but residual mass is seen on CT, RPLND is advocated
  ◊ 20% residual cancer
  ◊ 40% teratoma
  ◊ 40% fibrosis
- Some advocate RPLND even if there is no residual mass and the markers normalize because residual germ cell is seen in up to 10%
- Residual cancer is usually embryonal cancer, but malignant teratoma is seen in less than 5% and is unresponsive to chemotherapy (only 15% of patients survive following surgical excision)
- Relapse or residual cancer is treated with salvage chemotherapy (VIP X 4) (vinblastin, ifosfamide, cisplatin)
- Chance of cure is equal to the chance of death with autologous bone marrow transplant (ABMT)

Stage IIC-III

- Initial chemotherapy followed by surgery for residual disease
- Primary chemotherapy
  - BEP X 3 for stage IIc and BEP X 4 for stage III
  - In IIc disease with partial response, may proceed to RPLND
- Salvage chemotherapy or high dose chemotherapy with autologous bone marrow transplant
  - No response to first line chemotherapy
  - Incomplete resection after RPLND

Toxicity of Chemotherapy

Bleomycin: Pulmonary fibrosis
Etoposide (VP-16): Myelosuppression, alopecia, renal insufficiency (mild), secondary leukemia
Cisplatin: Renal insufficiency, nausea, vomiting, neuropathy

Prognosis

- Seminoma (at 5 years)
  - I: 98%
  - IIA: 92–94%
  - IIB-III: 33–75%
- NSGT (at 5 years)
  - I: 96–100%
  - IIA: >90%
  - IIB-III: 55–80%

Prognostic Factors

NSGCT

- Good prognosis group
  - Testis/retroperitoneal primary
  - No non-pulmonary visceral metastases
  - AFP <1,000 ng/mL
  - HCG <5,000 IU/L
  - LDH <1.5 times normal
- Intermediate prognosis group
  - Testis/retroperitoneal primary
  - No non-pulmonary visceral metastases
  - Normal AFP
  - Any HCG
  - Any LDH
- Poor prognosis group
  - Mediastinal primary
  - Non-pulmonary visceral metastases
  - AFP >10,000 ng/mL
  - HCG >50,000 IU/L
  - LDH >10 times normal

Seminoma

- Good prognosis group
  - Any primary site
  - No non-pulmonary visceral metastases
  - Normal AFP
  - Any HCG
  - Any LDH
- Intermediate prognosis
  - Any primary site
  - Non pulmonary visceral metastases
  - AFP >1,000 and <10,000 ng/mL or
  - HCG >5,000 and <50,000 Iu/L or
  - LDH >1.5 times and <10 times normal
- Poor prognosis group
  - Mediastinal primary
  - Non-pulmonary visceral metastases
  - AFP >10,000 ng/mL
  - HCG >50,000 IU/L
  - LDH >10 times normal

Leydig Cell Tumor

- Most common non-germ cell tumor
- 1–3% of all testis tumors
- Bimodal age distribution: Ages 5–9 years and 25–35 years
- Bilateral in 5–10%
- No association with cryptorchidism
- Prepubertal children may present with virilization and elevated urinary 17-ketosteroid levels; adults are usually asymptomatic (25% gynecomastia)
- Histology
  - Solid sheets of cells with oval nuclei
  - Reinke crystals (fusiform shaped cytoplasmic inclusion) are pathognomonic although rare
  - *Treatment:* Radical orchiectomy and RPLND for malignant tumors (10% malignant)
- Prognosis excellent for benign lesions and poor for patients with disseminated disease

Sertoli Cell Tumor

- Less than 1% of all testicular tumors
- Bimodal age of distribution: < 1 year and 20–45 years old
- 10% lesions are malignant
- Virilization seen in children and gynecomastia in adults
- Metastatic disease determined by presence of metastasis
- Radical orchiectomy with RPLND in malignant disease

Gonadoblastoma

- 0.5% of testicular tumors
- Seen in patients with gonadal dysgenesis
- 4/5 patients are phenotypic females with streak gonads
- Radical orchiectomy with gonadectomy of the contralateral gonad (bilateral in 50%)

58 | Hydrocele

Points to be noted in a scrotal swelling:

- Can I get the above swelling (If it is possible to get the above swelling then it is a purely scrotal swelling)
- Is fluctuation positive (In cystic fluid containing swellings fluctuations are positive)
- Is transillumination positive (transillumination is positive in presence of clear fluid)
- Are testis and epididymis palpable separate from the swelling (If not palpable separately then it is likely to be a case of primary vaginal hydrocele)

Differential Diagnosis

- Vaginal hydrocele
- Pyocele
- Chylocele
- Hematocele
- Epididymal cyst
- Spermatocele
- Varicocele
- Encysted hydrocele of the cord

Solid swellings of the scrotum

- Infective
  - Acute
    - ◊ Orchitis — pyogenic/viral
    - ◊ Epididymitis
  - Chronic
    - ◊ Nonspecific
    - ◊ Residual infection
- Trauma
  - Chemical exposure
  - Post vasectomy
  - Clotted hematocele
- Specific
  - Tuberculosis
  - Malakoplakia
- Neoplasms
  - Benign
  - Malignant

DEFINITION

Abnormal collection of fluid in some parts of the processus vaginalis usually in the tunica. It can be primary or secondary.

Primary Hydrocele

Primary hydrocele occurs without any underlying disease of the testis or epididymis. It is the most common form of vaginal hydrocele. It is commonly caused by:

- Defective absorption of fluid
- Excessive production
- Interference with drainage of fluid by lymphatics of the cord
- Direct communication with peritoneal cavity (Congenital hydrocele)

Types of Hydrocele

- Non-communicating hydrocele
- Communicating hydrocele
- Encysted hydrocele of the cord

Hydrocele Fluid

- Amber colored
- Specific gravity of 1022–1024
- Contains mainly water and inorganic salts
- 6% albumin, fibrinogen, cholesterol, tyrosine crystals (long standing cases)
- Long standing hydrocele fluid may contain cholesterol crystals
- Hydrocele fluid clots if a drop of blood is added to the fluid

Features of Primary Hydrocele

- Purely scrotal swelling
- Usually tense
- Fluctuation is positive
- Transillumination is positive. Transillumination will be negative if the hydrocele sac is thickened or calcified or hydrocele gets converted in to hematocele or pyocele
- Testis cannot be felt separate from the swelling

Secondary Hydrocele

- Associated with an underlying pathology like tumor trauma or infection
- Caused by excessive secretion
- Usually lax and small
- Testis is felt separately and may be tender
- The fluid may be sero-sanguinous and thus poorly transilluminant

Causes of Secondary Hydrocele

- Acute epididymo-orchitis
- Chronic epididymo-orchitis
- Torsion of the testis
- Post herniorrhaphy
- Testicular tumors

Congenital Hydrocele

- Due to patent processus vaginalis
- Appears on assuming erect position and disappears at rest
- Collection represents peritoneal fluid
- Can be emptied manually also

Infantile Hydrocele

- The tunica vaginalis and processus vaginalis are communicating with each other
- There is obliteration at the level of internal ring and hence no direct communication with peritoneal cavity
- Hydrocele is usually tense

Encysted Hydrocele of the Cord

- A segment of the processus vaginalis associated with the spermatic cord remains unobliterated and becomes filled with fluid
- Swelling is ovoid and smooth with a cystic consistency
- The swelling can be moved down with traction on the testis
- Commonly mistaken for a hernia or lipoma of the cord but is transilluminant

Clinical Features

History

- Duration of the swelling
- Residence or visit to area endemic for filariasis
- Associated pain or fever
- History of trauma
- Family history of testicular tumor

Examination

- Presents with scrotal swelling
- Rugosity of the scrotum is lost
- Swelling is non-reducible with no impulse on coughing
- Testis and epididymis are not felt separately
- It is possible to get above the swelling
- Cord structures are normal
- Transillumination is positive
  - It may be negative if:
    ◊ Hemorrhage or serosanguinous fluid present
    ◊ Wall is thick as in long standing hydrocele
    ◊ Secondary hydrocele
- Swelling is not reducible and usually non tender

Investigations

- Only hemoglobin and coagulation profile are required to proceed for surgery
- It is essentially a clinical diagnosis
- Secondary hydrocele or doubtful cases can be investigated further by ultrasonography

Complications

- Hematocele — due to trauma
- Pyocele — due to secondary infection
- Calcification
- Atrophy of the testis in cases of large long standing hydrocele
- Rupture
- Hernia of the hydrocele sac through the dartos muscle

Management

- Surgery
- Sclerotherapy
- Tapping of fluid

Surgical Procedures for Hydrocele

Eversion of sac (Jaboulay's procedure)
- The sac is everted inside out
- Cut margins are sutured behind the testis and epididymis
- In the early postoperative period the secretions of tunica vaginalis are absorbed by scrotal lymphatics and veins
- Later due to constant friction with subcutaneous tissue, secretory endothelium changes its character and gradually stops secreting

Excision of the sac
- Indications
  - Large redundant sac
  - Thick sac
  - Infected sac
  - Hematocele
- The hydrocele sac is opened, taking great care not to injure the spermatic cord
- The sac is simply excised, leaving room to oversew the edge of the excised sac

Lord's procedure
- Plication of the sac is done. It is commonly employed for small and thin sac.

- The lord plication technique (1964) is performed by opening the hydrocele, delivering the testis and cauterizing or oversewing the cut edges of the sac
- Use interrupted, radially placed chromic sutures to plicate the sac
- Closure is then performed

Herniotomy
- For congenital hydrocele

Sclerotherapy

Agents for Sclerotherapy
- Most commonly used sclerosing agent is tetracycline (500 mg)
- 2.5% phenol solution
- 95% alcohol
- Ethanolamine oleate

Epididymal Cyst

- **Retention cyst:** Spermatocele
- **Degeneration cyst:** May be solitary or multiple

Spermatocele

It is a uni-locular retention cyst due to distal obstruction of a part of epididymis. It is commonly located near the head of the epididymis and is filled with barley water fluid which contains sperms.

Clinical Features
- Soft scrotal swelling
- Arises above and behind the testis
- Testis is separately palpable
- Transillumination is positive

Transilluminant swellings of the inguino-scrotal region
- Vaginal hydrocele
- Epididymal cyst
- Spermatocele
- Encysted hydrocele of the cord

59 Hypospadias

DEFINITION

- Hypospadias results from arrested penile development resulting in a proximal urethral meatus
- A congenital condition in which the opening of the meatus lies on the under surface of the penis
- Usually combination of following features
  - Ventral meatus
  - Ventral curvature (chordee)
  - Dorsal "hood"; deficient foreskin ventrally. In a variant of hypospadias known as megameatus intact prepuce (MIP) there is normally formed foreskin which can conceal the glandular or distal shaft hypospadias. Diagnosis is made only when child undergoes elective circumcision or when the foreskin retracts
  - Patients can have ventrally deficient prepuce with ventral curvature with normally placed urethral opening. This condition is known as congenital ventral curvature

Classification

- Anterior (distal)
  - Glandular
  - Coronal
  - Sub-coronal
- Middle
  - Distal penile
  - Mid-shaft
  - Proximal penile
- Posterior (Proximal)
  - Peno-scrotal
  - Scrotal
  - Perineal

Embryology

- Normal development of urethra
  Urethral plate develops from extension of endoderm of cloaca in the ventral midline of genital tubercle. The proliferation of mesenchyme tissue on either side of the urethral plate gives rise to urethral folds and urethral groove. Fusion of urethral folds starts proximally and continues distally till glans. Glandular urethra develops from ectodermal ingrowth from tip of glans till urethral plate which later get canalised. Other theory is tabularisation of urethral plate to the tip of glans.
  Chordee is due to persistence of ventral curvature of the penis during its development as there is a developmental arrest in hypospadias. Prepuce forms from a cellular lamella which is located dorsally at the coronal sulcus and fuses ventrally at the frenulum. This ventral fusion does not occur if urethral development is arrested leading to a hooded prepuce.

Hypospadias and Syndromes

Nearly 200 syndromes are associated with hypospadias
Common syndromes are:

Smith-Lemli-Opitz Syndrome

- Results from autosomal recession of DHCR7 gene on chromosome 11 coding for 7- dehydrocholesterol reductase.
- Patient has mental retardation, facial dysmorphism, microcephaly, syndactyly, and hypospadias.

WAGR syndrome: There is deletion in chromosome 11 leading to Wilms tumor, aniridia, mental retardation and hyospadias. This is due to altered WT1 activity.

Other syndromes associated with hypospadias are

- Hand foot genital syndrome
- Optiz G syndrome
- Wolf Hirschhorn syndrome

Incidence

- 1:300 live male births
- Some genetic component
  - 8% of patients have father with hypospadias
  - 14% of patients have male siblings with hypospadias
  - If child with hypospadias, risk to next child
    ◊ 12% risk with negative family history
    ◊ 19% if cousin or uncle with hypospadias
    ◊ 26% if father or sibling
- More common in caucasians (Jews and Italians)
- Higher incidence in monozygotic twins (8.5x)

Other Association in Etiology

Placental dysfunction in early pregnancy predispose to hypospadias.

High risk is associated with low birth weight (<10 percentile), preterm birth (<37 weeks), prepregnancy maternal obesity, diabetes and maternal hypertension. Decreased maternal age (<24 years) and increased maternal age (>40 years is associated with increased incidence of hypospadias).

Associated reproduction is associated with an increased hypospadias risk which can be attributed to hormonal manipulation during and after the procedure.

Associated Anomalies

- Undescended testes 9% and inguinal hernia 9%
- Upper tract anomalies rare (1–3%)

- Utriculus masculinus
  - 10 to 15% in perineal or penoscrotal hypospadias
  - Incomplete Müllerian duct regression
- Rule out intersex, especially with cryptorchidism
  - Adrenogenital syndrome
  - Mixed gonadal dysgenesis
  - Incomplete pseudohermaphroditism
  - True hermaphroditism
- Hypospadias and cryptorchidism
  - High index of suspicion for an intersex state
  - Walsh reported the incidence of intersexuality in children with cryptorchidism, hypospadias, and otherwise nonambiguous genitalia to be 27%
  - Nonpalpable testis were at least threefold more likely to have an intersex condition than those with a palpable undescended testis (50% versus 15%)
  - The idea that evaluation for an endocrine abnormality and/or intersex state should be undertaken in those with posterior hypospadias, regardless of gonadal position or palpability, is controversial but is supported in the literature, because significant, identifiable, and treatable abnormalities are common
  - Further evaluation
    ◊ Only with severe hypospadias and sexual ambiguity
      ⇒ Includes testicular abnormalities
      ⇒ Up to 25% of these patients have enlarged utriclus or other female structures
    ◊ The incidence of abnormalities with other forms of hypospadias approximates that of the general population
    ◊ Therefore, no further evaluation is indicated

History of Procedures

- First in 100 to 200 AD
  - Heliodorus and antyllus
  - Amputation distal to meatus
- Dieffenbach 1838
  - Pierced glans to meatus and left stent in place
- Thiersch, 1869
  - Local tissue flaps

- Hook
  - Vascularized preputial flaps
- Multistage repairs
  - Release chordee
  - Urethroplasty
- One stage repairs
  - More feasible since the introduction of artificial erection, which has nearly eliminated inadequate chordee release

Treatment

- Meatoplasty and glanuloplasty
  - Multiple techniques
- Orthoplasty
  - Utilize artificial erection
  - Release urethra from fibrous tissue
  - Plicate dorsal tunica albuguinea
  - Ventral graft if needed
- Urethroplasty
  - Onlay vascularized flap
  - Tubularized flap
  - Free graft
- Skin cover
  - Mobilized dorsal prepuce and penile skin
  - Double faced island flap
- Scrotoplasty

Factors for Technical Success

- Use of vascularized tissues
- Careful tissue handling
- Tension-free anastomosis
- Non-overlapping suture lines
- Meticulous hemostasis
- Fine suture material
- Adequate urinary diversion

Technical Aspects

- Instruments
  - Fine instruments for delicate tissue handling
- Suture
  - Chromic— absorbs rapidly
  - 6–0 or 7–0 polyglycolic for buried sutures
- Hemostasis
  - Tourniquet
  - Lidocaine with epinephrine

- Low current Bovie, bipolar sticks to tissue
- Magnification
- Dressing
  - Immobilization and prevention of hematoma and edema
- Diversions
  - Stent secured to glans with open drainage into a diaper
- Bladder spasms
  - Oxybutinin
- Analgesia
  - Local penile block
  - Caudal block
- Age at repair
  - 6 to 18 months

Testosterone Cream

- May or may not be beneficial
- Considerable controversy surrounding the use of hormonal stimulation
- Whether to administer any adjunctive gonado-tropins or hormones and, if so, which agent, route, dose, dosing schedule, and timing of treatment is to be employed
- Gearhart and Jeffs (1987) administered testo-sterone enanthate intramuscularly (2 mg/kg body weight), 5 and 2 weeks before recons-tructive penile surgery. They noted a 50% increase in penile size and an increase in available skin and local vascularity in all patients.

Hypospadias Repair

- Over 150 operations have be described
- Distal hypospadias
  - Tubulization of the incised urethral plate (Snodgrass)
  - Meatal advancement (MAGPI)
  - Meatal-based flaps (Mathieu)
- Proximal hypospadias
  - Onlay grafts
  - Vascularized inner preputial transfer flaps (Duckett)
  - Free grafts (skin, buccal mucosa)

60 | Circumcision

- Practiced in west Africa for over 5000 years
- Inherited by Jews from Negroes or Babylonians
- Not effective in adults in reducing incidence of Penile carcinoma, but if carried out at birth it brings down incidence of penile carcinoma significantly

Indications of Circumcision

- Religious or social reasons like in Jews or Muslims
- Recurrent attacks of balanoposhtitis due to accumulation of smegma in prepuce sac
- Narrow opening causing obstructive symptoms in a child patient like ballooning of preuce or narrowing of stream or recurrent attacks of urinary tract infection
- Difficulty in having intercourse
- Tight frenulum
- Carcinoma penis confined to prepuce
- To facilitate in taking a biopsy from underlying growth of glans penis
- Warts confined to prepuce

Contraindications to Circumcision

- Bleeding disorder which is not controlled
- Hypospadias as the skin of the prepuce can be used for reconstruction of urethra at a later stage

Steps of Circumcision in Adults

- Adhesions between glans and prepuce carefully dissected
- Coronal sulcus exposed
- Prepuce dorsally slit up to coronal sulcus
- Distal 2/3rd of prepuce (both layers) excised all around leaving a cuff of 1 cm
- Inner layer further trimmed to 5 mm from coronal sulcus
- The artery of frenula is carefully ligated by figure of eight suture
- Cut margins of prepuce stitched together

In children as prepuce is long clamp and cut technique can be used.

61 Carcinoma Penis

- Poor personal hygiene
- Phimosis — Irritation by accumulated smegma
- Balanoposthitis
- Premalignant lesions
- Penile trauma — scarred penis
- Human papilloma virus infection
- Exposure to tobacco
- UV light exposure

Premalignant Lesions

- Cutaneous horn — develops over previous lesions
- Balanitis xerotica obliterans — lichen sclerosus
- Leukoplakia
- Keratotic balanitis

Site of Origin

- Inner surface of the prepuce (20%)
- Corona glans
- Glans penis (50%)
- Foreskin
- Shaft of the penis (rare)

Pathology

- Squamous cell carcinoma
- Adenocarcinoma from Tyson's glands
- Anaplastic carcinoma
- Basal cell carcinoma
- Malignant melanoma (rare)

Macroscopic Types

- Proliferative (Fig. 61.1)
- Ulcerative
- Flat infiltrating type—anaplastic

Microscopic Types

- Usual type
- Papillary

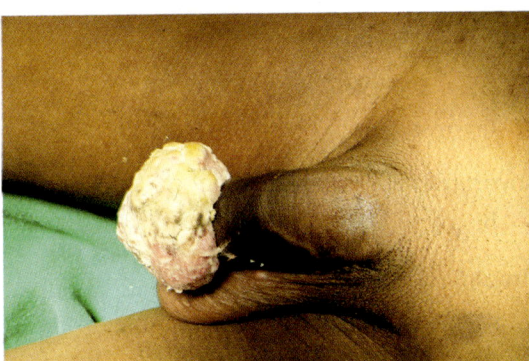

Fig. 61.1: Proliferative type of carcinoma penis

- Basaloid (Aggressive)
- Warty
- Verrucous (HPV Associated)
- Sarcomatoid (Aggressive)

Secondary Carcinoma of Penis

- *From local spread:* Bladder, prostate, rectum
- Retrograde lymphatic spread
- Retrograde venous embolism

Pathways of Spread

- *Direct spread:* From prepuce, glans, shaft. Urethra is not involved even in extensive growth.
- *Lymphatic spread:* Superficial and deep iliac nodes involved. Further spread occurs to pelvic nodes (External iliac, internal iliac and obturator) in advanced cases. Cross connections between two sides occur at many levels.
- *Venous spread:* Rare and involves the distant organs.

Clinical Features

- Common in age group usually >40 years, may present at earlier age as well
- Phimosis may be acquired due to narrowing of the prepuce following carcinomatous fibrosis
- Patient often does not see the growth
- Irritation occurs due to collection of discharge
- Bloody discharge may be present
- Growth may sometimes be visible after dorsal slit
- Inguinal lymph nodes may be palpable due to metastasis or inflammation
- Growth may be visible in later stages when it erodes the foreskin

Poor Prognostic Factors

- Older age of presentation
- Higher stage at diagnosis
- Involvement of lymph nodes

Investigations

- Biopsy which may be facilitated by dorsal slit.

Treatment

Radiotherapy

- Small growth
- Well differentiated
- Limited to glans
- Young patient

Advantages

- Avoids mutilating surgery

Disadvantages

- Inferior results with more chances of recurrence
- Shrivelled penis
- Painful erections
- Post radiation sterility

Contraindication

- Large growths >4cm
- Anaplastic growth
- Growth involving shaft
- Elderly patient

Surgery

- *Partial Amputation:* When growth is limited to the glans
- *Total Amputation:* When growth involves the shaft
- *Inguinal lymph nodes:*
  - ✓ If inguinal lymph nodes are not palpable dissection of groin lymph nodes is not indicated in T1 lesions if there is no lymph vascular invasion and the lesion is well differentiated.
  - ✓ If the lesion is T2 or higher without clinical involvement of lymph nodes, bilateral superficial groin dissection is performed and sent for frozen section.
  - ✓ On the side having metastatic deposits in superficial inguinal lymph nodes, complete groin dissection is carried out.
  - ✓ In case of palpable lymph nodes in low stage and low grade lesions a 6 weeks course of antibiotics is given. If lymph nodes disappear after course of antibiotics protocol similar to non-palpable lymph nodes is followed.
  - ✓ If lymph nodes persist after course of antibiotics complete dissection of groin lymph nodes on involved side and superficial dissection on opposite side is performed.

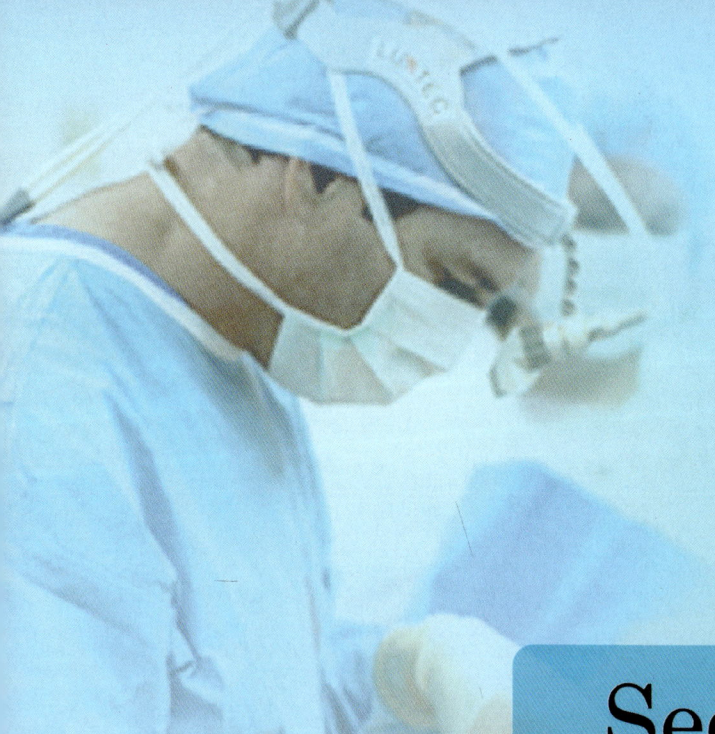

Section V

62 | Acute Abdomen

ACUTE ABDOMEN

- Challenge to surgeons and physicians
- Most common cause of surgical emergency admission
- Clinical course can vary from minutes to hours
- It can be an acute exacerbation of a chronic problem, e.g. chronic pancreatitis, vascular insufficiency

Definition

- Acute abdomen is a term used for an abdominal condition that needs immediate surgical intervention
- Presentation of previously undiagnosed abdominal pain
  - Lasting less than 1 week
  - Prior to a clinical encounter in primary or secondary care

Causes

  - Acute appendicitis
  - Acute cholecystitis
  - Small bowel obstruction
  - Perforated peptic ulcer
  - Pancreatitis
  - Diverticular disease
- Accounts for 20–40% of admission rates
- 50–65% rate of inaccurate initial diagnosis

Pathophysiology

- Visceral pain
  - Distension, inflammation or ischemia in hollow viscous and solid organs
  - Localization depends on the embryologic origin of the organ
    - ◊ Foregut to epigastrium
    - ◊ Midgut to umbilicus
    - ◊ Hindgut to the hypogastric region
- Parietal pain is localized to the dermatome above the site of the stimulus and is referred.
- Referred pain produces symptoms, not signs, e.g. tenderness

Differential Diagnosis

- Generalized abdominal pain
  - Perforation
  - Abdominal aortic aneurysm (AAA)
  - Acute pancreatitis
  - Diabetes mellitus (DM)
  - Bilateral pleurisy
- Central abdominal pain
  - Early appendicitis
  - Small bowel obstruction
  - Acute gastritis
  - Acute pancreatitis
  - Ruptured AAA
  - Mesenteric thrombosis
- Epigastric pain
  - Peptic ulcer

- Esophagitis
- Acute pancreatitis
- AAA
- Right upper quadrant pain
  - Gallbladder disease
  - Duodenal ulcer
  - Acute pancreatitis
  - Pneumonia
  - Subphrenic abscess
- Left upper quadrant pain
  - Gastric ulcer
  - Pneumonia
  - Acute pancreatitis
  - Spontaneous splenic rupture
  - Acute perinephritis
  - Subphrenic abscess
- Suprapubic pain
  - Acute urinary retention
  - Urinary tract infection (UTI)
  - Cystitis
  - Pelvic inflammatory disease (PID)
  - Ectopic pregnancy
  - Diverticulitis
- Right iliac fossa pain
  - Acute appendicitis
  - Mesenteric adenitis (young)
  - Perforated peptic ulcer
  - Diverticulitis
  - PID
  - Salpingitis
  - Ureteric colic
  - Meckel's diverticulum
  - Ectopic pregnancy
  - Crohn's disease
  - Biliary colic (low-lying gall bladder)
- Loin pain
  - Muscle strain
  - UTIs
  - Renal stones
  - Pyelonephritis
- Left iliac fossa pain
  - Diverticulitis
  - Constipation
  - Irritable bowel syndrome (IBS)
  - PID
  - Rectal cancer
  - Ulcerative colitis (UC)
  - Ectopic pregnancy

Assessment

- Well elicited history
- Proper examination
- Investigations are usually carried out only to
  - Support the clinical diagnosis, or
  - Narrow down the differential diagnosis.

History

- History of present illness
- Family history
- Past medical history
- History of medication, e.g. ingestion of certain toxic drugs or alcohol

Pain

Pain is the most common and important symptom. History of pain should include:

- Onset
- Severity
- Type of pain
- Radiation of pain
- Change in nature of pain
- Associated bowel and urinary symptoms
- Aggravating or relieving factors

Onset of Pain

- Sudden onset pain which wakes the patient from sleep
  - e.g. perforation or strangulation of bowel
- Slow insidious onset
  - Inflammation of visceral peritoneum.
  - Contained process such as evolving abscess.
- Crampy or colicky pain
  - Biliary colic, Ureteric colic or intestinal colic

Nature of Pain

- Colicky pain
  - Baseline of no pain in true colic
  - IBS
  - Bowel obstruction—ureteric colic
- Nagging and grumbling
  - Biliary colic
  - Cholecystitis
  - PID
  - UTI
- Stabbing
  - AAA leaking

- Burning or boring
  - Peptic ulcer disease
  - Esophagitis
- Gnawing
  - Pancreatitis
  - Pancreatic cancer

Progression of Pain

- *Progression from:* Dull, aching, poorly localized character; to sharp, constant and better localized pain; indicates involvement of parietal peritoneum

Associated Bowel Symptoms

- Constipation
  - Progressive intestinal obstruction from a neoplasm or inflammatory bowel disease
  - Paralytic ileus
  - Post-operative
  - Obstructed groin hernia
- Diarrhea
  - Diarrhea with pain is mainly medical
  - The following are the exceptions:
    ◊ Obstructed Richter's Hernia
    ◊ Gall Stone ileus
    ◊ Superior mesenteric vascular occlusion
    ◊ Intestinal obstruction associated with pelvic abscess
    ◊ Spurious diarrhea in chronic fecal impaction

Drug History

- Corticosteroids — mask pain
- Anticoagulants — can lead to an intramural hematoma of the gut causing obstruction
- Oral contraceptives — rupture of hepatic adenomas
- NSAIDs — erosive gastritis and peptic ulcers

Nausea and Vomiting

- Frequency of vomiting
- Character of vomiting
  - Projectile, non-projectile or self-induced
- Nature of vomiting
  - Bilious vomiting of small bowel obstruction
  - Non-bilious vomiting in obstruction proximal to ampulla of Vater
  - Feculent vomiting in distal small gut obstruction, large bowel obstruction and strangulation

- Pain first, followed by vomiting is usually surgical
  - The vomiting is due to 'reflex pylorospasm'
- Nausea and vomiting first, followed by pain is usually due to a medical condition
- Vomiting is very prominent in
  - Mallory-Weiss syndrome
  - Boerhaave syndrome (trans- mural esophageal tear)
  - Acute gastritis
  - Acute pancreatitis

Anorexia

- Anorexia or decreased appetite with pain is usually seen in acute appendicitis

Urinary Symptoms with Pain

- Ureteric colic
- Cystitis

Fever with Chills and Rigors

- Amoebic liver abscess
- Pyogenic liver abscess
- Perinephric abscess
- Intra-abdominal pus collection

Other History

- *Past surgical history:* Previous operations leading to adhesions
- *Past medical history:* Sickle cell disease, Diabetes, Cancer or Renal failure
- Menstrual history in females
  - Missed period—ectopic pregnancy
  - Mid of period—ovulation pain (Mittelschmerz)
  - With heavy periods—endometriosis
- Family history of colon cancer, any other malignancy or inflammatory bowel disease

Physical Examination
General Appearance

- Anxious patient lying motionless
  - Acute appendicitis
  - Peritonitis
- Rolling in bed and restless
  - Ureteric colic
  - Intestinal colic

- Writhing in pain
  - Mesenteric Ischemia
- Bending Forward
  - Chronic Pancreatitis
- Jaundiced
  - CBD obstruction
- Dehydrated
  - Peritonitis
  - Small bowel obstruction

Vital Charting

- Temperature, Pulse, BP, Respiratory rate
- Ruptured AAA or ectopic pregnancy can lead to
  - Pallor
  - Hypotension
  - Tachycardia
  - Tachypnea
- Low grade rise in temperature is seen with
  - Appendicitis
  - Acute cholecystitis
- High grade rise in temperature is seen with
  - Salpingitis
  - Abscess
- Very high grade temperature with increasing lethargy seen in imminent septic shock
  - Peritonitis
  - Acute cholangitis
  - Pyonephrosis

Systemic Examination

Cardiopulmonary Examination

- Check for
  - Possible MI
  - Basal pneumonia
  - Pleural effusion

Abdominal Examination

The abdomen is divided into nine regions for systematic examination and evaluation (Fig. 62.1)

Inspection

- Scaphoid or flat in peptic ulcer
- Distended in ascites or intestinal obstruction
- Visible peristalsis in a thin or malnourished patient (with obstruction)
- Erythema or discoloration
  - Peri-umbilical — Cullen sign
  - Inguinal — Fox sign
  - Flanks — Grey Turner sign

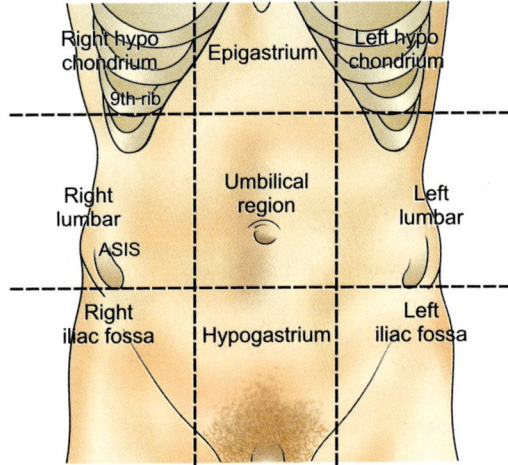

Fig. 62.1: Division of the abdomen into nine regions

  - Seen in hemorrhagic pancreatitis or any other cause of hemoperitoneum
- Any visible masses
- Any visible cough impulse at hernia site

Palpation

- Be gentle
- Start away from site of pathology then towards
- Check for hernia sites
- Tenderness
- Rebound tenderness
- Guarding — involuntary spasm of muscles during palpation
- Rigidity — when abdominal muscles are tense and board-like; indicates peritonitis
- Local right iliac fossa tenderness
  - Acute appendicitis
  - Acute salpingitis in females
  - Amebiasis of cecum
- Low grade, poorly localized tenderness
  - Intestinal obstruction
- Tenderness out of proportion to examination
  - Mesenteric ischemia
  - Acute pancreatitis
- Flank tenderness
  - Perinephric abscess
  - Retrocecal appendicitis

Some Importants Named Signs

1. Cullen's sign is bluish pariumbilical discoloration often seen in retroperitoneal hemorrhage.

2. Kehr's sign denotes severe left shoulder pain due to irritation of diaphragm is classically seen in splenic rupture.
3. *Grey Turner sign:* Discoloration of flank seen in retroperitoneal hemorrhage
4. *Chandelier sign:* Manipulation of cervix in female patient causes to lift her buttock off the table, seen in PID.
5. *Rovsing sign:* Pain in right iliac fossa on palpation of left iliac fossa is seen in acute appendicitis.
6. *Iliopsoas sign:* Hyperextension of right hip joint causes abdominal pain is seen in retrocecal appendicitis, perinephric abscess.
7. Thumbing tenderness over lower ribs is seen in inflammation of diaphragm, liver abscess or splenic abscess.

- Pulsatile abdominal mass with hypotension — leaking AAA
- Cutaneous hyperaesthesia indicates involvement of parietal peritoneum
- Per rectal examination
  - Tenderness
  - Induration
  - Mass (Blummer's shelf)
  - Frank blood
- Per vaginal examination
  - Bleeding
  - Discharge
  - Cervical motion tenderness
  - Adnexal masses or tenderness
  - Uterine size or contour

Auscultation

- Bowel sounds
  - Listen for >2 min to confirm absence
  - High pitched, hyperactive or tinkling
- Bruit in epigastrium

Surgical Myths

- Rebound tenderness, considered the clinical indicator of peritonitis, has a high (25%) false negative rate
- Rigidity, referred tenderness and pain on cough are sufficient evidence for peritonitis
- Except for detection of blood, routine PR exams add little to clinical assessment
- Administration of analgesics prior to surgical consultation does not obscure the diagnosis, but improves accuracy

Investigations

- Complete blood count with differential leukocyte count
  - Attention to the leukocyte count as a screening test only if substantially elevated
  - 25% of patients with elevated leukocyte count do not have different outcomes from those with a normal leukocyte count
- C-reactive protein estimation is more sensitive
- Electrolyte, blood urea, creatinine
- Urine dipstick to rule out diabetes
- Amylase or lipase for acute pancreatitis
- Liver function test
- Pregnancy test (when appropriate) as in young females.

Radiology

- Upright X-ray chest for
  - Basal pneumonia
  - Ruptured esophagus
  - Elevated hemidiaphragm
  - Free gas under diaphragm
- Abdominal X-ray film
  - Air-fluid levels
  - Stones
  - Ascites
  - Eggshell calcification in AAA
  - Air in biliary tree
  - Obliteration of psoas shadow in retroperitoneal disease
  - Right lower quadrant sentinel loop in acute appendicitis
- Other investigations
  - USG
  - CT abdomen for AAA, pancreatic disease or ureteric colic (noncontrast)
  - Mesenteric angiography for ischemia, hemorrhage

Laparoscopy

- Early diagnostic laparoscopy may result in
  - Accurate
  - Prompt and
  - Efficient management of acute abdominal pain
- Reduces the rate of unnecessary laparotomy
- Increases the diagnostic accuracy
- May be a key to solving the diagnostic dilemma of non-specific abdominal pain

63 | Abdominal Trauma

- Penetrating trauma
- Blunt trauma
- Iatrogenic injuries

Penetrating Trauma

- Stab wound
- Gun shot injury
- Blast injuries

Blunt Trauma

- Road traffic accidents
- Fall from height
- Crush injuries
- Sports injuries
- Violence

Iatrogenic Injuries

- Trauma during endoscopic procedure, e.g. colon perforation during colonoscopy or duodenum perforation during ERCP
- During external cardiac message
- During insertion of peritoneal dialysis catheter
- While performing liver biopsy
- Rectal perforation during insertion of rectal catheter in barium enema examination

Anatomical Considerations

Abdomen can be divided into four areas:
- Intra thoracic abdomen contains part of liver, spleen, fundus of stomach, intra-abdominal esophagus and diaphragm. As these organs are protected by rib cage they are less likely to get involved in blunt trauma until unless injury is of severe magnitude
- True abdomen contains intra-abdominal organ
- Pelvic abdomen contains urinary bladder, rectum and genital organs in females
- Retroperitoneal abdomen

Initial Management

Trauma Protocol

- Immobilize cervical spine by cervical collar or braces till the time cervical spine fracture has been ruled out by imaging, e.g. X-ray cervical spine or CT
- 100% oxygen by face mask
- 16–18 wide bore IV line preferably two are inserted
- Blood samples are withdrawn for grouping and cross matching and for base line investigations
- Crystalloid/colloid infusion is started
- Trauma series X-ray — chest, cervical spine and pelvis

Primary Survey

A-Air way management

B-Breathing

C-Circulation

D-Disability

E-Exposure

Abdominal Trauma: Examination

Inspection

- Abdominal distension
- Movement of abdominal wall with respiration
- Record all external marks of injury
- Record entry and exit site of bullet injury
- Discoloration of skin

Palpation

- Look for tenderness/rigidity/guarding
- Spine tenderness
- Pelvic compression test and compression of lower chest wall
- Per rectal examination

Percussion

- Look for free fluid

Auscultation

- Bowel sounds
- Bruit

Investigations

Lab Investigations

- Hematocrit estimation
- Urine analysis
- Serum amylase estimation
- Other routine lab tests for base line

Radiological Investigations

- X-ray chest erect for fracture ribs and free gas under diaphragm
- X-ray abdomen supine for bowel gas pattern and psoas shadow

Diagnostic Peritoneal Lavage (DPL)

Indications

- Unconscious patient
- Patients with high energy transfer with equivocal physical signs
- Multiple injuries with unexplained shock
- Patients with spinal cord injury
- Intoxicated patients
- Patients with suspected abdominal injury undergoing surgery for other conditions

Contra-indications

- Previous abdominal surgery
- Pregnancy
- Obesity
- Patient with obvious surgical abdomen

Positive Diagnostic Peritoneal Lavage (DPL)

- Aspiration of gross blood
- RBC count >100,000/cumm (for stab wound >1000 RBC/cumm)
- WBC count >500/cumm
- Amylase >200 units
- Presence of bile, feces or bacteria

Limitations

- False positive in 20% of cases mainly in pelvic fractures
- Does not differentiate between solid organ and hollow viscus injuries

CT Abdomen

Indicated in hemodynamically stable patients

- To identify and grade solid organ injuries
- To diagnose retroperitoneal injuries
- To follow patients of solid organ injuries treated conservatively

Drawbacks

- Expensive
- Requires radiological dependence and subject to availability of CT
- Low sensitivity to diagnose bowel or diaphragmatic injuries

Diagnostic Laparoscopy

- To identify peritoneal violation in anterior or flank stab wounds
- To identify diaphragmatic injuries

Ultrasonography (FAST)

- To evaluate presence of hemoperitoneum in blunt abdominal trauma
- FAST means focused abdominal sonotomography
- Positive FAST in unstable trauma patients indicates the need for laparotomy without any further tests
- Negative FAST means source of bleed is from other than abdomen
- Advantages
  - Rapid, fast, cheap
  - Non-invasive, no radiation
  - Can be performed at bed side
  - No need to shift patient to radiology

- Limitations
  - Obesity
  - Gas interposition
  - Subcutaneous emphysema
  - Operator dependent

Management

Conservative management by observation
- Hemodynamically stable patients with blunt abdominal trauma with mild to moderate grade of solid organ injuries
- Hollow viscus injuries must have been ruled out
- Managed in ICU setting
- Blood grouped and cross matched
- OT is informed and directed to receive the patient if conservative management fails

- Monitoring by vital parameters, hematocrit and serial CT/Imaging
- Exploration done if clinical or radiological deterioration or >4 units blood transfusion in 24 hours is required

Operative Management

- Indications of laparotomy
  - Signs of peritoneal irritation
  - Unexplained shock
  - Evisceration of viscus
  - Positive DPL
  - Deterioration during observation
  - Gunshot wounds
  - Stab wound with penetration of peritoneum
  - Blast injuries

64 Dysphagia

SWALLOWING

- The act of swallowing involves three phases: Oral, pharyngeal, and esophageal.
- Swallowing takes about 8–10 seconds.

Evaluation of Dysphagia

History

- Duration of dietary changes, weight loss
- Odynophagia means painful swallowing most commonly due to infective pathology
- Dysphagia for solids, liquids or even for patient's own saliva
- Level of sensation of dysphagia
- Past surgery to head and neck, trauma, ingestion of corrosive substances
- Associated symptoms such as with GERD, voice changes, nasal leakage, otalgia
- Common systemic processes associated with dysphagia:
  - Tobacco/alcohol
  - Medications — antihistamines, anticholinergics, antidepressants, antihypertensives
  - Osteoarthritis
  - Systemic neuromuscular disorders
  - Autommune disorders
  - Psychiatric state

Physical Examination

- *General:* Body habitus, mental status, drooling of saliva, wheezing, dyspnea, voice quality
- Cranial nerves examination to rule out neurological cause
- Inspection of the tongue and palate for strength/symmetry
- *Laryngeal examination:* Pooled secretions, vocal fold movement, interaretynoid area
- Examination of cervical lymph nodes especially left supraclavicular group to rule out any secondaries
- Examine hepatomegaly or free fluid in the abdomen which may point towards esophageal malignancy

Imaging Studies

Plain Film — X-Ray Soft Tissue Neck (AP and Lateral views)

- Identifies suspected infectious cause of dysphagia with gross displacement of structures, but as such do not have much role.

Barium Swallow

- Identifies structural disorders, e.g. dysphagia for solid foods and the level of obstruction.
- Advantages
  - Good anatomical detail
- Disadvantages
  - Radiation
  - Cannot be done in bedridden patients
  - Cannot detect dynamic disorders

Esophageal Manometry

- Helps in diagnosis of disorders in which intraluminal pressures must be measured (achalasia, esophageal spasm, etc.)
- Advantages
  - It is the only test based on pressure wave physiology
- Disadvantages
  - Cannot diagnose visible lesions
  - Unpleasant for patient
  - Technically demanding.

Bolus Scintigraphy

- It helps to follow improvement in a patient with history of aspiration, patient with achalasia.
- Advantages
  - Less radiation
  - Quantitative counts of particles
- Disadvantages
  - No anatomic details can be delinated
  - Single bolus, no different consistency used

Fiberoptic Endoscopic Evaluation of Swallowing

- It is the investigation of choice
- Advantages
  - Portable
  - Allows assessment of sensation
  - Cheap
  - Can be used for patient teaching
  - No radiation
- Disadvantages
  - Cannot evaluate cricopharyngeus directly
  - Cannot evaluate esophagus

Differential Diagnosis

- Foreign body
- Tracheostomy balloon obstructing esophagus
- Cricopharyngeal achalasia
- Zenker's diverticulum
- Cervical spine disease — osteophytes pressing on esophagus

- Esophageal webs and rings
- Esophageal stricture — caustic ingestion
- Achalasia cardia
- Diffuse esophageal spasm
- Gastroesophageal reflux disease, especially with stricture
- Esophageal malignancy
- Systemic disorders
  - Stroke — present in up to 47% of cases
  - Amyotrophic lateral sclerosis
  - Parkinson's disease
  - Multiple sclerosis
  - Muscular dystrophy
  - Myasthenia gravis
- Autoimmune disorders
  - Systemic sclerosis
  - Systemic lupus erythematosis
  - Dermatomyosits
  - Mixed connective tissue disease
  - Mucosal pemphigoid, epidermolysis bullosa
  - Sjögren's syndrome (xerostomia)
  - Rheumatoid arthritis (cricoarytenoid joint fixation)
- Aging
  - Dysphagia is present in 2% > 65 years
  - Poor dentition
  - Loss of tongue connective tissue
  - Increased pharyngeal transit time
  - Globus hystericus
  - Imagined dysphagia
  - Somatization

Dysphagia in Children

- Nasal obstruction
- Oral lesions — clefts, ranulas, mucoceles
- Laryngomalacia, laryngeal clefts, TD fistula
- Vascular rings, foregut malformations
- Tumors — hemangiomas, lymphangiomas, papillomas, leiomyomas, neurofibromas

65 | Esophagus

ANATOMY

1. The esophagus starts at the level of sixth cervical vertebra corresponding to cricoid cartilage and ends in front of the T12 vertebra.
2. Esophagus is by enlarge a midline structure except at the following three places
   a. At the base of the neck where it lies on left
   b. At the level of T7 where it lies to the right of midline
   c. At the level of T12 where it lies left of spine
3. Three anatomical divisions, i.e. (i) Cervical, (ii) Thoracic, (iii) Abdominal
4. Three functional divisions, i.e. (i) Upper esophageal sphincter (UES) is a high pressure zone at the inlet of the Esophagus, (ii) Lower esophageal sphincter (LES) at the end.
5. From oncological point of view it can be divided into two parts (i) Proximal, (ii) Distal
6. It is 22 to 28 cm in length (24 cm with variation of 5 SD). Length depends upon the height of the person. Abdominal esophagus is 3–4 cm in length
7. There are three areas of constriction, i.e. (i) At the start, (ii) In the chest where it crossed by left bronchus/aortic arch, (iii) At the hiatus of diaphragm
8. Cervical esophagus is 5 cm long and extends from sixth cervical vertebrae to the suprasternal notch
9. Thoracic esophagus is 18–20 cm long
10. Mucosal lining is squamous epithelium except in the abdominal part where it is columnar type
11. Muscle consists of two distinct layers, i.e. inner circular and outer longitudinal. In the upper one third of the esophagus these two layers are striated, but in lower two third these two layers are smooth muscle. In between the two layers of muscle, lies loose connective tissue, blood vessels and interconnected network of ganglia known as Auerbach's plexus
12. *The blood supply* is
    a. From inferior thyroid artery for cervical portion
    b. The thoracic portion is supplied by bronchial arteries and direct branches from aorta
    c. The abdominal portion is supplied by ascending branch of left gastric and inferior phrenic artery
13. *The venous drainage* is
    a. The cervical portion drained by inferior thyroid veins
    b. The thoracic portion is drained by bronchial azygos or hemi azygos veins
    c. The abdominal portion is drained by coronary veins
14. *The lymphatic drainage:* There is dense sub mucosal plexus which extends longitudinally

throughout the length. The cervical portion drains in to deep cervical nodes. The upper thoracic portion drains in to para-tracheal nodes. The lower thoracic portion drains in to sub-carinal nodes, nodes in the inferior pulmonary ligament and in to superior gastric nodes. The abdominal portion drains in to superior gastric nodes.

Investigations for Esophagus

1. *Barium swallow study:* This study is very good for anatomical delineation, to find out any stricture, filling defect or any external compression. It will give information about the type of narrowing of lumen like eccentric narrowing or smooth tapering.
   Indications of barium swallow:
   a. Initial investigation for dysphagia of any origin
   b. In evaluation of GERD to exclude hiatus hernia and esophageal shortening
   c. In evaluation of esophageal symptoms who has undergone previous surgery of esophagus or esophago-gastric junction
   d. In patients with known benign or malignant strictures who are planned for surgery or endoscopic intervention
2. *Upper GI endoscopy:* It helps in defining the exact pathology, in taking biopsy and for therapeutic purposes like sclerotherapy or balloon dilatation of stricture.
3. *Esophageal manometry:* This investigation is useful in diagnosis of motility disorders, e.g. achalasia cardia. Pressure recording is done with multi-lumen catheter attached with transducers. The mechanical function of the esophageal musculature and sphincters by recording intra-luminal pressure changes caused by contraction is evaluated.
4. 24 hour pH monitoring is useful for diagnosis of gastro-esophageal reflux. The pH measuring electrode is inserted through trans nasal route 5 cm above the manometrically defined LES. A reflux episode is defined as pH drop below 4.

Esophagitis

It can be reflux esophagitis due to reflux of acid or non reflux esophagitis.

Etiology of Non-reflux Esophagitis

a. Corrosive poisoning, e.g. Lye, acids, sodium hydrochloride
b. Infections, e.g. Candida infection, Herpes virus
c. Drug induced, e.g. tetracycline , NSAID, doxycycline
d. Radiation if combined with adriamycin or actinomycin D
e. Aphthous esophagitis
f. Crohn's disease
g. Bullous dermatosis

Reflux Esophagitis

Factors preventing reflux of acid in to esophagus
a. Lower esophageal sphincter
b. Positive Intra-abdominal pressure
c. Pinch cock like action of left crus of diaphragm
d. Acute angle of His (Esophago-gastric angle)
e. Phreno-esophageal membrane fixes the esophago-gastric junction to diaphragm
f. Rosette like lower esophageal mucosal fold which closes the esophageal gastric junction

Clinical Features

a. Heart burn which is aggravated by posture, large meals, bending stooping
b. Regurgitation of stomach contents in mouth at night
c. Dysphagia can be due to edema, spasm, fibrosis or stricture
d. There can be pain on swallowing due to esophagitis
e. Patient can have chest pain due to sudden reflux of acid and can mimics cardiac event
f. Patient can have respiratory symptoms, e.g. dry cough, changes in voice, choking episode, chest infection
g. Patient can present with anemia due to repeated hematemesis

Complications

a. Ulcers
b. Stricture
c. Columnar metaplasia

Investigations

- 24 hour pH monitoring and manometry
- Endoscopy

Management

1. Life style modifications
2. Dietary management

3. Drugs — Proton pump inhibitors and prokinetic drugs are useful
4. Surgical management is indicated in following circumstances:
   a. Failure of medical therapy
   b. Development of complications
   c. Reflux after previous abdominal surgery
   d. Atypical symptoms, e.g. respiratory, pharyngeal or dental problems
   e. If there is a need for long term medical therapy proved by rapid recurrence of symptoms within a day or two of stopping medical therapy
   f. Patients need increasing dose of Proton Pump Inhibitors (PPI) to control their symptoms
   g. Patient showing poor compliance to taking drugs or changing their lifestyle which is an essential component of medical therapy

Contraindications to Anti-reflux Surgery

1. Medically complicated morbid obesity patients with BMI >35 Kg/m^2 should be treated by Roux-en-y gastric bypass or sleeve gastrectomy
2. Patients with Barrett's esophagus and high grade dysplasia should be treated by esophageal resection
3. Severe peptic strictures if the esophagus cannot be dilated up to 16 mm (48 Fr) should be treated by esophageal resection
4. Patients who have previously undergone gastric surgery, gastric bypass or vertical banded gastroplasty

Achalasia Cardia

Etiology and Pathology

1. It is the commonest primary esophageal motility disorder with an incidence of 0.4 to 0.6 per hundred thousand and prevalence of 8 per hundred thousand.
2. Etiology and pathogenesis is not known.
3. There is decrease or loss of myenteric ganglion cells with variable degree of neural fibrosis and chronic inflammation in the myenteric plexus. There is paucity of nerve fibers in the distal smooth segment of the esophagus.
4. Manometric profile shows absence of peristalsis in the esophageal body with incomplete relaxation of high pressure LES in response to swallowing. Resting pressure in the LES is elevated and usually more than 25 cm of Hg.

5. Esophageal carcinoma develops in 3–5% of cases in long standing cases of achalasia cardia usually after an average of 20 years.
6. Leukoplakia of esophagus mucosa is commonly seen.
7. Esophagitis and mucosal ulceration usually occurs due to stasis and bacterial proliferation.

Clinical Features

a. Key features are dysphagia, regurgitation and chest pain.
b. Dysphagia is mainly for solid food, is intermittent initially and is of variable severity. It can get aggravated by emotional distress and cold liquids.
c. Dysphagia usually have gradual onset and plateau within two years. Majority of patients present after two years.
d. Swallowing improves after drinking liquids, after Valsalva maneuver, eating in upright posture or after breath holding as all these increases intra-esophageal pressure and helps to overcome the resistance at LES.
e. Initially there are episodes of odynophagia and chest pain associated with dysphagia when esophageal dilatation is minimal. Chest pain can mimic angina pain.
f. With the onset of esophageal dilation chest pain and odynophagia becomes less prominent and gradually disappear.
g. Later on around 80% of patient starts having spontaneous and postural regurgitation of foamy saliva which contains mucus. However, patients do not lose their weight.
h. Patients may seek advice on account of halitosis and persistent eructation's of foul smell.
i. Heart burn is seen in long standing cases due to development of esophagitis resulting from bacterial fermentation of retained food in dilated esophagus.
j. Advanced cases may present with severe dysphagia, nutritional anemia, repeated troublesome regurgitation, weight loss and respiratory complications like pneumonia, lung abscess, bronchiectasis, and lung fibrosis.
k. The diagnosis is essentially confirmed by barium swallow study, endoscopy, manometry and chest X-ray.

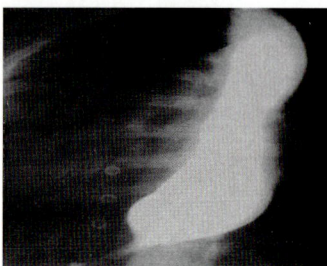

Fig. 65.1: Achalasia cardia

l. Contrast study usually reveals massively dilated esophagus with smooth beak like tapering of esophagus at GE junction and absence of gastric air bubble in 50 % of cases.

m. Endoscopy is performed to rule out any stricture, malignancy of GE junction or any other mechanical cause of stenosis. LES usually appears puckered and do not open with air insufflations, however scope can be negotiated easily across GE junction in achalasia cardia.

n. Manometry is investigation of choice for diagnosis of achalasia cardia with classical findings of absence of primary peristalsis in the body of esophagus with increased pressure in LES which fails to open in response to swallowing.

Treatment

1. Medical treatment in the form of long acting nitrates may be beneficial in 50 to 70 percent of cases initially, however due to development of tachyphylaxis less than 50% of patients have sustained response. Calcium channel blockers have been tried, but has not proven to be beneficial in controlled trial.

2. Injection of botulinum toxin in LES has shown immediate results in 90 percent of cases in terms of symptomatic improvement and reduction of resting LES pressure by 40%. However, there is no improvement in terms of esophageal emptying and benefit is not long lasting as there is need of repeated injections. Botulinum toxin binds to pre-synaptic receptors and inhibits the release of acetylcholine from axons. It is a safe therapy and can be used in elderly patients who are at high risk of surgery or in patients with atypical symptoms when diagnosis is not very certain.

3. Pneumatic dilation or surgical myotomy are definite methods of treatment which give long lasting cure.

4. Pneumatic dilation done is using polyethylene balloons with 30–40 mm diameter. Dilation is done up to diameter of 3 cm. The balloon is placed at GE junction and inflated to its maximum diameter under fluoroscopy control. There is risk of esophageal perforation in 13% of patients and the response rate is 60 to 80%.

5. Surgical treatment is indicated in following situations:

   a. After failure of botulinum toxin injection or pneumatic dilatation. The failure is indicated by reappearance of symptoms after short period of treatment

   b. A patient who has associated pathology which needs surgical treatment for their correction or because of associated pathology non operative treatment becomes risky. These conditions are epiphrenic diverticulum which makes non operative management risky. Associated hiatus hernia is an indication for surgery itself

   c. If surgery is patient's choice in the beginning itself

   d. In young adults and pediatric age group patient surgery is preferred as repeated non operative procedures carry morbidity

Operation which is carried out is Heller's cardiomyotomy which comprises of division of musculature on anterior aspect of esophagus up to the mucosa. The mucosa bulges out through divided muscle. The extent of division of muscle is up to 5 cm proximally on esophagus from GE junction and 1 cm distally on stomach from GE junction. The aim is to make GE junction incompetent. In order to avoid future problems of GE reflux the procedure is combined with partial (180 degree) anterior (Dor) or posterior (Toupet) fundoplication.

Malignant esophageal neoplasm

1. Majority of them are carcinoma and carry very poor prognosis

2. It is the disease of old persons (more than 60 years) with overall incidence of 10–20 per hundred thousand of population per year in western countries. In China and South Africa its incidence is 160 per 1,00000

3. Adenocarcinoma is infrequently seen before the age of 40

4. Squamous cell carcinoma is rarely seen before the age of thirty

5. Male to female ratio for squamous cell carcinoma is 3:1, but this ratio for adenocarcinoma is 15:1
6. The etiology of carcinoma of esophagus is multi-factorial and following factors have been incriminated:
   a. Consumption of alcohol in excess increases the risk by five fold
   b. Smoking also increases the risk by five times
   c. The combination of smoking and alcohol consumption increases the risk of developing esophageal cancer by 25–100 times
   d. Consumption of fewer amounts of fruits and green vegetables leading to deficiency of antioxidants
   e. Presence of excess amount of exogenous carcinogens and promoting factors
   f. Tylosis palmaris et plantaris is an autosomal dominant disorder in which there is hyperkeratosis of skin of palms and sole in the second or third decade and by seventh decade majority of patients develop esophageal carcinoma
   g. Patients with Plummer-Vinson syndrome has very high risk of developing esophageal carcinoma. In this condition there is deficiency of iron and vitamins leading to atrophy of esophageal mucosa with increased risk of developing cancer of cervical esophagus
   h. Patients with achalasia cardia and Barrett's esophagus have intermediate risk of developing carcinoma esophagus. The risk of carcinoma in achalasia cardia is not reduced by myotomy. Patients with achalasia cardia carry 16 fold increased risk of developing esophageal malignancy in the long term
   i. Patients with Barrett's esophagus have 40 times more chances of developing adenocarcinoma of lower third of esophagus
   j. Patients who have received radiotherapy for Hodgkin's and non Hodgkin's lymphoma are at high risk of developing carcinoma of esophagus
   k. Patients who have been treated for squamous cell carcinoma of head and neck are at high risk of developing esophageal carcinoma
   l. Patient who have ectopic gastric mucosa in esophagus also have high risk of developing esophageal malignancy
   m. Stricures developing after lye ingestion also carry very high incidence esophageal malignancy risk

Pathology

Various histopathological types of esophageal malignancy are
1. Squamous cell carcinoma (95%)
2. Adenocarcinoma (1–2%)
3. Squamous cell variants
   – Verrucous carcinoma although a low grade malignancy carries a very poor prognosis. Esophageal resection is the treatment of choice as verrucous type of esophageal carcinoma does not respond to radiotherapy
   – Basaloid type is a locally aggressive neoplasm with late metastasis. Resection of esophagus is the treatment of choice
   – Carcinosarcoma presents as polypoidal mass and has both squamous cell and spindle cell components
   – Adenoid cystic carcinoma behaves biologically similar to their counterpart in salivary gland. They are slow growing tumor and arise from intramural sub mucosal salivary glands
4. Adenocarcinoma variant: They have mucin secreting component and includes mucoepidermoid carcinoma and adenosquamous carcinoma. They arise from glands situated in the sub mucosa of esophagus.
5. Leiomyosarcoma arise from muscularis propria of esophagus usually in the lower two third of esophagus. They are usually slow growing with low potential for metastasis. They are usually radio resistant and surgical resection is the treatment of choice.

Symptoms

a. Early stage cancer may be asymptomatic or present with symptoms of GERD like heartburn, regurgitation of food and heaviness in the chest.
b. Most common and striking feature is dysphagia. As the esophagus is distensible tubular structure, dysphagia do not appear till the lumen is narrowed to 1/3 rd of original size.
c. Normal diameter of esophagus in an adult is 24 mm. Dysphagia is noted for solids only when the lumen get narrowed to 12 mm and for liquids when diameter is narrowed down to 8 mm.
d. With the onset of dysphagia weight loss starts appearing.
e. Advanced causes can present with symptoms due to trachea-esophageal fistula like choking, coughing, aspiration

f. Local invasion of recurrent laryngeal nerve can lead to hoarseness of voice and vocal cord paralysis.

g. Some patients can present with cervical lymph nodes enlargement.

Diagnosis

a. Barium meal swallow study is done in all cases presenting with dysphagia. It is an initial screening test which can differentiate between intra-luminal and intramural lesions as well as intrinsic and extrinsic lesions.

b. Endoscopy is performed for biopsy and to note the location of lesion from incisor teeth. The length of lesion is also noted.

c. Further staging investigations include CT abdomen, chest, PET scan and endoscopic ultrasonography.

Treatment

The treatment depends upon staging of disease and the condition of the patient.

If the tumor is confined to esophagus without lymph node involvement, removal of tumor with adjacent lymph nodes may be curative. In this subgroup of patient if the tumor is *in situ* or intra-mucosal endoscopic resection of tumor may be tried.

In locally advanced tumors, i.e. tumor which has gone out of esophageal wall or involvement of lymph nodes, multimodality treatment, i.e. chemotherapy followed by surgery or radiation and chemotherapy followed by surgery is under taken.

For disseminated tumors' treatment is aimed at palliation of symptoms. For palliation of dysphagia placement of expandable esophageal stents by endoscopic method is carried out.

Presence of palpable cervical lymph nodes is taken as M1a disease and these patients receive only palliative treatment.

Treatment by Tumor Location

Cervical Esophagus

Cervical esophageal cancers are mostly squamous in nature and are generally unresectable due to early involvement of larynx, great vessels, or trachea. Radiation therapy with concomitant chemotherapy is the usual treatment as only few patients are diagnosed at the stage when they are fit for radical resection.

Tumors of Middle Third of Esophagus

T1 and T2 (T1 is tumor confined to sub mucosa and T2 is tumor invading muscularis propria) tumors without lymph node involvement are treated by resection. Transmural tumors (T3) or tumor having lymph node involvement are treated by neoadjuvant chemotherapy followed by resection. Esophageal resection of thoracic portion can be through trans-hiatus route or by VATS (Video assisted thoracoscopic surgery) or with open thoracotomy.

Tumor of lower esophagus and cardia are adenocarcinoma, resection within continuity, lymph node dissection is the treatment of choice until unless preoperative staging demonstrates that tumor is unresectable. At least 10 cm of normal esophagus above tumor should be removed because there are chances of skip lesions and tumor spread submucosally in longitudinal direction.

Contraindications to esophageal resection are:

a. Recurrent nerve palsy

b. Presence of Horner's syndrome

c. Presence of paralysis of diaphragm

d. Persistent spinal pain

e. Fistula formation

f. Presence of malignant pleural effusion

g. Tumor more than 8 cm in length

h. More than 4 lymph nodes enlargement on CT

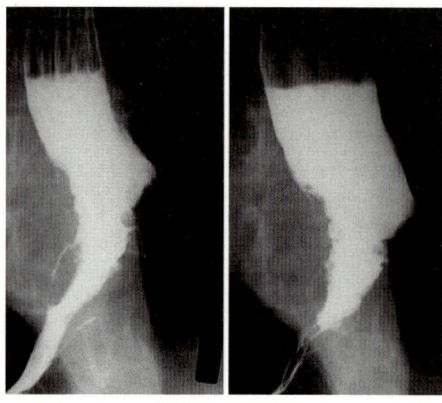

Fig. 65.2: Malignancy of the esophagus

Applied Anatomy and Physiology of Stomach

- Roughly J shaped at rest
- Size and shape varies with
  - Volume of food or fluid it contains
  - Position of body
  - Phase of respiration
- High and transverse in obese and short persons
- Elongated in thin persons

Parts of the Stomach

- **Stomach has**
  - **Two surfaces:** Anterior and posterior
  - **Two curvatures:** Greater and lesser
  - **Two orifices:** Cardia and pylorus
- **Cardia:**
  - Gastro-esophageal junction

  - 2.5 m left of midline
  - T10 level
- **Fundus:**
  - Above the horizontal line from cardiac notch to greater curvature
  - In contact with left dome of diaphragm
  - Full of swallowed air
- **Incisura:**
  - Junction of horizontal and vertical part of lesser curvature
  - Clearly seen from inside at endoscopy
- **Pyloroduodenal junction:**
  - Identified by the vein of Mayo externally
  - Right of midline at L-1

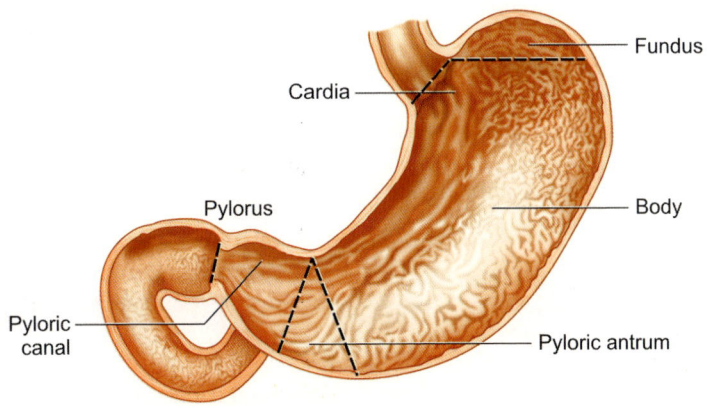

Fig. 66.1: Parts of the stomach

Stomach Bed

- Left crus and dome of diaphragm
- Body of pancreas
- Splenic artery
- Transverse mesocolon, left flexure
- Part of left kidney, left suprarenal
- Coeliac plexus, ganglion and lymph nodes

On Upper GI Endoscopy

- Body and fundus recognized by thick vertical mucosal folds
- Incisura seen as transverse ridge
- Antrum by flat mucosa

On Ultrasound

- Stomach wall thickness is 5–6 mm
- On endoluminal or laparoscopic ultrasound it is seen as 5 layered structure
- Endolumuinal USG is the most sensitive method in assessing 'T component' of gastric malignancy

Histology

- Three layers
  - Mucosa
  - Submucosa
  - Muscularis propria

Mucosa

- Mucus secreting epithelial cells lining the surface and gastric pits
- Lamina propria containing gastric glands of specialized cells
- Muscularis mucosa dividing mucosa from submucosa
- *Muscularis Mucosa:* Lymphatics cross the muscularis mucosa in the stomach to reach lamina propria in contrast to colon, where lymphatics do not cross muscularis mucosa.
- Three types of mucosa in stomach
  - *Cardiac mucosa:* Simple mucus secreting glands, circular or oval shaped
  - *Body and fundus:* Gastric glands are elongated; test tube shaped and contain pareital and chief cells
  - *Antral mucosa:* Gastric glands are branched and secrete mucus and gastrin

Histological Division

- Between antrum and body does not correspond to anatomical division

- A tongue of antral mucosa extends up the lesser curvature
  - Extend increases with age leads to high gastric ulcers in elderly
- Foci of gastric metaplasia commonly seen in 1st part of duodenum

Histological difference between Ulcer and Erosions

- Erosion
  - Mucosal defect which does not penetrate muscularis mucosa
- Acute ulcer
  - Penetrates the muscularis mucosa for a variable distance
  - No changes of repair
  - No fibrous tissue seen
- *Chronic ulcer*
  - Fibrous tissue has formed
  - Normal architecture cannot be restored

Cardiac Sphincter

- Not to a distinct anatomical sphincter
- Competence maintained by
  - Rosette like mucosal fold at gastroesopha-geal junction (plugging action)
  - Acute angle of entry of lower esophagus into stomach (Valve like effect)
  - Fixation of gastro-esophageal junction by phreno-esophageal ligament
  - Presence of lower 3 cm of intra-abdominal esophagus which is compressed by positive intra-abdominal pressure
  - Circular muscles of the lower esophagus which are thickened
  - Right crus of diaphragm acts as a "Pinch Cock" to the lower esophagus

Pyloric Sphincter

- Well defined anatomical structure with a physiological mechanism
- Comprises of outer longitudinal and inner circular muscle layer
- Circular muscle in the shape of inverted V
- Limbs spread to greater curvature for up to 5 cm
- Longitudinal muscle continuous with the longitudinal muscle of duodenum

Blood Supply

Arterial Supply

- *Left gastric artery* — branch of celiac axis

- *Right gastric artery* — branch of common hepatic artery
- *Right gastroepiploic artery* — branch of gastroduodenal artery and anastomoses with the left gastroepiploic artery to form an arcade
- Left gastroepiploic artery — branch of splenic artery
- Short gastric arteries from splenic artery

Clinical Importance

- Gastroduodenal artery passes behind duodenum and often gets eroded by overlying duodenal ulcers leading to severe hemorrhage
- Left gastric lymph nodes lie near the origin of the left gastric artery, so during radical gastrectomy, left gastric artery should be flush ligated to attain total clearance of lymph nodes

Venous Drainage

- Veins mainly accompany arteries
- Left gastric or coronary vein is of surgical importance, as it receives branches from esophagus
- This vein must be divided specifically in operations for bleeding esophageal varices

Microcirculation

- Vessels to the mucosa of the lesser curvature arise directly from left or right gastric arteries instead of submucosal plexus
- These small vessels take a long course to reach mucosa by piercing serosa, muscle and lamina propria
- Long course of these vessels and lack of submucosal plexus are responsible for the development of lesser curvature ischemia more often

Nerve Supply

- Anterior/left vagus nerve
- Posterior/right vagus nerve

Anterior Vagus Nerve

- At diaphragmatic hiatus, anterior vagus lies behind peritoneum and phreno-esophageal ligament
- Closely applied to anterior surface of esophagus
- Usually single large trunk
- In 30% more than one trunk
- Easily identified by palpation with slight tension on esophagus

- Often a branch passes to stomach on left side at a point 5–7 cm from cardio-esophageal junction

Posterior Vagus Nerve

- Not approximated to the esophagus
- Separated from it by 10 mm, lies more to the patient's right
- Thicker than anterior vagus
- May present as more than one trunk in 10% of cases

Vagotomy

- Several cms. of vagal trunk should be excised during vagotomy in view of marked capability of regeneration of the autonomic nervous system
- A small branch from left gastric artery accompanies the posterior vagus nerve
- Both ends of divided vagus should be ligated while doing posterior truncal vagotomy to avoid troublesome bleeding
- Nerve of Grassi
  - Often culprit for incomplete vagotomy
  - It is a branch of posterior vagus, passes behind esophagus to supply gastric fundus
  - Originate at gastro-esophageal junction or upto 5–7 cm from gastro-esophageal junction
  - 5–7 cm of nerve must be mobilized and then branch to the left identified
- Nerve supply of pyloric antrum
  - At 7 cm from pylorus, anterior vagus usually divides into branches
  - Appearance of this division has been described as "Crow's foot"

Test for Completeness of Vagotomy

- Intra-operative tests
  - Burge test:
    ◊ Described by Burge and Vane (1958)
    ◊ Stomach is converted into closed system by occlusion of cardia and pylorus
    ◊ Rise in intragastric pressure recorded after electrical stimulation of vagi by ring electrodes placed around esophagus
    ◊ Results of tests correlate well with postoperative acid secretion
    ◊ Provides a useful form of quality control in surgical training centers

- Grassi test:
  ◊ Devised by late professor Grassi of Rome in 1971
  ◊ Gastric acid secretion is stimulated by intravenous injection of pentagastrin during operation
  ◊ pH of gastric mucosa mapped after pentagastrin infusion
  ◊ If vagotomy complete, pH > 5.5
  ◊ Before vagotomy, it is less than 2.5
- *Congo red test:*
  ◊ Congo red dye is sprayed on to the gastric mucosa through the endoscope
  ◊ It turns black in the presence of acid
  ◊ It is used:
    ⇒ To delineate the extent of parietal cell mass while performing highly selective vagotomy
    ⇒ To define a subgroup of patients with acid antrum
    ⇒ To check the completeness of vagotomy
- Post-Operative tests
- Insulin test:
  ◊ Depends upon vagal response to insulin induced hypoglycemia
  ◊ Contraindicated in :
    ⇒ Epilepsy
    ⇒ With ischemic heart disease
    ⇒ Patients over 65 years of age
  ◊ Not useful in diabetic patients
  ◊ *Before vagotomy:* There is a strong acid response
  ◊ *One week after complete vagotomy:* There is no or little response with recurrent ulcer rate of less than 5 percent
  ◊ *Positive response:* 5–10 days after vagotomy indicates incomplete vagotomy with risk of recurrent ulceration of 6 to 50%
- Sham feeding test:
  ◊ Derived from Pavlov's work
  ◊ Presently regarded as a useful research tool

Types of Vagotomy

- *Truncal vagotomy:*
  - Both trunks are divided above celiac and hepatic branches adjacent to the hiatus
- *Selective vagotomy:*
  - Anterior and posterior vagi are divided distal to the celiac and hepatic branches

  - Extragastric gastrointestinal vagal innervation preserved
  - Risk of gallstone formation and diarrhea is less
- *Highly selective vagotomy:*
  - Branches of the anterior and posterior nerves of Latarjet to the body of stomach are divided at lesser curvature
  - Terminal branches to pylorus and antrum are preserved

Lymphatic Drainage

Lymph nodes were classified in relation to primary tumor from N1 to N4

- N1 — lymph nodes within 3 cm of primary tumor
- N2 — lymph nodes which are more than 3 cm from edge of primary tumor or nodes along left gastric, common hepatic, splenic arteries or celiac axis
- N3 — lymph nodes in hepatoduodenal ligament, retropancreatic lymph nodes, lymph nodes near diaphragm or in root of mesentry
- N4 — para-aortic lymph nodes or lymph nodes around middle colic artery

However this classification is no more followed, but still useful in deciding extent of gastric resection.

Functions of Stomach

Three major functions
- Motor
- Secretory
- Endocrine

Motor Functions

- Vagal mediated and gastrin induced receptive relaxation
- Mixing and grinding of food to form chyme
- Emptying of food at regular intervals

Secretory Functions

- Secretion of acid, pepsin, mucus, intrinsic factor, water and electrolytes

Endocrine Functions

- Gastrin, serotonin, somatostatin are released into blood

Physiological Functions of Gastric Exocrine Secretions

- Initiation of peptic hydrolysis of dietary proteins and triglycerides (H^+, pepsin, gastric lipase)

- Liberation of vitamins B_{12} from dietary proteins (H^+, pepsin)
- Binding of vitamin B_{12} for subsequent uptake (intrinsic factor)
- Facilitation of duodenal inorganic Fe^{++} and Ca^{++} absorption (H^+)
- Stimulation of pancreatic HCO_3^- secretion via secretion release (H^+)
- Suppression of antral gastrin release (H^+)
- Killing or suppression of growth of ingested microrganisms (H^+)
- Protection against noxious agents (mucin, mucus gel)

Mechanism of Acid Secretion (Fig. 66.2)

- When stimulated, parietal cells can secrete HCl at a concentration of roughly 150 mM (pH 0.8)
- Acid is secreted in to large canaliculi, which are continuous with the lumen of the stomach
- H^+ ion is concentrated in parietal cells 3 million fold higher than in blood
- Chloride is secreted against both concentration and electrical gradient
- H^+/K^+ ATPase (proton pump) located in the canalicular membrane is the key player in H^+ ion secretion
- This ATPase is Magnesium dependent
- Types of receptors on parietal cells which stimulates acid secretion
  - Histamine receptors (H2) for histamine released from enterochromaffin (ECL) and mast cells
  - Muscarinic (M3) type of cholinergic receptors for acetylcholine released from postganglionic neurons
  - Cholecystokinin (CCKB) receptors for gastrin released from G Cells
- Inhibitors of acid secretion
  - Cholecystokinin
  - Somatostain
  - Secretin
  - Prostaglandin esp. PGE2
  - Glucagon, e.g. peptides
  - Gastric inhibitory peptides
  - Peptide YY and enteroglucagon
- Steps of acid secretion in parietal cell
  - Hydrogen ions are generated within cells from dissociation of water
  $$H_2O \rightarrow H^+ + OH^-$$
  - Hydroxyl ions so formed combine with carbon dioxide to form bicarbonate. This is catalyzed by carbonic anhydrase
  $$OH^- + CO_2 \rightarrow HCO_3^-$$

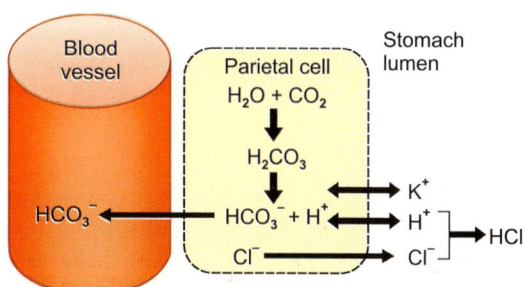

Fig. 66.2: Mechanism of acid secretion

Site	N1 nodes	N2 nodes
Upper third	Left paracardial	Supra and suppyloric
	Right paracardial	Common hepatic
	Lesser curvature	Left gastric
	Greater curvature	Splenic artery and hilum
		Celiac axis
Middle third	Right paracardial	Splenic artery and hilum
	Right gastric	Left paracardiac
	Lesser and greater curvature	Left gastric
	Suprapyloric and subpyloric	Common hepatic
		Celiac axis
Lower Third	Lesser curvature	Right paracardial
	Greater curvature	Left gastric
	Supra and infra pyloric	Common hepatic
		Celiac axis

Table 66.1: Classification of various nodal stations of the stomatch

- HCO$_3^-$ is transported out of basolateral membrane in exchange for Cl$^-$
- Outflow of HCO$_3^-$ from gastric mucosa to blood results in "alkaline tide"
- Cl$^-$ and K$^+$ transported in to lumen of canaliculus by Conductance channels
- H$^+$ ion exchanged with K$^+$ from cell into lumen of canaliculus through the action of proton pump

Tests for Gastric Acid Secretion

- Basal acid output (BAO)
  - Quantity of HCl secreted per hour by the stomach in the unstimulated basal state
  - Expressed as meq of HCl/hour
  - Normal range 1–5 meq/hour
  - Acid output = Volume of gastric juice in litres/hour × Conc. of H$^+$ ion (in meq/litre)
- Maximal acid output (MAO):
  - Total acid put during the hour after stimulation with pentagastrin (6 mg/kg SC and or histamine (10 mg/kg SC)
  - Value is calculated by adding the results of either four 15 minute or six 10 minute sample collections after stimulation
  - Normal range 25–55 meq HCl/hour
- Peak acid output:
  - Two highest consecutive 15 minute periods of stimulated output, are multiplied by a factor of 2 to yield a value for one hour period
- Gastric secretary studies are useful:
  - In patients with suspected gastric hyper-secretion
  - In evaluation of medical and surgical therapy in acid peptic disorders
  - In suspected Zollinger-Ellison syndrome

Effects of Truncal Vagotomy

- Lower esophagus:
  - Pressure in the lower esophageal sphincter is reduced
  - 10% patients can have transient dysphagia and heart burn
- Stomach:
  - Basal acid output reduced by 70–80%
  - Maximal acid output reduced by 50–60%
  - Response to standard dose of pentagastrin reduced
  - Loss of receptive relaxation of stomach leading to feeling of post-prandial epigastric fullness
  - Gastric mucosal blood flow decreased
  - Reduced rate of gastric emptying for solids, due to decreased force of contraction of antral pump
  - Increased rate of gastric emptying for liquids, due to increased intragastric pressure due to loss of receptive relaxation of stomach, leading to increase in pressure differential between stomach and duodenum
- **Biliary system:**
  - Increased fasting gallbladder volume and decreased contractility
  - Increased tendency to gall stone formation due to bile stasis
- Pancreas
  - Reduced pancreatic enzyme secretion by 50–70%
  - Increased production of glucagon
- Small intestine:
  - Abnormal proliferation of bacteria in the small intestine
  - Reduced absorption of iron and calcium
  - Diarrhea

67 Peptic Ulcer

- Craters extending to below the muscularis mucosa of stomach (gastric ulcer) or duodenum (duodenal ulcer).
- A product of self-digestion.

Epidemiology

- *Estimated life time prevalence:* 10%
- *Male:* Female = 3 – 4:1
- *Duodenal ulcer:* Gastric ulcer = 3:1
- Duodenal ulcer emerges 10–20 years earlier than gastric ulcer

Etiology and Pathogenesis

- *Helicobacter pylori* infection
- NSAIDs and aspirin
- Acid/Pepsin
- Smoking
- Genetics
- Psychological factors

The peptic ulcer occurs if the aggressive factors increase or defensive factors decrease or both.

Aggressive Factors

- Acid/pepsin
- *Helicobacter pylori* infection
- NSAID
- Smoking

Defensive Factors

- Mucus-bicarbonate barrier
- Barrier of apical membrane
- Mucosal blood flow
- Prostaglandins
- Epithelial cell restitution

Clinical Feature of Peptic Ulcer

It is difficult to differentiate between duodeual and gastric ulcer on the basis of symptoms. Age group of two groups are although different, but it is not usually possible to differentiate between duodenal and gastric ulcer on the basis of clinical features.

Main clinical features are:

1. **Pain:** Pain is usually in the upper mid abdomen, may radiate to back. Pain is usually intermittent and eating may relieve the pain.
2. **Periodicity:** Symptoms of peptic ulcer may disappear at constant intervals due to spontaneous healing of ulcers.
3. **Vomiting:** Vomiting is not regular feature, it may be self induced to relieve pain. However, if a constant feature there is a pylortic stenosis.
4. **Weight loss:** Patients with gastric ulcer often loose weight because they are afraid to eat due to pain.
5. **Bleeding:** All ulcers are prove to bleed, which may be acute or chronic.

Clinical Examination

There may be epigastric tenderness.

Investigations

Upper GI endoscopy is the investigation to diagnose peptic ulceration. In gastric ulcer, four quadrant property should be taken to rule out malignancy.

Treatment

Medical treatment

- H$_2$ receptor and proton pump inhibitors are commonly used as medical management.
- *H. pylori* eradication is routinely given to patterns with peptic ulceration, as *H. pylori* is the principle aetiological agent in peptic ulcer which is not induced by NSAID.

Surgical Treatment

Indications

Surgery is mainly reserved for complications of peptic ulcer.

Complications of Peptic Ulcer are

1. Perforation of ulcer leading to peritonitis
2. Bleeding from ulcer which can be
   a. Acute
   b. Chronic — occult blood loss
3. Stenosis leading to gastric outlet obstruction
4. Penetration into a solid organ
5. Malignant change in gastric ulcer

PERFORATION

Perforation: The ulcer perforates into the peritoneal cavity with spillage of contents. In chronic ulcer there is increasing dyspepsia prior to the perforation.

- Penetration or erosion into a solid organ: liver or pancreas
- In perforation of an acute ulcer there may not be any pre-existing symptoms
- Anteriorly situated ulcers perforate but posterior ulcers penetrate

Risk Factors

- *Drugs:* Long term use of steroids, NSAID, aspirin
- *Situations of stress:* Burns, multiple injuries, sepsis, chemotherapy, radiotherapy
- Smoking

Clinical Features of Perforated Ulcer

- Starts as an excruciating epigastric pain

- The intensity of pain depends on the degree of peritoneal soiling and whether the perforation becomes sealed
- The spillage can track along the right paracolic gutter leading to signs of acute perforated appendicitis with clinical signs mainly localized to the right iliac fossa
- Vomiting occurs in delayed cases and is due to paralytic ileus

Physical Signs of Perforated Ulcer

There is severe constant pain in upper abdomen or whole of abdomen which increases on deep inspiration and coughing. There is board like rigidity of the abdomen. Abdominal wall does not move with respiration.

The patient lies still in the bed as any movement will exacerbate the pain.

Investigations in Perforated Ulcer

- Plain abdominal X-ray in erect position will show pneumoperitoneum, i.e. free air visible in the right subdiaphragmatic space
- Multiple air/fluid levels in advanced cases due to paralytic ileus
- If no pneumoperitoneum, then sealed perforation or acute pancreatitis likely
- USG of the abdomen will reveal fluid within peritoneal cavity

Management of Perforated Ulcer

- Correction of hypovolemia, electrolyte disturbances, low urinary output
- In severe cases monitoring is done by CVP measurement and hourly urine output
- Colloids and crystalloids are both equally effective
- Nasogastric aspiration is started to take care of bowel distension
- Intra venous proton pump inhibitors are given (PPI)
- Planning for operation is done
- In sealed perforated ulcer Taylor's method of conservative management is done
- Taylor's method comprises of NG aspiration, IV fluids, antibiotics, intravenous proton pump inhibitors
- *Indication:* Young patients with short history of perforation of acute ulcer and with minimum of air and fluid under liver. Close clinical observation is required.

- Operative procedure:
  - Simple closure of the perforation with omental patch
  - Peritoneal lavage
  - Multiple drains

Pyloric Stenosis

- Chronic scarring from ulceration in the pyloric region leads to gastric outlet obstruction or pyloric stenosis.
- It mainly occurs in a patient with long-standing ulcer disease ignored, neglected or badly treated.
- One should be aware that pyloric stenosis might be due to a malignant antral tumor. In every case of pyloric stenosis, upper GI endoscopy should be performed to rule out malignancy.

Clinical Features

- Pain in the upper abdomen, relieved by vomiting
- Vomiting is effortless, projectile with partially digested food and bile is absent
- Nasogastric aspiration reveals only gastric fluid with thick partially digested food
- On examination patient is generally malnourished and underweight
- Patient is dehydrated with loose skin folds
- Patient may be anemic
- Gastric stasis is revealed by succussion splash on percussion
- Visible peristalsis may be seen passing across the upper abdomen from left to right

Metabolic Features

- The patient becomes progressively dehydrated and hyponatremic
- In an attempt to conserve circulatory volume, sodium is retained by the kidneys and hydrogen plus potassium is excreted preferentially
- Alkalosis becomes more severe and hypokalemia more marked
- Hypocalcemia can manifest as disturbance of consciousness and tetany
- Electrolyte disturbances in patients with severe pyloric stenosis are termed DARROW'S SYNDROME.

Investigations

- Lab investigations will reveal hyponatremia, hypokalemia, hypochloremia, metabolic alkalosis, hypocalemia and raised blood urea level.

- Barium meal upper GI study will reveal hugely dilated stomach with narrowing at antrum with deformed first part of duodenum suggestive of pyloric stenosis.
- Upper GI endoscopy with multiple biopsies from antrum should be performed in every case.

Pyloric Stenosis Management

- The priority is correction of fluid and electrolyte abnormalities.
- For rehydration normal saline infusion is started and once urine output is adequate, potassium supplements are given to correct hypokalemia.
- Provision of adequate sodium allows excretion of alkaline urine so that the alkalosis becomes correctable by itself.
- Clinical improvement is indicated by increased urine output and normalization of blood urea and electrolytes.
- Gastric lavage is done until fluid is clear.

Surgical Treatment

- Partial gastric resection with gastro-duodenal anastomosis (PEAN-BILROTH I)
- Partial gastric resection with gastro-Jejunal anastomosis (BILROTH II or REICHEL-POLYA)
- For old, frail patients bypass operation like gastro-jejunostomy is carried out.

BLEEDING PEPTIC ULCER

- Acute bleeding is the commonest complication
- It carries the highest mortality
- Bleeding results from erosion of the ulcer into a blood vessel
- The most common sign is malena +/– hematemesis
- One out of three pts. have no history of ulcer
- In major bleeding GI transit is so rapid that stool is bright red
- Peptic ulcer is the most common cause of acute hemorrhage in the upper GI tract accounting for more than 50% of cases
- Although hospitalization and surgery for uncomplicated peptic ulcer (PU) has decreased over the past 30 years, the number of hospital

admissions for hemorrhage associated with PU has remained relatively unchanged.

Severity of Acute Bleeding is Assessed by

BP, pulse rate, fall in Hb
Systolic BP < 100, PR > 100 with the patient supine, suggest major blood loss (>1 l).

Adverse Clinical Factors on Outcome

- Severe, continuing bleeding
- Early re-bleeding within 3–5 days of initial stabilization
- Age greater than 60
- Associated diseases: cardiovascular and liver diseases

The differential diagnosis includes:

- Rupture of esophago-gastric varices
- Hemorrhagic gastritis
- Mallory-Weiss laceration
- Ulcerated benign and malignant gastric tumors
- Vascular anomalies (angiodysplasia)
- Aorto-enteric fistula in pts. with a prosthetic aortic graft

Bleeding Peptic Ulcer—Endoscopic Classification for Severity of Bleeding

Forrest's Classification of Bleeding Activity

Forrest Ia-active bleeding—arterial spurting
Forrest Ib-active bleeding—oozing
Forrest II-bleeding ceased—clot lying on ulcer or visible vessel stump
Forrest III-bleeding ceased—no signs of recent bleeding.

Three Phases in the Management of the Bleeding

- Resuscitation
- Diagnosis
- Definitive treatment

Resuscitate hemorrhagic shock—ICU care might be required

Do not sedate patient for endoscopy

- Rapid transfusion
- BP, pulse rate, urine output monitoring
- Confusion and restlessness demand attention for oxygenation

Diagnosis

- History—dyspepsia, liver disease, intake of alcohol, aspirin, NSAID
- Endoscopic examination is done to find out the source and the gravity of bleeding
- Endoscopic criteria for early surgery:
  - Arterial spurter
  - Visible vessel in base of ulcer
  - Adherent clot

Indication For Surgery

- Continuing bleeding
- Re-bleeding

Check coagulation parameters before surgery.

Surgery in Bleeding Ulcer

- Partial gastrectomy but morbidity and mortality high
- Under-running of the bleeding ulcer, followed by the treatment with antiulcer drugs

68 | Gastric Cancer

1. It is the 14th most common malignancy and cause of cancer death in the US, however, in India it is the fifth most common cancer in males and seventh most common cancer in females
2. Highest incidence of gastric cancer in India is seen in Mizoram
3. It is the most common cancer in Japan
4. Gastric carcinoma is a disease of elderly with incidence in the seventh decade and carries a very dismal prognosis with an average overall 5 years survival rate of 10 percent
5. More than 60 percent of newly diagnosed cases occur in males
6. A better survival rate is seen in Japan due to active screening resulting in early diagnosis
7. There is an overall decline in the incidence of gastric cancer during the last three decades
8. The decreased incidence is due to increased consumption of fresh fruits and vegetables. The protective vegetables include green leafy vegetables. Increased uptake of carotene, vitamin C and calcium is also protective
9. Cancer of stomach is more common in semi-skilled or unskilled people in comparison to professionals or executives

Etiology

The known risk factors for development of gastric cancer are:

1. **H. pylori gastritis:** The risk of gastric cancer is three times more common in patients with persistent chronic H. pylori infection.
   a. Corpus predominant H. pylori gastritis leads to hypochlorhydria and predisposition to gastric ulcer and cancer
   b. Role of bone marrow derived stem cell has been incriminated in the development of gastric cancer in chronic *H. pylori* gastritis
   c. Gastric cancer develops in 2.9 percent of patients who are seropositive for *H. pylori* but in none of the case who are seronegative
   d. *H. Pylori* infection leads to atrophic gastritis which in turn progresses to intestinal metaplasia, dysplasia and intestinal type of gastric cancer
   e. Development of gastric cancer in *H. pylori* gastritis is related to virulence of *H. pylori*
   f. Patients infected with positive cytoxan associated gene A (Cag A) are more likely to develop gastric cancer
2. Consumption of pickled, salted, or smoked food carries high risk of gastric cancer. This type of food contains high level of nitrates. Gastric bacteria which are more commonly seen in conditions of achlorhydria convert nitrates to nitrites. Nitrites are known carcinogens. Preserved food and canned food are rich in nitrates
3. There is likely a synergistic effect between *H. Pylori* infection and dietary factors causing

gastric cancer. *H. Pylori* increases the growth of bacteria which causes carcinogen production and inhibits its removal. *H. Pylori* also decreases the production of ascorbic acid which has scavenging effect on oxygen free radicals

4. Gastric cancer is more common in following subgroup of patients:
   a. Atrophic gastritis and pernicious anemia
   b. Previous partial gastrectomy after 10 years
   c. *Adenomatous and hyperplastic gastric polyps:* Patients with these types of polyps have 10 times more chance of developing gastric cancer
   d. Familial polyposis
   e. *Hypogammaglobulinemia:* There is 50 times more chances of developing gastric cancer
   f. *Blood group A:* Diffuse gastric cancer is more common

5. *Genetic factor:* Most gastric cancers are aneuploid. More than two third of gastric cancers have deletion or suppression of tumor suppressor gene p53 and overexpression of COX-2 gene. Gastric cancers which over express COX-2 gene are more aggressive. Germ line mutation in CDH1 gene which encodes E-cathedrin is associated with hereditary diffuse gastric cancer and prophylactic total gastrectomy should be considered in these patients as there are 80 percent life incidences of developing gastric cancer

6. *Smoking:* Cancer especially of gastric cardia with a hazard ratio (HR) of 4:10

7. *Obesity:* 2.3 fold increased chances

Genetic alterations in gastric cancer:

a. Activation of oncogene: There is overexpression of c-met proto-oncogene which is a receptor for hepatocyte growth factor, k-ras gene and c-erb B2 oncogene.

b. Inactivation of tumor suppressor genes p-53 and p-16

c. Reduction of cellular adhesions

d. Reactivation of telomerase

e. Presence of microsatellite instability is seen in 20–30 percent of intestinal type of gastric cancer

Pathology

Various pathological types of gastric malignancy are
a. Adenocarcinoma (95%)
b. Lymphoma (4%)

c. Malignant GIST (1%)
d. Other rare types include carcinoid, squamous cell carcinoma, blood borne metastasis from other sites, e.g. melanoma or breast carcinosarcoma

Borrmann's Classification

This classification divides gastric cancer in to five types based on gross appearance. It was described way back in 1926, but still used these days for describing endoscopic findings.

Five types are:

a. *Protruding type or polypoidal type:* The lesion is elevated above the surrounding mucosa (type 1)

b. Ulcerated type with sharply demarcated margins (type 2)

c. Ulcerated without definite limits with infiltration in to surrounding walls (type 3)

d. Diffusely infiltrating without significant ulceration (type 4)

e. Non classifiable (type 5)

Lauren's Classification

Lauren in 1965 classified gastric cancer in to two types, i.e. intestinal and diffuse. These are two are distinct entities in terms of pathology, epidemiology and prognosis.

Intestinal Type

a. Majority of cases are associated with intestinal metaplasia

b. Commonly occurs in the setting of environment with precancerous condition like gastric atrophy

c. Males are more commonly affected

d. Involves older age group of patients

e. Usually they are well differentiated with glandular structure formation

f. Blood borne metastasis leading to distant spread is more common

g. Genetic abnormality common seen in intestinal type of gastric cancer are microsatellite instability and mutation of genes like APC and inactivation of tumor suppressor gene like p53 or p16

Diffuse Type

a. Usually not associated with intestinal metaplasia

b. Most of the time genetic factors play a major role in its causation and familial in nature

c. Females are more commonly affected

d. Occurs in younger age group in comparison to intestinal type

e. There is no glandular structure formation and is poorly differentiated with lot of signet ring cells

f. Metastasis is mainly lymphatic and transmural

g. There is decreased E-cadherin formation

Signs and Symptoms

1. Signs and symptoms in initial stages are non specific and includes recent onset 'A"s, i.e. anemia, Anorexia, Asthenia in a middle aged person and malignancy itself remain silent

2. Recent onset of non specific dyspepsia may be present which is insidious in onset

3. Patient may present with epigastric lump which is a late feature. This palpable lump is either due to bulky antral tumor or due to omentum involvement with secondary lymph nodes in it known as omentum caking

4. Patient may present with obstructive symptoms like dysphagia in carcinoma of cardia or gastric outlet obstruction in pyloric cancer

5. Distant metastasis, e.g. ascites, umbilical nodule (Sister Joseph nodule), left superaclavicular lymph node enlargement (Virchow's lymph node)

6. A bulky antral tumor or lymph node enlargement may lead to jaundice due compression of common bile duct in hepato-duodenal ligament.

Early Gastric Cancer

• Early gastric cancer is defined as cancer confined to mucosa or sub mucosa irrespective of lymph node involvement

• Prognosis is very good in early gastric cancer as the incidence of lymph node involvement is very low in comparison to late carcinoma

• Incidence of lymph node involvement is 10–15% in early gastric carcinoma

• The 5 years survival rate after adequate resection is 80 percent

• Early gastric cancer can be classified as protruding, superficial or excavating type on the basis of endoscopy

• Superficial type can be of elevated type, flat type or depressed type

Pre-operative Staging

Following investigations are performed for pre-operative staging

a. Flexible endoscopy and endoscopy ultrasonography:

  a. It provides complete visualization of tumor, tissue diagnosis.

  b. It can be used therapeutically in treatment of early gastric cancer confined to mucosa by performing endoscopic mucosal resection known as EMR.

  c. If patient presents late with gastric outlet obstruction and is not fit for surgery endoscopic dilatation and stent insertion can be done to relieve obstruction

  d. Endoscopic ultrasound is the investigation of choice for accurate T staging and for assessment of peri-gastric lymph nodes.

  e. On endoscopy ultrasound is performed using 7 .5 to 12 MHz transducer with stomach distended with water. The stomach appears as five alternating hypo echoic and hyper echoic layers.

b. *Computed tomography:* It is a mainstay for evaluation of intra-abdominal metastatic disease. It can also be used for loco regional staging; however its accuracy is less than endoscopic ultrasonography.

c. *Positron emission tomography (PET):* In patients with advanced disease who are given neoadjuvant chemotherapy, PET can be used to monitor the response of neoadjuvant chemotherapy if they were positive for PET initially.

d. *Laparoscopy:* Staging laparoscopy is a part of standard protocol for the pre-operative work up of carcinoma stomach. It can detect peritoneal deposits and secondary liver not picked up on CT.

Treatment

• Curative surgical resection remains the main stay for treatment

• Recently addition of adjuvant or neoadjuvant chemotherapy or in combination with radiotherapy has been shown to increase the cure rate and disease free survival in appropriately selected cases.

• NCCN guideline recommends neoadjuvant chemotherapy for any patient without metastatic disease if node positive or staged T2 or more on pre-operative staging.

• Chemotherapy which has been used is epirubicin, cisplatin, and 5 fluorouracil. This pre-operative chemotherapy leads to significant increase in survival and reduced disease progression as shown in MAGIC (Medical research council adjuvant gastric infusional chemotherapy) trial

- *Adjuvant chemotherapy:* There is clear advantage of 5FU based adjuvant chemotherapy in R1 resection or R0 resection with T2 or greater disease or node positive disease
- The principal of surgical resection is removal of tumor with 5 cm of normal stomach beyond the palpable margins with R0 resection which means resected margins are free on microscopic examination. R1 resection means whole of the disease has been removed macroscopically, but resected margin are not tumor free microscopically
- For nodal dissection all peri-gastric lymph nodes should been removed and resected specimen should contain at least 15 lymph nodes

69 | Acute Intestinal Obstruction

Acute intestinal obstruction is defined as a partial or complete interference with passage of stools distally in the small intestine.

Types

Pathologically

- Dynamic or mechanical
  - Hyperperistalsis proximal to obstruction
- Adynamic or paralytic (Absent or infective peristalsis)
  - No organic block
  - Functional obstruction
  - Absence of peristaltic activity
  - Failure of neuromuscular mechanism
  - Spastic paralytic ileus seen in lead poisoining.

Clinically

- Acute (usually in small gut)
- Chronic (usually in large gut)
- Acute on chronic — onset of acute obstruction in patient of chronic obstruction

Etiology

Lesions Outside the Wall

- Adhesions
  - Post-operative or inflammatory
  - Responsible for 60% of bowel obstruction
  - More common after pelvic operations or lower abdominal procedures
- Bands

- Hernia
  - External
  - Internal
- Neoplastic
- Intra-abdominal abscess

Lesions in the Intestinal Wall

- Congenital
  - Malrotation
  - Duplication cyst
- Inflammatory
  - Crohn's disease
  - Tuberculosis
  - Actinomycosis
  - Diverticulitis
- Neoplastic
  - Primary neoplasm
  - Metastatic neoplasm
- Traumatic
  - Hematoma
  - Ischemic stricture
- Miscellaneous
  - Intussusception
  - Endometriosis
  - Post radiation stricture

Causes in the Lumen

- Gall stone ileus
- Enterolith

- Bezoar
- Foreign body

Pathological Types of Small Gut Obstruction

Simple Obstruction

- Non-strangulated

Strangulated

- Obstruction with impaired blood supply.

Closed Loop Obstruction

- Segment of gut closed from both above and below, i.e. obstructed on either side.

Management of Intestinal Obstruction

It depends on three things:
- Whether the obstruction is mechanical or paralytic
- Its probable level
- Whether there is any element of strangulation.

Mechanical vs Paralytic

See Table 69.1

Level of Obstruction

High Small Bowel

- Onset of symptoms is sudden
- Upper abdominal pain with variable severity, colicky in nature usually
- Extreme degree of dehydration
- Abdomen is non-distended
- X-ray abdomen shows gasless abdomen or dilated duodenum (double bubble) or first jejunal (triple bubble) loop

Low Small Gut

- Onset of symptoms is more gradual
- Is associated with severe upper abdominal colicky pain
- Dehydration is less marked
- Distension is moderate and central in position

- X-ray of abdomen shows air-fluid level in erect film with no gas in colon.

Large Gut

- Usually insidious onset
- Pain is central/lower abdominal. It is colicky in nature or the patient may have generalized discomfort due to distension
- Patient may be slightly dehydrated
- Abdominal distension is progressive and peripheral
- X-ray shows gas in colon proximal to the site of obstruction

Pathology and Effects of Obstruction

Distal

- Normal for first few hours with normal peristalsis
- Later collapse

Proximal Loop

- Shows progressive distension due to gas and fluid accumulation
- Gas
  - Swallowed air
  - Diffusion from blood into the lumen
  - Bacterial action/digestion producing gas
- Fluid
  - 8 litres of fluid is secreted into the gut lumen per day
  - In intestinal obstruction this fluid is not reabsorbed due to
    - ◊ Fluid does not reach colon
    - ◊ Occlusion of veins due to distension of gut (and resulting increased intra-abdominal pressure).

Cause of Death

- Fluid and electrolyte loss
- Absorption of intestinal toxins leading to toxenis.
- Cardiorespiratory embarrassment caused by massive distension.
- Strangulation of gut leadings to gangrene.

Table 69.1: Differences between mechanical and paralytic obstruction

	Mechanical	Paralytic
Pain	Colicky pain is present	Absent
Vomiting	Less profuse	Profuse vomiting
Abdominal distension	Absent in high; central abdominal in low and peripheral in large gut obstruction	Generalized
Bowel sounds	Exaggerated	Absent (silent abdomen)

Clinical Features

Intestinal obstruction presents with four cardinal signs – pain, vomiting, distension and constipation.

Pain

- Usually the first symptom
- Colicky, severe, sudden onset
- Periumbilical in small gut
- Lower abdominal in large gut
- May be absent in post-operative adhesive obstruction and in paralytic ileus

Vomiting

- Initially digested food, then bilious, the feculent (with overgrowth of bacteria). Frequent vomiting usually seen in late obstruction or strangulation of gut.

Distension

- May be present in mesenteric vascular occlusion, paralytic ileus, low small gut or large gut obstruction

Constipation

- Not present in (i.e. often present with diarrhea)
  - Gall stone ileus
  - Obstructed Richter's hernia
  - Mesenteric vascular occlusion
  - Obstruction with pelvic abscess
  - Inpartial obstruction due to fecal impaction or colonic neoplasm

Pyrexia in the Presence of Obstruction Indicates

- Onset of ischemia
- Intestinal perforation
- Inflammation associated with obstructing disease

Investigations

Biochemistry

- Usually normal in early stages
- Later on there is
  - Decreased serum levels of sodium, potassium and chloride
  - Increased levels of bicarbonate and creatinine
  - Increased hematocrit due to hemoconcentration
  - WBC count >15000/cumm or metabolic acidosis should suggest strangulation

Radiology

X-Ray Abdomen — Supine and Erect

- Dilated loops of small bowel in ladder-like pattern
- Multiple air fluid levels
- No gas in colon in complete small bowel obstruction
- Air-fluid level absent in
  - Early obstruction
  - Proximal obstruction
  - Closed loop obstruction
- Strangulation is suggested by
  - Loss of mucosal pattern
  - Presence of gas in the wall of gut (Pneumatosis intestinalis)
  - Gas in intrahepatic branches of portal vein (Pneumobilia)

Contrast Studies

- To exclude colonic obstruction water soluble contrast is used.

CECT Abdomen

Indicated in cases of obstruction due to
- Intestinal malignancy
- Inflammatory bowel disease
- Extrinsic cause of obstruction

Strangulation should be Suspected if

- Irreducible external hernia is tense and tender
- If pain becomes constant/localized or becomes more severe/infrequent spasms
- Elevation of temperature/tachycardia
- Rigidity/rebound tenderness present
- State of shock exists inspite of adequate fluid resuscitation
- If pain persists for more than 2 hours after Ryle's tube suction has been established

Treatment

Three mainstays of the treatment of intestinal obstruction:
- Gastrointestinal suction
- Fluid and electrolyte disturbance
- Relief of obstruction by surgery

Gastrointestinal Suction by Nasogastric Tube

- Removal of fluid and gas from stomach and upper intestine

- Abolishes vomiting
- Progressive relief of pain and distension
- Facilitates operation
- Reduces risk of aspiration during anesthesia induction
- Suction is carried out by plastic or red rubber tubes of any of the type
  - Ryle's tube
  - Miller-Abbott tube
  - Cantor's tube

IV Fluid Replacement and Correction of Metabolic Abnormality

- Third space loss due to pouring of fluid of intestinal secretion into distended gut above obstruction
- Replaced by 1L of normal saline and 1L of 5% dextrose over 2–3 hours
- Maintain a urine output of 50 ml/hour
- CVP can also be monitored
- Combination of gastrointestinal suction and IV fluids may relieve obstruction in cases of
  - Obstruction due to simple kinking of gut
  - Obstruction due to bands and adhesions
  - Partial small bowel obstruction

Early Surgery is Indicated in case of

- Obstructed or strangulated hernia
- Intestinal strangulation
- Acute obstruction, when no response to conservative management within 24 hours

Operations for Intestinal Obstruction

- Usually exploratory laparotomy except due to hernia
- Obstruction can be relieved by
  - Division of bands
  - Lysis of adhesions
  - Resection and anastomosis of gut in strangulation, infarction, tumor, long stricture
  - Stricturoplasty in short stricture
  - Bypassing the obstruction
  - Drainage of bowel to exterior

Obstructive Jaundice: Pathophysiology, Clinical Features and Investigations

CHOLESTASIS

- Cholestasis is reduction or stoppage of bile flow, which can be intrahepatic or exahepatic
- Intrahepatic chestasis can be
  - Non obstructive (disorders that impair the body's ability to eliminate bile)
  - Obstructive (widespread blockage of small ducts)
- Extrahepatic cholestasis (obstructive jaundice).

Obstructive Jaundice

- Failure of the normal amount of bile to reach intestine due to mechanical obstruction of the extra hepatic biliary tree or within the porta-hepatis.

Physiological Facts

- *Total Bile flow:* 600 ml/day (500–1000 ml/day)
- Hepatocyte component — 450 ml/day, which can be bile salt dependent or bile salt independent due to biliary glutathione and ductular bicarbonate secretion.
- Cholangiocyte component — 150 ml/day, it depends upon secretin stimulation
- Total serum bilirubin 0.3 to 1.2 mg per dl
- With conjugated bilirubin <15 percent
- 1 mg/dl of bilirubin = 17mmol/L.

Types of Biliary Tract Obstruction

- Complete obstruction
- Intermittent obstruction
- Chronic incomplete obstruction
- Segmental obstruction.

Complete Obstruction

- Presents as jaundice.

Causes

- Head of pancreas carcinoma
- Common bile duct ligation
- Cholangiocarcinoma
- Parenchymal liver tumors.

Intermittent Obstruction

- Symptoms and typical biochemical changes
- Clinically jaundice may or may not be present.

Causes

- CBD stones
- Periampullary tumors
- Duodenal diverticulum
- Biliary parasites
- Hemobilia.

Chronic Incomplete Obstruction

- With or without classical symptoms or bio-chemical changes
- Pathological changes in bile ducts or liver.

Causes

- Strictures of common bile duct

- Stenosis of biliary - enteric anastomosis
- Chronic pancreatitis
- Cystic fibrosis
- Sphincter of Oddi stenosis.

Segmental Obstruction

- One or more segment of intrahepatic biliary tract obstructed.

Causes

- Traumatic
- Intrahepatic stones
- Sclerosing cholangitis
- Cholangiocarcinoma.

Physical Effects of Obstruction

- Normal secretary pressure of bile is 15–25 cm of water
- At 35 cm of water there is suppression of bile production
- High pressure leads to cholangiovenous and cholagiolymphatic reflux of bacteria
- Dilatation of bile duct and intra-hepatic biliary radicals (IHBR)
- IHBR dilatation absent if there is secondary hepatic fibrosis or cirrhosis.

Pathophysiology

- Increase in biliary pressure leads to
  - Disruption of tight junctions between hepatocytes and bile duct cells with increased permeabilty leading to reflux of bile contents in liver sinusoids, leading to neutrophil infiltration, increased fibrinogenesis and deposition of reticulin fibers in portal triad
  - Reticulin fibers gets converted in to type 1 collagen
  - Laying down of collagen fibers leads to hepatic fibrosis , obstruction of sinusoids and secondary biliary cirrhosis and portal hypertension.
  - Fibrosis can also lead to atrophy of obstructed liver.

Changes in Liver Blood Flow

- *Acute obstruction:* Increase in hepatic arterial blood flow
- No change in portal venous blood flow
- Chronic bile duct obstruction leads to decrease in total liver blood flow, dilation of sinusoids and elevation of portal pressure.

Effecton Wound Healing

- Delayed wound healing
- High incidence of wound dehiscence
- Decreased activity of enzyme Propyl hydroxylase in the skin
  - Which helps in incorporation of proline in collagen leading to defective synthesis of collagen.

Cardiovascular Effects

- Decreased cardiac contractility
- Reduced left ventricular pressure
- Impaired response to beta agonist drugs
- Decreased peripheral vascular resistance
- Net result
  - Hypotensive patient
  - Exaggerated hypotensive response to bleeding
  - More prone to postoperative shock

Renal Failure

- 10% incidence with 70% mortality
- Factors responsible
  - Depressed cardiac function
  - Increased levels of ANP resulting in Hypo-volemia
  - Direct effect of bile salts on kidney mediated by increased prostaglandin E2
- Endotoxemia (50%) leads to
  - Renal vasoconstriction
  - Shunting of blood from cortex
  - Activation of complement system-peritubular and glomerular fibrin deposition
- Leading to tubular and cortical necrosis.

Immune System

- Defects in cellular immunity
  - Impaired T cell proliferation
  - Decreased Neutrophil chemotaxis
  - Defective bacterial phagocytosis
  - Depressed function of RE system, i.e. Kupffer cells.

Coagulation Factor Defects

- Prolongation of Prothrombin time
- Loss of calcium
- Endotoxin induced damage to factor XI and XII, platelets
- Low grade DIC with increased fibrin degradation products
- Thrombocytopenia from hypersplenism.

Biochemical Effects

- Bilirubin Rise by 25–43 micromol/litre/day
- Mechanism of hyperbilirubinemia:
  - Biliary venous and biliary lymphatic regurgitation due to disruption of tight intracellular junction
  - Trans-hepatocytic regurgitation due to reversal of the secretory polarity of hepatocytes
  - Rupture of dilated canaliculi in to sinusoids due to necrosis of hepatocytes.

Alkaline Phosphatase

- Most sensitive indicator of biliary obstruction
- Factors responsible are
  - Biliary compartment regurgitation
  - Increase in hepatic synthesis.

Clinical Features

History

- Previous dyspepsia, fat intolerance
- Jaundice: Onset, course, itching
- Pain suggest biliary colic.
- Pyrexia is suggestive of cholangitis
- Weight loss suggest malignancy.
- Dark urine and clay colored stools
- Travel to endemic area
- Contact with jaundice patient
- History of upper abdominal operation
- History of plasma or blood transfusion
- Drug intake, i.e. anti-tubercular drugs
- History of injection in preceding six months.

Jaundice

- Yellowing of sclera occurs at 3 mg%
- Yellowing of skin and mucous membrane at 6 mg%
- *Differential diagnosis:* Beta carotenemia, quinacrine therapy, malingering with picric acid
- Bilirubin level rise up to three weeks then stabilize
- **Why bilirubin levels plateau:**
  - Increased excretion of bile pigments through by products other than bilirubin not giving diazo reaction
  - With increasing levels of conjugated bilirubin a portion gets covalently bonded to serum albumin and this protein bound bilirubin (Delta bilirubin) is not measurable by routine technique.

Itching

- Retained bile salts in subcutaneous tissue
- Levels does not correlate well with itching
- Itching disappears in terminal liver failure but bile salt level still remain increased.
- Other theory of itching:
  - Due to endogenous opiate peptides inducing opioid receptor mediated scratching activity of central origin.

Clinical Examination

- *Anemia:* Hemolysis, cancer or cirrhosis
- Gross weight loss - Malignancy
- Hunched up position- Chronic pancreatitis or cancer head of pancreas.
- Fetor hepaticus, flapping tremors, personality changes suggest - impending hepatic coma
- Skin changes - Bruising, purpuric spots, vascular spiders, palmar erythema, white nails, and loss of secondary sexual characters suggest stigmata of chronic liver disease
- Scratch marks, finger clubbing, xanthoma on eyelids, palmar creases
- Malignant skin nodules at umbilicus
- Ankle edema — cirrhosis or IVC obstruction due to hepatic or pancreatic malignancy.

Abdominal Examination

- Dilated peri-umbilical veins - cirrhosis and portal collateral circulation
- Ascites - Cirrhosis or malignant disease
- Nodular liver suggest secondaries liver and smooth enlargement of liver is due to hydro-hepatosis.

Spleen enlargement in obstructive jaundice can be seen in following conditions:

1. In a haemolytic anemia which can have pigment stones leading to obstructive jaundice and spleenomegaly due to haemolytic anemia itself.
2. Left sided portal hypertension due to splenic vein thrombosis in carcinoma head of the pancreas, which will also give rise to obstructive jaundice.

- **Courvoisier's law** - Palpable non tender gall bladder in jaundice patient – malignant biliary obstruction
- Exceptions
  - Double impaction of stones

- Impaction of pancreatic calculus at ampulla of Vater
- Oriental cholangio-hepatitis
- Mirizzi's syndrome.

Investigations

1. Liver function test: Liver function test will reveal
   a. Conjugated hyperbilirubinemia
   b. Raised alkaline phosphatare (more than 1.5 times the upper limit of normal)
   c. AST and ALT are either normal or mildly raised (less than 10 times of normal)

2. Ultrasonography (USG) is the initial investigation. USG will reveal size of CBD, any echogenic shadow within the lumen of CBD, any mass lesion in head of pancrease, gall stones or any mass lesion in the gall bladder. Secondaries in the liver can be detected.

3. If USG is suggestive of stone disease, then next imaging should be MRCP, which will exactly reveal size of CBD, number and size of stones in CBD and location of stones in the CBD.

4. If USG is suggestive of malignancy, then contrast enhanced spiral CT (CECT) should be performed, which will accurately stage the malignancy. CT guided biopsy from the primary tumour can be taken.

71 | Portal Hypertension

- "Porta" in Latin means gate or passage
- Portal pressure gradient 12 mmHg or more is often associated with varices and ascites
- Many conditions are associated with it, the most common being **cirrhosis** of the liver
- Normal pressure in portal vein is 5–7 mm of Hg.

Embryology

- Portal vein develops from
  - Post duodenal plexuses of embryonic vitelline veins
  - May form from pre duodenal plexuses which will lead to anterior portal vein which is associated with annular pancreas, malrotation and biliary tract anomalies

Anatomy of Portal Vein

- 8 cm long, no valves, 8 mm diameter
- Begins at L2 behind neck of pancreas in front of IVC.
- The superior mesenteric vein and splenic vein join behind the pancreas to form the portal vein.
- Portal vein drains blood from the small and large intestines, stomach, spleen, pancreas and gallbladder.
- Tributaries of portal vein
  - Splenic (short gastric, left gastro-epiploic, pancreatic, inferior mesenteric)
  - Superior mesenteric (jejunal, ileal, ileocolic, right colic, middle colic)

  - Left gastric
  - Right gastric
  - Para-umbilical
  - Cystic veins
- The portal trunk divides in to 2 lobar veins, the right drains the cystic vein, the left receives umbilical and paraumbilical veins that enlarge to form the caput medusae. The coronary vein drains the distal oesophagus, which also enlarge in portal hypertension. Oesophageal varices is collaterals between left gastric and short gastric (portal venous system) and the azygs vein (systemic vein).

Physiology

- Portal circulation
  - 1 to 1.2 litres per minute
  - 40 ml/min O_2 (72 % of total O_2 supply)
  - 80 % of total blood supply to liver
- Portal Pressure Gradient is defined by
  - PV pressure – IVC pressure
  - Normal 5 mm Hg
  - 6–10 mmHg sub clinical portal hypertension
  - >10 mm Hg oesophageal varices
  - >12 mm Hg variceal bleeding /ascites

Pathophysiology

- P = FR, where P is pressure gradient through the portal system, F is the volume of blood flowing through the system, R is the resistance to flow
- Changes in either F or R affect the pressure

- In most types of portal hypertension, both flow and resistance are altered.

Increase in Resistance

- Liver disease is responsible for a decrease in portal vascular radius, producing an increase in portal vascular resistance
- In cirrhosis, the increase occurs at the micro-circulation (sinusoidal) level.
- The resistance is also due to active myofibroblasts or vascular smooth muscle cells in the intrahepatic veins

Increase in Flow

- The increase in blood flow is caused by splanchnic arteriolar vasodilatation caused by release of endogenous vasodilators
- The increased flow aggravates the increase in portal pressure and contributes to Portal hypertension despite the formation of portosystemic collaterals that divert as much as 80% of portal flow

Manifestations of Splanchnic Vasodilatation

- Increased cardiac output
- Arterial hypotension
- Hypovolemia
- The above explains rationale for treating patients with low sodium diet and diuretics to attenuate the hyperkinetic state

Mortality/Morbidity

- Variceal hemorrhage is the most common complication
- 90% with cirrhosis develop varices
- 30% of these bleed
- The first episode is estimated to carry a mortality of 30–50%

Sites of Collateral Circulation

- Lower end of esophagus and fundus of esophagus
- In rectal haemrrhoids
- Around umbilicus
- Natural porto systemic shunts (NPSS) opens at
  - Gastro-adrenro-renal
  - Lienorenal

  NPSS more common in extra hepatic portal vein obstruction

Clinical Features

History

- Directed towards determining the cause and the presence of complications of portal hypertension
- Jaundice, transfusions, IV drug abuse, pruritis, hereditary liver disease
- Hematemesis, melena, mental status, abdominal girth, pain, fever, hematochezia

Physical Examination

- Signs of portosystemic collateral formation:
  - Dilated veins in abdominal wall
  - Caput medusa
  - Rectal hemorrhoids
  - Ascites
  - Umbilical hernia
- Signs of chronic liver disease
  - Ascites
  - Jaundice
  - Palmar erythema
  - Asterixis/flapping tremors
  - Testicular atrophy, gynecomastia
  - Muscle wasting, Dupuytren's contracture
  - Splenomegaly

Causes of Portal Hypertension

Prehepatic

- Portal vein thrombosis
  - Neonatal umbilical sepsis
  - Hypercoagulable state
- Splenic vein thrombosis
  - Pancreatitis
  - Carcinoma head of pancreas
- Banti syndrome - splenomegaly, normal liver, portal hypertension
- Increased portal flow
  - Arteriovenous fistula
  - Massive splenomegaly (primary hematologic disease)

Hepatic

- Presinusoidal
  - Schistosomiasis
  - Congenital hepatic fibrosis
  - Primary biliary cirrhosis
  - Chronic active hepatitis
  - Hepatocellular carcinoma

- Secondaries liver
- *Toxins:* Vinyl chloride, Arsenic, copper
- Other periportal disorders e.g. primary biliary cirrhosis, sarcoidosis, congenital hepatic fibrosis)
- Idiopathic portal hypertension
- Sinusoidal
  - *Hepatic cirrhosis:* Alcoholic or post viral
  - Non cirrhotic acute alcoholic hepatitis
  - Cytotoxic drugs
  - Vitamin A intoxication
- Postsinusoidal
  - Veno-occlusive disease

Posthepatic

- Hepatic vein thrombosis (Budd chiari syndrome)
- Membranous obstruction of inferior vena cava
- Cardiac causes (e.g. constrictive pericarditis, restrictive cardiomyopathy)

Common Causes of Portal Hypertension in India

- Cirrhosis < 50%
- Non cirrhotic portal fibrosis 10–25%
- Extra hepatic portal vein obstruction 30–40%
- Budd –Chiari syndrome 8–26%

Non Cirrhotic Portal Fibrosis

- Northern and Eastern part of India
- 30–50 years commonly involved.
- Peri-sinusoidal fibrosis seen.
- Obliteration of peripheral portal venule
- Normal sized liver
- Nodular type or non-nodular type
- Progressive loss of liver function

Natural History of Portal Hypertension

- In cirrhotic patients progressive and early liver failure
- In NCPF non nodular variety liver failure occurs late
- Nodular type of NCPF early liver failure
- IN EHPVO liver perfusion maintained.

Investigations

- Liver function test (LFT)
- Prothrombin time
- Albumin level
- Hepatitis serology
- Platelets

- Anti nuclear antibodies (ANA), antimito-chondrial antibodies
- Alpha 1-antitrypsin deficiency.

Imaging Studies

- Duplex Doppler is safe and non invasive. Demonstrates portal flow, portal vein thrombosis, splenic vein thrombosis
  - Nodular liver surface, splenomegaly, presence of collateral circulation.
  - Portal flow in portal hypertension can be
    ◊ Hepatopetal (10–30 cm/sec) (towards liver) in EHPVO
    ◊ Stagnant flow/thrombosis
    ◊ Hepatofugal (away from liver) seen in cirrhosis
  - *Hepatic artery:* Resistivity index (RI) is increased in
  - Obstruction of IVC or hepatic veins
  - Patency of shunts
  - Limitations include meals, medications and sympathetic nervous system affects flow.
- CT scan when USG is inconclusive
  - Look for collaterals from portal system
  - Dilatation of the vena cava suggests portal hypertension
  - Limitations include not being able to use IV contrast in allergic patients or with renal failure.

Invasive Procedures

- Hemodynamic measurement of pressure, usually not performed due to invasive nature
- Measures hepatic venous pressure gradient (HVPG) by a similar to Swan Ganz catheter, where balloon is inflated measuring wedged hepatic venous pressure, minus the unoccluded pressure in the HVPG.
- Endoscopy is performed to screen for varices
  - Gastroesophageal varices confirms diagnosis of portal hypertension, absence does not rule it out
  - Many times an incidental finding when scoped for something else
- Portovenography
  - Done if intervention contemplated
  - Splenoportography
  - Arterioportogram
  - Transjugular venography
  - Spiral CT angiography.

Treatment

Medical Treatment

Treatment is directed at cause

- Emergent treatment
- Primary prophylaxis
- Elective treatment.

Emergent Treatment

- Bleeding from varices ceases spontaneously in 40%. Rebleed in 40% within 6 weeks
- Following resuscitation, treatment includes control of bleeding, prevention of recurrence, blood replacement, avoid over expansion of volume status
- Upper GI endoscopy to diagnose source of bleed and for specific treatment of bleeding lesion
- All patients with cirrhosis and upper GI bleed are at risk for severe bacterial infections, which are associated with early rebleed
- Use of antibiotics has shown to increase survival, decrease rate of infection
- Thus prophylactic use of antibiotics in acute bleeding is recommended.

Pharmacologic Therapy

- Somatostatin - decreases portal flow, splanchnic vasoconstriction
- Octreotide - 50mcg/h shown to reduce complications of bleeding after sclerotherapy
- Vasopressin - reduces blood flow to all splanchnic organs, decreases portal pressure, venous blood flow. Use nitro-glycerine with it. It's the most potent splanchnic vasoconstrictor.

Endoscopic therapy – endoscopic sclerotherapy and variceal ligation (EST, EVL)

- Hemostasis in 80%, declines to 70% at day 5 due to very early rebleeding
- No more than 2 sessions before deciding on TIPS or surgery
- Complications include fever, stricture, perforation, mediastinitis, ulceration, pleural effusion
- EVL and EST comparable in control of bleeding
- EST associated with more complications.

Minnesota tube

- Balloon tamponade only in massive bleeding as a temporizing measure
- Complications – Esophageal rupture, rebleed, mediatinitis

- Has 4 lumens -1 for gastric aspiration, 2 to inflate the balloons, 1 above the esophageal balloon to prevent aspiration
- Usually only need to inflate gastric balloon.

Prophylaxis

- Beta-blockers (propanolol, nadolol) are non-cardio-selective; reduce portal and collateral blood flow. Also reduces cardiac output, splanchnic vasoconstriction
- Bleeding rates significantly reduced and mortality rates are lowered.
- No role for sclerotherapy in primary prophylaxis
- EVL is more effective than no treatment to prevent first bleed but similar efficacy to beta-blockers, with more adverse effects. EVL not recommended for primary prophylaxis except perhaps in patients with very large varices.

Elective Treatment

- This is for prevention of rebleeding (2 year recurrence rate of 80%)
- Propanolol and nadolol, reduce rebleed, increase survival
- Beta blockers vs sclerotherapy have comparable rates of prevention
- EVL is considered treatment of choice in prevention of rebleeding, may combine with drugs.

Surgical Treatment (Shunts)

- Total portosystemic shunts include any shunt larger than 10mm between portal vein and IVC. Includes (end to side) and side to side portocaval shunts.
  - Side to side controls bleeding and ascites, but encephalopathy a problem (40–50%).
- Partial portal systemic shunts reduce the size to 8 mm in diameter.
  - Use an interposition graft between portal vein and IVC.
  - 90% control of bleeding, decreased incidence of encephalopathy and liver failure.
- Selective shunts aim to decompress varices whilst maintaining portal hypertension to maintain portal flow to liver.
  - Warren distal splenorenal shunt, the most commonly used for patients with refractory bleeding and good liver function. Decompresses gatroesophageal varices through short gastrics, splenic vein to left renal vein.

Lower incidence of encephalopathy (15%), preserves some liver function. It does produce ascites.

- Types based on anatomy
  - Direct bypass
    ◊ Porto-caval
    ◊ Distal spleno-renal
    ◊ Proximal spleno-renal
  - H type bypass
    ◊ Porto-caval
    ◊ Meso-caval
    ◊ Spleno-renal
    ◊ Atypical derivations
- Risks
  - Shunt thrombosis - risk is low. If the shunt thromboses, then portal hypertension recurs.
  - Liver failure - creation of a shunt reroutes the blood away from the liver and deprives partly the liver of the portal flow and this can lead to liver failure mostly in patient with advanced cirrhosis. This is avoided by proper selection of the candidates
  - Encephalopathy - Re-routing the blood flow directly to the heart also carries some risk of encephalopathy and other problems at long term.
- Indications
  - Well compensated cirrhosis
    ◊ Bleeding ectopic varices
    ◊ Unsuccessful sclerotherapy/banding
    ◊ Untractable ascites

- Non-cirrhotic portal hypertension
  ◊ Inadequate local medical support
  ◊ Refractory/recurrent bleeding

Devascularization Procedures

- Include splenectomy, gastroesophageal devascularization, and esophageal transection.
- Incidence of encephalopathy is low, because of maintenance of portal flow.
- Used in patients who are not candidates for decompression in whom 1st line therapy has failed. This includes patients with splenic or portal vein thrombosis in addition to cirrhosis
- Splenectomy- the spleen is a major inflow path to GE varices. Splenectomy gives better access to fundus and distal esophagus to complete the devascularization.
- Complicated by portal vein thrombosis and ascites.
- Sugiura procedure - devascularizes whole greater curve from pylorus to esophagus, upper two thirds of lesser curve. The esophagus is devascularized a minimum of 7 cm.

Liver Transplant

- The ultimate operation, as it relieves portal hypertension, prevents bleeding, manages ascites and encephalopathy by restoring liver function.
- *Child class A:* Shunt surgery
- *Child class B:* Shunt or TIPS
- *Child class C:* TIPS or liver transplant

Table 71.1: Comparison of effectiveness of various techniques			
	Disconnection	*Splenectomy*	*Shunt*
Portal pressure	—	—	+
Esophageal varices	+	—	+
Hypersplenism	—	+	+

Table 71.2: Child classification			
	Class A	*Class B*	*Class C*
Ascites	None	Slight	Moderate
Encephalopathy	None	I and II	III and IV
Albumin (g/L)	> 35	28–35	< 28
Bilirubin (mg/dl)	< 2	2–3	> 3
PT (INR)	1–4	4–6	> 6

Transjugular Intrahepatic Portosystemic Shunt (TIPS)

- For continued bleeding despite medical and endoscopic treatment in patients with Child C disease and selected Child B disease.
- It is only useful in portal hypertension of hepatic origin.
- From internal jugular to hepatic vein and thru hepatic parenchyma to portal vein. Tract dilated and stented.
- Accepted Indications
  - Active bleeding despite endoscopic or pharmacologic treatment
  - Recurrent variceal bleeding despite adequate endoscopic treatment.
  - Potential indications include bleeding gastric fundic varices, refractory ascites
  - Preparation to transplant
- Complications of TIPS
  - Hematoma, cardiac arrhythmias, bacteraemia
  - Perihepatic hematoma, rupture of liver capsule
  - Extrahepatic punture of portal vein
  - Arterioportal fistula, portobiliary fistula
  - Encephalopathy (30%)
  - Liver failure

Gastro-Intestinal Bleeding

Emergency Therapy of Variceal Hemorrhage
- Fluid resuscitation
- Platelet transfusion (if Platelet count< 50,000/ mm^3)
- Vit. K/Fresh frozen plasma
- Upper GI endoscopy (diagnostic + variceal obliteration)

- Pharmacologic intervention
  - Somatostatin
  - Vasopressin
- Rescue therapy
  - Balloon compression
  - TIPS
  - Shunt surgery

Sclerotherapy/Banding

- Limits:
  - Ectopic varices
  - Recurrence
- Complications of sclerotherapy
  - Ulcer
  - Stricture
  - Mediastinitis
  - Esophageal dysmotility
  - Gastroesophageal reflux

Guidelines for Management of Portal Hypertension

• Compensated liver disease	
• No complications yet	• Wait and see
• Minor/moderate risk of bleeding	
• Compensated liver disease	• Medical treatment
	• B-Blockers
• Previous bleeding, banding	• Diuretics
	? TIPS
• Ascites	? Shunt surgery
• End-stage liver disease	
• Recurrent varices and bleeding	• Transplant
• Refractory ascites	

72 Liver Abscess

- First description of hepatic abscess dates back to the days of Hippocrates (4000 B.C.)
- Open surgical drainage of liver abscess was carried out by Ochsner (1938)
- Percutaneous drainage and antibiotic therapy for solitary liver abscess was first proposed by McFadzean (1953)

Types of Liver Abscess

- Liver abscess can be
  - Amoebic liver abscess (ALA)
  - Pyogenic liver abscess (PLA)
  - Tubercular liver abscess
  - Fungal liver abscess
  - Hepatic ascariasis and infections by liver flukes (*Fasciola hepatica* and *Clonorchis sinensis*) are rare causes
- In west, majority are pyogenic (80%)
- In India majority are amoebic (80%)

Amoebic Liver Abscess

- An invasive form of amoebiasis
- Caused by *Entamoeba histolytica*
- The liver is the most common extra-intestinal site of amoebiasis

Epidemiology

- Common in subtropical and tropical countries with poor standards of sanitation
- Endemic form in developing countries
- *Bimodal age distribution:* Peaks at 2–3 years and >40 years
- Third most common parasitic cause of death

Hepatic Amoebiasis

- Amoebiasis affects 40–50 million people annually
- Majority of infections occur in developing countries with "poor socioeconomic and sanitation level"
- High rates of infection occur in India, Africa, Central and South America

Epidemiology

- Commonly seen in:
  - Persons of lower socioeconomic status
  - Institutionalized patients
  - Military personnel
- More common in the third and fourth decade of life
- 90% develop in men (may be low levels of available free iron in females prevent infection in them)
- Higher incidence in individuals having exogenous iron supplementation

Pathogenesis

- Trophozoites of *Entamoeba histolytica* invade the mucosa of large gut
- Reach portal radicles
- Once in liver, they cause extensive necrosis

Pathology

- Commonly involves right lobe of liver possibily because of following reasons:

There is streaming of blood in the portal vein with flow from right side of the colon drains mainly in to the right lobe of liver via superior mesenteric vein and amoebiasis most commonly affects the right side of the colon

- Right hepatic lobe involved in 70–90%
- Left hepatic lobe involved in 13%.
- Liver capsule serves as a barrier to growth of ALA
- Preponderant on postero-superior surface of liver as this portion is devoid of liver capsule and offer less resistance.
- ALA contains fluid, lined by an inner wall and a connective tissue capsule
- Liver cells undergo liquefaction necrosis to produce a cavity filled with blood and liquefied liver cells without any acute inflammatory cells
- Pus in ALA
  - Anchovy sauce
  - No odour
  - Sterile–contains hepatocytes, dead RBC.
- Secondary infection
  - Alter the colour and consistency of pus
  - May impart it an odour

Clinical Features

History

- Ten times more common in adults than in children
- Three to ten times more common in men
- Peak incidence between 20–60 years
- Complications and mortality more common in
  - Neonates
  - Pregnant women
  - Postpartum ladies
  - Immuno-compromised patients
  - Alcoholics
- History of active diarrhoea in less than one third of patients.
- Cultures of stool positive in more than 75%
- Pain and fever is present in > 90%
- Pain
  - Abrupt in onset,
  - Localized to right upper abdomen, can radiate to right shoulder or scapula.

- In epigastrium or retrosternal region in left lobe abscess.
- Fever
  - High grade
  - With chills and rigors
- Anorexia, nausea and vomiting
- Diarrhea (present in 25% of cases only)
- Cough, if ruptures into pleural cavity
- Pruritis (rarely)

Physical Examination

- Tender, soft hepatomegaly with sharp margin
- Intercostal tenderness
- Mild icterus often seen
- Right basal lung signs often present
- Pericardial rub can be heard in left lobe abscess.
- May present with ascites and jaundice

Differential Diagnosis

- Acute cholecystitis
- Viral hepatitis
- Pyogenic liver abscess
- Necrotic adenoma
- Hydatid cyst

Laboratory Investigations

- Leukocytosis in 70% of cases.
- Eosinophilia may be seen in 10–15% of patients.
- 50% have low hemoglobin
- Hyperbilirubinemia in 10%
- Mild elevation of SGOT and SGPT in 35–45%
- Alkaline phosphatase elevated in 50%
- Prolonged prothrombin time
- Wet mount of stool positivity for trophozoites in:
  - 70% of patients with concurrent colitis (if 3 stool samples are tested)
  - 40–50% patients with only liver abscess

Imaging

X-Ray Chest

- X-ray chest PA view erect is abnormal in 60% of patients and may reveal
  - Elevation of right diaphragm
  - Right basal atelectasis
  - Right pleural effusion
  - Extraluminal air-fluid level

Ultrasonography

- > 90% accuracy
- Simple, inexpensive and easily available

- Abscess can be clearly defined from surrounding liver
- Distal acoustic enhancement appearing as "white out" of structures distal to abscess cavity
- *Contents:* Hypoechoic, heterogenous and have internal echoes
- Serial scanning unwarranted in patients with clinical improvement
- Resolving abscess acquires a more echogenic and fibrous wall in 8 to 16 weeks
- Single abscess in the right lobe in 75–80%
- Left lobe abscess in 10%
- Caudate lobe abscess in 6%

Computed Tomography

- Sensitivity >95%
- Does not add to diagnostic accuracy of ultrasonography
- May have a role in the evaluation of imminent rupture, atypical case or a chronic case

Magnetic Resonance Imaging (MRI)

- May have a role in follow up of a treated case and in differentiation from hepatic neoplasms
- Appear as hypointense, heterogenous on T1 image and hyperintense on T2 image

Gallium scanning

- Can help in differentiation between amoebic (cold spot) and pyogenic liver abscess (warm spots)

Amoebic Serology

- Ninety to 95% of patients have serum antiamoebic antibodies. It can be detected by indirect hemagglutination (IHA) or enzymelinked immunosorbent assay (ELISA)
- Antibody response detectable 7–10 days after the onset of symptoms
- Titres reach a peak by the second and third
- IHA test is considered positive if dilution exceeds 1:128
- IHA highly specific for invasive amoebiasis.

Diagnostic Aspiration

- To rule out pyogenic abscess when serology is negative
- Fluid is odourless, has an anchovy sauce appearance with a negative Gram's stain and culture

- Trophozoites recovered in 33–90% of aspirates (higher yield if wall scrapings are stained)

Complications

Risk Group

- Neonates
- Pregnant women
- Postpartum women
- Immuno-compromised patients
- Alcoholics.

Peritoneal or Visceral Involvement

- Spontaneous intraperitoneal rupture in 2.7 to 17% of cases
- Treated by percutaneous drainage of liver abscess and the extravasated pus
- Indications for laparotomy:
  - Doubtful diagnosis
  - Concomitant hollow viscous perforation
  - Failure of conservative management.

Thoracic and Pleuro-Pulmonary Involvement

- Right sided effusion
- Rupture of abscess in to pleural cavity
- Rupture into bronchial system
- Treatment
  - Thoracocentesis
  - Intercostal tube drainage

Pericardial Involvement

- Rupture in to pericardium with cardiac tamponade
- Pericardial effusion

Various Directions in Which an Amoebic Liver Abscess can Rupture

- Right pleural cavity from right lobe
- Left pleural cavity from left lobe
- Peritoneal cavity
- Pericardium from left lobe
- Right lung
- Left lung
- Colon

Metastatic Abscess

- Pulmonary amoebiasis
  - Primary- without concomitant hepatic abscess
  - Secondary- arises as a complication of hepatic abscess

- Cerebral amoebiasis
- Cutaneous amoebiasis
- Splenic amoebiasis

Treatment

- Medical management
- Therapeutic aspiration
- Percutaneous drainage

Medical Management

- Mainstay of treatment
- Metronidazole is the drug of choice
  - Oral dose of 800 mg TDS for 10 days cures approximately 95% of patients with amoebic liver abscess
  - Serious side effects rare
  - Common side effects, i.e. nausea, vomiting, metallic taste in the mouth, dark brown discoloration of urine, disulfiram like reaction leading to alcohol intolerance
  - Contraindicated in the first trimester of pregnancy
  - 5 to 15% of patients are resistant to metronidazole
- Newer imidazoles, e.g. Tinidazole or secnidazole are equally effective
- Emetine, dehydroemetine and chloroquine
  - For complicated amoebic liver abscess
  - When metronidazole therapy fails
  - Act only on trophozoites
  - Emetine is a potentially toxic drug with narrow therapeutic range
  - Important side effects include hypotension, tachycardia, chest pain, dyspnea, and changes in the ECG

Therapeutic Aspiration

- Indications for performing therapeutic aspiration:
  - Failure to respond to medical treatment after 72 hours
  - If abscess cavity > 250 ml, to decrease the risk of rupture
  - Left hepatic lobe abscess
  - If bacterial super infection is suspected or for a suspected pyogenic liver abscess
  - Lesions associated with marked tenderness and diaphragmatic elevation
  - Impending rupture

  - When metronidazole is contraindicated as in pregnancy
- Routine aspiration of amoebic liver abscess does not decrease resolution time, but can increase the secondary bacterial infection rates
- Percutaneous drainage by catheter indicated for management of peritoneal, pulmonary or pericardial complications
- Catheter drainage often eliminates the need for operative intervention

Laparotomy

- Laparotomy indicated if
  - Increasing signs of peritonitis in spite of catheter drainage
  - There is fistulisation into hollow viscous
  - There is secondary bacterial infection with septicemia.

Prognosis

- Overall 4% mortality
- Risk factors for mortality include:
  - Serum bilirubin > 3.5 mg%
  - Encephalopathy
  - Serum albumin < 2 mg%
  - Multiple abscess cavities
  - Total volume of abscess > 500 ml
  - Pulmonary involvement
  - Rupture or extension
  - Late presentation
- In ruptured amoebic liver abscess (occurring in 2 to 17% of patients) mortality increases from 6 to 50%.

Pyogenic Liver Abscess (PLA)

- May be of biliary, portal, arterial or traumatic origin
- Disease of biliary system currently account for approximately 40% of pyogenic liver abscess
- Biliary manipulations have also become an important cause of pyogenic liver abscess
- Portal venous source arising from intestinal pathology is found in 20% of patients

Etiology

Potential Sources of Infection

- Bile ducts- ascending cholangitis (35–40%)
- Portal vein- pylephlebitis (e.g. from appendicitis/diverticulitis/perforated colon cancer) (20%)

- Direct extension from a contiguous disease (e.g. perforated ulcers/gangrenous cholecystitis/subphrenic abscess)
- Trauma (blunt/penetrating/following ablation for hepatic tumours) (4%)
- Via hepatic artery (e.g. septicemia, IV drug abuse, chemoembolization for malignancy, umbilical artery catheterization) (12%)
- Cryptogenic (10–45%)- etiology unknown

Predisposing Factors

- Young children with host defense abnormalities, sickle cell disease or immunological disorders
- Traumatic liver injury in young adults
- In adults diabetes mellitus, jaundice, cirrhosis, chronic pancreatitis, chronic pyelonephritis, inflammatory bowel disease, leukemia and lymphoma
- Patients on chemotherapy and steroids, patients with AIDS and other malignancies.

Pathology

- The etiology serves as best predictor of size, number and location of abscesses
- May be single or multiple
- Single abscesses are larger and located on right side in 70% of cases
- Multiple abscesses occur on right side in 50% cases
- Usually portal, traumatic and cryptogenic pyogenic liver abscesses are solitary and large
- Biliary and arterial pyogenic liver abscesses are multiple and small.

Clinical Presentation

- Early symptoms are nonspecific
- Malaise, nausea, anorexia and weight loss, headaches, myalgia and arthralgia
- More specific symptoms appear later
- Fever, chills and abdominal pain
- Fever most common of these is present in >80% of cases, and is of a sustained nature
- On examination, right upper quadrant tenderness, hepatomegaly/jaundice, ascites or pleural effusion/rub may be found
- Septic shock may occur in few, especially with an obstructed biliary tract
- Uncommonly patients may present with peritonitis.

Diagnosis

Laboratory Investigations

- Elevated WBC count
- Elevated transaminases, alkaline phosphatase and gamma-glutamyl transpeptidase in 90% of cases
- Elevated bilirubin may or may not be present.
- Hypoalbuminemia
- Prolonged prothrombin time.

Plain Radiographs of Chest and Abdomen

- Too nonspecific
- Gas forming organisms may give rise to an air fluid level
- Presence of right side pleural effusion, atelectasis or an elevated hemidiaphragm.
- Portal venous gas (in pylephlebitis) may be seen.

USG

- Appearance varies according to the stage of evolution of abscess
- Initially hyperechoic and later becoming hypoechoic
- Sensitivity varies from 75–95%
- Can only identify lesions >2 cm in diameter.

CT scan

- More accurate than USG in differentiating pyogenic liver abscess from other liver lesions with a sensitivity of 95%.
- Also helps in diagnosing the concurrent and causative pathology
- Can pick up abscesses >0.5 cm in size.

MRI

- Does not have any advantage over USG or CT
- MRCP helps in identifying the nature and size of biliary pathology and guide intervention
- Pyogenic abscesses have variable signal intensity on T1 and T2 weighted images, depending on protein content, but characteristically have:
  - High signal intensity on T2 weighted images
  - Rim enhancement after injection of gadolinium
  - Perilesional edema
- It may pick up abscesses as small as 0.3 cm in diameter.

Invasive Biliary Studies

- Endoscopic retrograde cholangio-pancreatico-graphy (ERCP) or per-cutaneous cholangio-graphy (PTC) may be indicated in patients with biliary system as the source of PLA.

Microbiology

- Organisms are related to the etiology and are isolated from aspirates of the abscesses (culture positive in 80–97%) and blood cultures (positive in 50–60%)
- Most common organisms are the gram negative aerobes *E. coli* and *Klebsiella sp.*
- **Most common anaerobes:** *Bacteroides*, anaerobic *Streptococci, Fusobacterium*
- *Candida* abscess are commonly seen in post chemotherapy patients
- An abscess secondary to biliary tract disease or GIT origin is more likely to be polymicrobial
- *M. tuberculosis* is commonly seen in AIDS patients
- Hematogenous abscess are mostly mono-microbial
- *Staphylococci* and *Streptococci* are the most common bacteria
- Negative cultures occur in 15%.

Principles of Treatment

- Drain the pus
- Institute appropriate antibiotics
- Deal with underlying source of infection when present
- Percutaneous drainage and antibiotics has become first line of treatment for most pyogenic liver abscesses.

Medical Management

- Broad spectrum antibiotics covering gram negative aerobes and anaerobes.
- Broad spectrum synthetic penicillin (ampicillin/amoxicillin) + An aminoglycoside + Metroni-dazole
  OR
  3rd generation cephalosporin + Metronidazole
- Modifications may be done once culture reports are available.
- Initially 2 weeks of parenteral therapy followed by 4 weeks of oral therapy may be appropriate.

Percutaneous Drainage (PCD)

- Performed under USG or CT guidance

- Either complete aspiration or insertion of a drain can be done
- Abscess that is unilocular and <5 cm is likely to respond with Percutaneous Needle Aspiration
- Failure is more likely with thick pus, non-collapsible walls or multiloculated PLA, where PCD may be done
- Primary PCD is also advised for abscesses > 5 cm
- Percutaneous drainage contraindicated in:
  – Multiple large abscesses
  – Known intra-abdominal source requiring surgery
  – Abscess of unknown etiology
  – Ascites
  – Requiring trans-pleural drainage.

Surgical Management

- Failure of non-operative treatment
- Complication of PCD such as bleeding or intraperitoneal leakage of pus
- Primary surgical treatment in intraperitoneal rupture
- Localization of abscess can be aided by intra-operative USG
- Isolated references of hepatic resections for pyogenic liver abscess are present but not a standard of care.

Prognosis

- Improvements in supportive therapy have brought down the mortality of uncomplicated pyogenic liver abscess from 100% to 2%
- Prognosis now depends on the etiology of pyogenic liver abscess and the comorbid conditions
- Risk factors associated with a grave prognosis:
  – Septic shock
  – Jaundice
  – Coagulopathy
  – Leukocytosis
  – Intraperitoneal rupture
  – Malignancy
- The mortality for patients with multiple pyogenic liver abscesses is higher compared to those with a single abscess

Tubercular Liver Abscess

- The first description by Bestowe in 1858
- The liver is an unusual target for formation of tuberculous abscesses

- An increase in incidence of tuberculosis of the liver has occurred in patients with AIDS

Pathology

- Usually secondary to pulmonary or gastro-intestinal involvement
- Diffuse form reflected in miliary tuberculosis predominates
- Focal or nodular form presenting as tuberculoma or abscess is uncommon

Clinical Presentation

- Symptoms and signs are non-specific
- Clinical manifestations include weight loss, anorexia, fever, abdominal pain, and jaundice
- Fever, hepatomegaly, right-sided hypochondrium pain, and icterus are usual clinical findings.

Diagnosis

- Clinical diagnosis difficult
- Ultrasonography and CT scan are very helpful
- *Differential diagnosis:* Amoebic or pyogenic abscesses and necrotic primary and metastatic neoplasms
- Confirmation of the diagnosis depends on demonstration of acid-fast bacilli in the aspirated pus, pus culture showing *Mycobacterium tuberculosis*, positive ELISA and PCR for *Mycobacterium tuberculosis* and histological examination of the abscess wall.

Treatment

- Anti-tubercular therapy alone

- Percutaneous aspiration along with anti-tubercular therapy
- Surgery reserved for cases in which percutaneous aspiration is not successful or not possible because of site, size and multiseptate nature of the abscess and lesions refractory to medical treatment
- The prognosis with anti-tubercular treatment is good.

Fungal Liver Abscess

- Usually arise in patients with immunocompromised states, leukemia and lymphoma or patients with other malignancies receiving chemotherapy
- Mycotic colonization of biliary tract is also quite common in patients with biliary stents who are receiving prolonged courses of antibiotics
- *Candida albicans*, *Cryptococcus* and *Aspergillus sp.* are the most common fungal isolates
- Requires special staining procedures and selected culture media

Treatment

- Systemic antifungal agents such as amphotericin B and fluconazole
- Treatment options include simple aspiration, percutaneous and open drainage
- Mortality with antifungal treatment is 20% vs. 62% untreated
- Outcome is directly related to treatment before fungemia ensues

73 Gallstone Disease

- Lies in the right upper quadrant, under the costal margin at the level of the 9th costal cartilage
- The level of the 9th costal cartilage can be palpated as a distinct notch.

Anatomy and Physiology

Parts of Gall Bladder

- Fundus
- Corpus or body
- Neck
- Cystic duct

Cystic duct joins with common hepatic duct to form common bile duct, which drains into second part of duodenum at ampulla of Vater

Function

- Stores bile in fasting state
- Mechanisms that help in the function are
  - Epithelial transport process – concentrates bile to keep volume small
  - Smooth muscle receptive relaxation – relaxation accommodates the bile entry
  - Neurohumoral excitation – Sphincter of Oddi tone (tonic contraction in fasting state)
- Components of bile
  - Primary bile salts – cholates, chenodeoxycholates
  - Secondary bile salts – deoxycholates, ursodeoxycholates, lithocholates
  - Phospholipids
  - Cholesterol
  - Protein
  - Electrolytes
  - Bilirubin

Mechanism and Factors of Cholesterol Gallstone Formation

- Hepatic cholesterol hypersecretion
  - Obesity
  - Females (estrogen and progesterone)
  - Age (middle age)
- Mucin hypersecretion
- Gall bladder hypomotility
- Increased intestinal conversion to deoxycholates

Gallstones

- Common (20% population)
- Cholesterol stones in West
- Female preponderance (3:1)
- Risk factors
  - Obesity
  - Oestrogen
  - Hypercholesterolemia
  - Increasing age

Clinical Manifestations

- Asymptomatic: Majority remains asymptomatic and diagnosed on USG

- Cholecystitis: Can be acute or chronic cholecystitis
- Biliary colic: Occurs due to obstruction by stone at neck of gall bladder.
- Complications
  - Jaundice
  - Pancreatitis
  - Cholangitis
  - Gallstone ileus
  - Carcinoma of gall bladder

Acute Cholecystitis

- Acute inflammation of the gallbladder
- Usually associated with calculi (stones)
- Calculus causes obstruction at Hartmann's pouch or cystic duct
- Less commonly with biliary sludge
- Acalculus (no-stone) cholecystitis rare
- Bacterial infection in 50% only
- Recurrent attacks result in fibrosed thickened gallbladder (chronic cholecystitis).

Clinical features
- Pain
  - Sudden onset, usually after fatty meal
  - Right upper quadrant — reaching up to back
  - Constant associated nausea and vomiting
  - May last several hours to days
  - Recurrent attacks common
- Signs
  - Pyrexia (37.5–38.5 degree celsius)
  - Associated jaundice signifies CBD blockage, CBD stone or Mirrizi's syndrome
  - Abdominal tenderness localized to RUQ
  - Murphys' sign positive - Inspiratory arrest with manual pressure below the gall bladder at the tip of 9th castal cartilage.

Biliary Colic

- Pain associated with obstruction of neck of gall bladder.
- Usually not colicky but constant (a misnomer)
- Presents as cholecystitis but not associated with fever/leucocytosis and positive Murphys' sign
- Usually resolves after minutes - few hours

Complications

- Empyema/mucocele
- Obstructive jaundice
- Ascending cholangitis
- Pancreatitis

- Ascending cholangitis
  - Charcots' Triad – Pain, Fever, Jaundice
- Courvoisiers' Law
  - *In the presence of jaundice a palpable gallbladder is most likely due to malignant obstruction of the bile duct*
  - Based on presumption that patients with gallstones have chronically inflamed, fibrosed gallbladders incapable of distension
  - Does not always hold true, e.g. Mucocele + CBD stone, or due to extrinsic compression of CBD by stone impacted at neck of gall bladder or due to pancreatic duct calculus impacted at ampulla of Vater.

Investigations

- Bloods
  - WBC reveals leucocytosis
  - LFT's (Bilirubin, GGT, Alk Phos)
  - Amylase estimation to rule out pancreatitis.
- Imaging
  - Ultrasound
  - MRCP in case of obstructive jaundice due to CBD stone.
- Special tests
  - Endoscopic retrograde cholangiopancreatico-duodenography (ERCP) for
    ◊ Therapeutic intervention

Management
Acute Cholecystitis
- Restrict oral intake (NPO)
  - Intravenous fluids
  - NG tube aspiration (for vomiting)
- Analgesia
  - NSAID, e.g. Inj. Diclofenac sodium.
- Intravenous antibiotics
  - Gram negative cover (Co-amoxiclavulinic acid—gentamicin—piperacillin)
- Cholecystectomy after 6 weeks.
- Early cholecystectary can be done if performed within 72 hours.

Biliary Colic
- Acute attack usually resolves spontaneously
- Analgesia
- Investigations as for cholecystitis
- Prolonged attacks treated as cholecystitis
- Elective cholecystectomy.

Ascending Cholangitis

- Resuscitation (IV fluids)
- Antibiotics (Broad spectrum)
- Intensive monitoring
- Definitive management
  - ERCP and stone removal +/– stent insertion
  - Cholecystectomy after resolution.

Gallstone Pancreatitis

- Commonest cause of pancreatitis
- More severe than alcohol Pancreatitis
- Due to CBD stones irritating pancreas
  - Obstruction at ampulla of Vater
  - Irritation in pancreatic portion of CBD
- Supportive
  - Fluid resuscitation
  - Antibiotics
  - Analgesia
- Definitive
  - ERCP and stone retrieval
  - Elective cholecystectomy.

Laparoscopic Cholecystectomy

- Commonest elective surgical procedure
- Standard treatment for gallstone disease
- May be performed as day care surgery
- Converted to open in a small number of cases
- Steps
  - Paint and drape
  - Use 4 ports – umbilical (camera), epigastric (working), right hypochondriac (holding Hartman's pouch), right lumbar (holding fundus)
  - Calot's triangle dissection first
  - Posterior dissection
  - Identify and divide cystic artery between clips
  - Identify and divide cystic duct between clips
  - Separate gall bladder from liver bed
  - Ensure hemostasis
  - Deliver the gall bladder (along with stones) through epigastric/umbilical port site
  - Port closure

- Modifications
  - Single port technique – all instruments through single custom made port inserted through umbilicus
  - Multiple ports inserted through a single umbilical incision
  - Use of needle instruments for retraction
  - Robotic cholecystectomy
  - (Natural orific translumenal endoscopic surgery) NOTES – through normal orifices (transgatric/transvaginal).

Complications

- Trauma
  - Common bile duct (CBD)
  - Intestine
  - Liver
- Hemorrhage
  - Vessel injury
  - Liver injury
  - Cystic artery clips
- Infection
  - Biliary peritonitis
- Post cholecystectomy syndrome
  - Rare
  - Pain
  - Occasionally due to stones in the biliary tree
- Port site hernia
  - Usually umbilical
  - 10 mm port sites are more predisposed.

Endoscopic Retrograde Cholangio Pancreatography (ERCP)

- Usually performed by gastroenterologists
- Diagnostic and therapeutic
- Indicated in jaundiced patients
- Ampulla of vater cannulated
- Demonstrates ductal anatomy
- Allows biopsy of malignant lesions
- Therapeutic in relieving obstruction
  - Stone retrieval or stenting.

74 | Pancreas

- 15 cm long
- Four parts – Head, neck, body and tail.

Head

- In the C-loop of duodenum, over renal veins and inferior vena cava
- Has an uncinate process.

Neck

- At the point of formation of portal vein.

Body

- Behind the lesser sac and transverse mesocolon
- In front of aorta, left renal vein, left kidney.

Tail

- Reaches upto splenic hilum and lies in close contact.

Arterial Supply

- Superior and inferior pancreaticoduodenal arteries
- Splenic artery.

Venous Drainage

- Head drains into portal and superior mesenteric veins
- Rest of pancreas drains into splenic vein.

Lymphatic Drainage

- Head – Celiac lymph nodes
- Uncinate process – Superior mesenteric lymph nodes/Pre-aortic nodes
- Rest of gland – Retroperitoneal nodes.

Direct Imaging Tests

- Ultrasonography is the initial imaging modality
- CT scan is investigation of choice for staging carcinoma pancreas
- MRI is useful for ductal anamoly.
- Endoscopic retrograde cholangiopancreatography (ERCP) can be used for cannulating pancreatic duct and CBD. In carcinoma pancreas, pancreatic duct may be narrowed or completely obstructed at the side of tumour or distal bile duct may be narrowed. In chronic pancreatitis, there is chain of lake appearance.

Tests of Exocrine Pancreatic Function

- Direct stimulation of pancreas by secretin followed by collection and measurement of contents
- Indirect stimulation of pancreas by amino acids, fatty acids and peptides and assay of proteolytic, lipolytic and aminolytic enzymes
- Measurement of fecal pancreatic enzymes such as elastase
- **NBT-PABA (Nitroblue Tetrazolium Para-amminobezoic acid) test:** The substance is administered orally and degraded in the gut by pancreatic enzyme and PABA is absorbed and excreated in urine. Levels of PABA in urine will decrease in case of pancreatic insufficiency.

Pancreatitis

- Acute pancreatitis:
  - Interstitial
  - Odematous
  - Necrotising which may be infected or non-infected
- Chronic pancreatitis:
  - Persistent
  - Progressive
  - Residual damage.

Acute Pancreatitis

- Spectrum of inflammatory lesions in the pancreas and peripancreatic tissues, ranging from edema, necrosis, hemorrhagic necrosis and fat necrosis
- Characterized by pancreatic inflammation and auto digestion.

Incidence

- 3% of all cases of abdominal pain
- World wide incidence ratio is 5 to 50 per 100000.

Etiology

- Alcohol
  - In 50% of cases
  - Alcohol stimulates pancreatic secretions rich in proteins → protein plugs → obstruction of pancreatic duct
  - Alcohol also causes
    ◊ Activation of trypsinogen
    ◊ Spasm of sphincter of Oddi
- Biliary tract disease
  - Stone in the gall bladder → migration to CBD → obstruction of ampulla of vater → stasis of pancreatic secretions.
  - Seen in 20–30% of cases of pancreatitis
- Collagen vascular disease
  - Polyarteritis nodosa
- Iatrogenic (ERCP, sphincterotomy, removal of stone from CBD, operation)
- Trauma (blunt, penetrating)
- Drugs (thiazides, steroids, estrogens, pzathioprine)
- Metabolic (hypercalcemia, hyperlipidemia)
- Infections (Mumps, Coxsackie B, Mycoplasma)
- Vascular (ischaemia, vasculitis)
- Congenital (pancreas divisum)
- Hyperparathyroidism → hypercalcemia
- Hyperlipdemia
- Hypotension, hypothermia
- Pancreatic duct obstruction (tumor)

- Toxin (scorpion bite)
- Malnutrition
- Idiopathic.

Pathogenesis

Initiating Event

- Causes activation of trypsinogen to trypsin
- Initiating event can be due to
  - Reflux of bile into pancreatic duct, due to the fact that biliary and pancreatic duct can terminate in a common channel
  - Incompetent ampulla, due to passage of stone → reflux of duodenal contents
  - Blockage of pancreatic ducts due to precipitation of calcium salts.

Autodigestion

- After activation of trypsinogen into trypsin, it acts and stimulates
  - Lipase which cause splitting of fats into fatty acids and glycerol
  - Elastase which digests elastic fibres
  - Lysolecithinase cause tissue necrosis
  - Prostaglandins, bradykinins, etc. act as inflammatory mediators.
- Extensive necrosis of pancreas
  ↓
  Myocardial depressant factors
  ↓
  Cardiac failure
  ↓
  Multiorgan failure

Pathology

- Interstitial edematous pancreatitis
- Necrotizing hemorrhagic pancreatitis.

Epidemiology

- Can occur at any age
- Rare in children and very young adult (infection, trauma, drugs, hereditary, parasites)
- *Alcohol - related pancreatitis:* young adult
- *Biliary tract disease:* Middle age and elderly.

Clinical Features

- Pain (>90%), develops quickly, reaching maximum within minutes, 50% radiate to back, relieved by stooping and bending forward
- Nausea

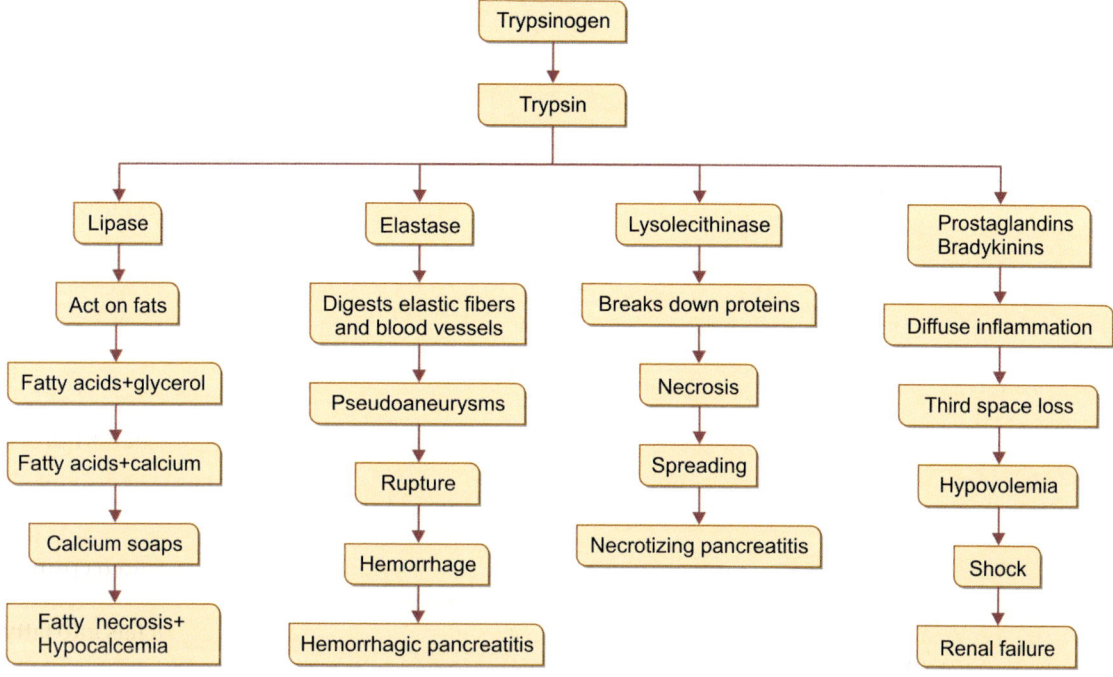

Fig. 74.1: Flowchart showing various steps in the etiopathogenesis of pancreatitis

- Vomiting – frequent and effortless due to pylorospasm
- Retching
- Hiccoughs
- Low grade fever
- Hematemesis and malena due to necrosis of duodenum.

Physical Signs

- Signs minimal relative to symptom
- Sick look
- Fever
- Features of shock – Tachycardia, low volume pulse, hypotension, cold extremities
- Cyanosis
- Faint jaundice
- Epigastric tenderness
- Abdominal distension with guarding and rigidity
- Paralytic ileus
- Shock
- Grey-Turner's sign (bluish discoloration in loin)
- Cullen's sign (bluish discoloration in periumbilical region)
- Fox's sign (bluish discoloration in inguinal region).

Diagnosis

- Serum amylase
    - Normal = 40 – 80 somogyi units
    - >400 SU is Suggestive and >1000 SU diagnostic
- Lipase – more specific but difficult to measure
- Urine amylase (elevation persists several days after normalization of serum amylase)
- Amylase/creatinine clearance 4x normal
- Other enzymes – Isoamylase, Trypsin, Ribonuclease
- Tumor markers – Pancreatic oncofetal antigen (POA), CA19–9.

Hyperamylasemia can also be seen

- Sialadenitis
- Peptic ulcer peforation
- Biliary disease
- Intestinal obstruction
- Mesenteric infarction
- Ruptured ectopic pregnancy
- Ruptured abdominal aortic aneurysm.

Blood Tests

- Hemogram - Leukocytosis, Fall in haematocrit suggest hemorrhagic necrosis

- Blood sugar - Hyperglycemia
- Serum calcium - Hypocalcemia
- Lipid profile - Hyperlipidemia
- Renal function tests – derranged in renal failure
- Serum albumin - Hypoalbuminemia.

Radiological Investigations

- Plain X-Ray Abdomen
  - Sentinel Jejunal loops
  - Colonic cut-off
  - Duodenal ileus
  - Generalized ileus
  - Retroperitoneal fluid accumulation: obliteration of psoas outline
  - Pleural effusion
  - Basal atelectasis
  - To rule out perforation
- USG
  - Non-invasive
  - Readily available
  - Can be done at bedside
  - Can reveal gallstone and dilated biliary system
  - *Disadvantage:* Poor visualization of pancreas, cannot diagnosis pancreatic necrosis, limited by gas in distended bowel
- CT
  - Pancreas
    ◊ Parenchymal enlargement (diffuse or focal)
    ◊ Parenchymal edema
  - Necrosis
    ◊ Peripancreatic change
    ◊ Blurring of fat planes
    ◊ Thickening of fascial planes
    ◊ Presence of fluid collection
  - Nonspecific
    ◊ Bowel distension, pleural effusion, mesenteric edema
  - CT grading of severity and Balthazar's Grading
- Endoscopic ultrasound to rule cut CBD stones.
- MRCP
- ERCP
  - Indicated in severe pancreatitis associated with biliary sepsis or obstruction
  - Done within 24 hours
  - Endoscopic sphincterotomy +/– stone extraction
  - Decrease morbidity and mortality
  - Procedure related complications are present

Complications

- Hypoxia with respiratory failure
- Shock
- Renal failure
- Hypocalcemia
- Hyperglycemia
- Gastrointestinal haemorrhage
- Subcutaneous nodules
- Intramedullary fat necrosis in bones
- Pseudocyst of pancreas
- Pancreatic abscess
- Pancreatic necrosis.

Course of Disease

- Wide variation in severity
- Mild self-limiting disease to rapidly progressing fatal disease
- Overall mortality 10–15%
- Severe group: up to 40%
- Death
  - *Early:* Multiple organ failure
  - *After 1st week:* Septic complication
- How to identify the severe group?
  - Scoring systems.

Scoring Systems

Ranson criteria (*see* Table 74.1)

Glasgow's Grading

• PaCO$_2$	<60 mmHg
• Age	>55 years
• Leukocytosis	>15000/cumm
• Hypocalcemia	<2 mmol/L or 8mg%
• Blood Urea	>16 mmol/L or 50mg%
• Enzymes (LDH and AST)	>600U/L
• Hypoalbuminemia	<32 g/L
• Hyperglycemia	>10 mmol/L or 180 mg%

Patients with three or more positive criteria have severe disease.

CT Grading

Grade of pancreas morphology

• Normal pancreas	0
• Pancreras enlargement only	1
• Obliteration of peripancreatic fat planes	2
• One peripancreatic fluid collection	3
• Two or more peripancreatic fluid collection	4

Table 74.1: Ranson's criteria

On admission	Non biliary	Biliary
Age	>55 years	> 70 years
WBC	> $16 \times 10^3/mm^3$	> $18 \times 10^3/mm^3$
Fasting sugar	> 200 mg%	> 220 mg%
LDH	> 350 IU/L	> 400 IU/L
SGOT	> 250 IU/L	> 250 IU/L
With in 24 hrs		
Fall in Hematocrit	> 10%	> 10%
BUN elevation	> 5 mg%	2 mg%
Serum calcium	<8 mg%	< 8 mg%
Arterial PO_2	< 60 mm Hg	< 60 mm Hg
Base deficit	> 4meq/L	> 5 meq/L
Estimated fluid sequestration	> 6L	4L

Degree of pancreatic necrosis

- No necrosis — 0
- Necrosis of <1/3rd of pancreas — 2
- Necrosis of ½ of pancreas — 4
- Necrosis of >1/2 of pancreas — 6

If score is >7–10, it indicates a prognosis of 17% mortality and 92% morbidity.

- Score mortality
  - <3 — 0.9%
  - 3–4 — 18%
  - 5–6 — 50%
  - >6 — 90%

Biochemical markers for severity of pancreatitis

- Trypsin activated peptide (TAP)
  - 5-aminoacid peptide
  - Released by activation of trypsinogen
  - If positive in urine s/o severe pancreatitis
  - Sensitivity 80% and specificity 90%.
- Serum trypsinogen – 2
  - 91% sensitivity
- C-Reactive Protein
  - If >100 mg% indicates necrotising pancreatitis
- Elevated levels of Neutrophil Elastase
- IL-6 and IL-8 are elevated in severe pancreatitis
- Alpha macroglobulin levels are raised in severe pancreatitis

Management

Management of Mild Pancreatitis

- Nil orally – Role of nasogastric tube aspiration is controversial.
- IV fluid – to correct volume deficit (third space losses)
- Analgesic – opiods may be required
- No need for antibiotic
- No need for CT scan
- Search for underlying cause
- Treat the underlying cause to prevent recurrent attack.

Management of Severe Pancreatitis

- Fluid resuscitation
- Oxygen therapy
- Intensive care support
- *Monitoring:* Urine output, central venous pressure, pulmonary artery wedge pressure, cardiac output, systemic vascular resistance
- Respiratory monitoring by arterial blood gas analysis and respiratory support
- Stress ulcer prophylaxis
- Nutrition
- Antibiotics only in severe cases or in pancreatic necrosis. Only Imipenem has been found to penetrate into pancreatic tissue in adequate concentrations.
- Somatostatin analogues, e.g. Octreotide reduce mortality.
- Peritoneal dialysis – prevent complications of severe pancreatitis

Surgical Intervention

- Diagnosis in doubt
- Failed medical treatment
- Biliary pancreatitis
- Pancreatic debridement in cases of infected pancreatic necrosis
- Management of complications
  - Pseudocyst
  - Abscess
  - Hemorrhage.

Biliary Pancreatitis

- Need to remove gallbladder and possible stones in CBD after attack over to prevent recurrence
- Pancreatitis resolves if pain subsides and serum amylase returns to normal
- Premature feeding can lead to recurrent attack
- ERCP for management of CBD stones.
- Laparoscopic cholecystectomy within same admission if possible, otherwise after 6–8 weeks.

Systemic Complications

- Respiratory failure, ARDS: Mechanical ventilation, PEEP
- *Heart failure:* Ionotropes support needed.
- *Renal failure:* Hemodialysis
- *GI failure:* Proton pump inhibitors
- *Coagulopathy:* FFP, platelet concentrate
- Neurological (irritability,confusion)
- Metabolic (hypocalcemia, hyperglycemia).

Antibiotics

- Infective complication usually occurs after 1st week
- Translocation of enteric organisms
- *E. Coli, Klebsiella, Enterococcus, Staphylococcus, Pseudomonas*
- Prophylactic antibiotics beneficial in severe cases, must be broad spectrum like 3rd generation cephalosporin or imipenem
- Early enteral feeding and gut decontamination may be beneficial.

Other Drugs

- *Somatostatin analogues:* Controversial
- *Anticholingeric agents, protease inhibitors, glucagon:* not useful

Nutrition

- Indicated in patients not expected to eat for 1 week or more
- Enteral feeding (nasogastric, nasojejunal or jejunostomy tubes placed after operation) is safe and beneficial, can be given in early stage
- Total parental nutrition in cases of paralytic ileus and duodenal obstruction

Local Complications

- Acute fluid collection
  - Early in the course of disease, located in or near the pancreas, wall encompassing the collection is ill defined
- Pseudocyst
  - Collection of pancreatic juice enclosed in a wall of fibrous or granulation tissue that arises following an attack of acute pancreatitis
  - Formation of a pseudocyst requires 4 weeks or more from onset of acute pancreatitis
- Pancreatic necrosis
  - A diffuse or focal area of nonviable parenchyma which is typically associated with peripancreatic fat necrosis
- Pancreatic abscess
  - Collection of pus, in proximity to pancreas containing little, or no pancreatic necrosis
- Pancreatic effusion
- Pancreatic ascites
  - Chronic generalized peritoneal enzyme-rich effusion usually associated with pancreatic duct disruption.

Diagnosis of Necrosis

- Contrast CT scan
  - Necrotic areas do not enhance
- Diagnosis of infected necrosis
  - Clinically increase abdominal pain, fever, leukocytosis and/or organ failure
  - Air bubbles in necrotic area
  - CT or USG guided FNA for smear and culture.

Surgery for Necrosis

- Non-operative treatment for sterile necrosis
- Infected necrosis needs surgical intervention
- *Operation:* Necrosectomy (devitalized pancreatic parenchyma and retroperitoneal fat)+/– drainage, lavage, re-laparotomy, zip closure, laparostomy
- *Minimal invasive:* Endoscopic/percutaneous
- *Pancreatic resection:* High morbidity and mortality.

Pseudocyst

- Drainage indicated if persists for 4–6 weeks and size >6 cm or symptomatic
- *Complications:* Rupture, hemorrhage, infection, obstruction
- Internal drainage is preferable to external drainage
- External drainage for infected or ruptured cysts or acute cysts with thin, friable walls.

- Internal drainage depends on location
  - *Retrogastric cyst:* posterior cystogastro-stomy
  - Cyst around head of pancreas: cystoduo-denostomy
  - Cyst bulge to transverse mesocolon: Roux-en-Y cystojejunostomy
  - Cyst in tail or body of pancreas: distal pancreatectomy + splenectomy.

Chronic Pancreatitis

- Uncertain pathogenesis
- Unpredictable clinical course
- Unclear treatment
- Spectrum of clinical features form silent disease to unexplained abdominal pain which eludes all diagnostic aids.

Etiology

- Alcoholic
- Trauma
- Obstruction (stricture, stone, tumor, pseudocyst)
- Hyperparathyroidism
- Hereditary
- Tropical pancreatitis
- Cystic fibrosis
- Idiopathic
- Hyperlipidemia
- Toxic substances.

Clinical Picture

- 3 leading symptoms
  - Pain (painless in 5–20%)
  - Exocrine insufficiency
  - Endocrine insufficiency
- Weight loss
- General debility
- Occasional acute attacks
- *Physical sign:* Tenderness.

Pathogenesis

- Hypersecretion of protein, plug formation, $CaCO_3$ precipitation
- Chronic inflammation
- Increased parenchymatous and ductal pressure
- Compartment syndrome
- Neural alteration/neuritis.

Morphology

- *Pancreas:* Atrophic or enlarged
  - Chronic change: fibrosis, inflammation, loss of exocrine tissue
  - *Acute change:* Edema, acute inflammation, necrosis
- *Pancreatic duct:* Dilatation, obstruction or shortening (chain-of-lakes)
- Acute pancreatits does not lead to chronic pancreatitis unless complications occur such as duct stricture, pseudocyst.

Investigation

- Blood tests
- *X-ray abdomen:* Pancreatic calcifications (up to 70%)
- USG
- CT
- EUS
- ERCP
- MRCP
- Pancreatic function tests.

Complications

- Pseudocyst
- Abscess
- Stenosis of CBD, duodenum, colon
- Pseudoaneurysm (splenic, Gastroduodenal, Pancreaticoduodenal)
- Fistula
- Pleural effusion
- Ascites
- Splenic vein thrombosis.

Treatment

- Eliminate etiology
- Pain relief
- Diabetes control
- Enzyme supplement
- *Intervention radiology:* Cyst, abscess, collection
- Endoscopic treatment (temporising role)
  - Biliary stent, pancreatic stent, remove stone
- Surgical treatment
  - *Drainage:* Longitudinal pancreatojejuno-stomy (Puestow's procedure)
  - *Resection:* Whipple, duodenum-preserving pancreatic head resection, distal pancreatec-tomy
  - *Combination:* Pancreatic head resection + longitudinal GJ.

75 Mesentery

- Acute non specific
- Tubercular

Acute Non Specific

- Aetiology not known
- Some associated with Yersinia infection
- Preceded by respiratory infection in 25%
- Self-limiting disease
- Never fatal
- May be recurrent.

Pathology

- Free peritoneal serous fluid
- Enlarged ileocecal peritoneal lymph nodes
- Red, size of walnut
- Nodes near root largest
- Free from peritoneal covering

Clinical Features

- Common during childhood
- Unusual after puberty
- Can be seen in teenage girls
- Attacks of central abdominal pain
- More when patient is tired
- Circumoral pallor
- No alteration of bowel habits
- Vomiting may be present
- Spasm of abdominal muscles during colic
- Does not look ill
- Elevated temp in > 50%
- Shifting tenderness
- P/R tenderness in 30%
- Other group of lymph nodes enlarged? Brucellosis.

Investigations

- Leuckocytosis - Especially on first day.

Treatment

- Bed rest
- Exclude appendicitis.

Tuberculosis of Mesenteric Lymph Nodes

- Usually Bovine type but can be human type
- Through ingestion of raw milk
- One to several lymph nodes can be involved with massive enlargement
- Entry through Peyer's patches.

Presentation

- Calcified lymph node along the line of attachment of mesentery
- Change position on repeated X-ray
- Round oval , mottled shadow with boss elated outline, i.e. black berry
- Generalised symptoms, i.e. loss of appetite, loss of weight, evening rise of temp
- Abdominal pain chronic or acute
- Intestinal obstruction
- Pseudo-mesenteric cyst due to careation of lymph node
- Palpable lymph node mass.

Mesenteric Cyst

- Chylolymphatic cyst
- Enterogenous cyst
- Cyst arising from urogenital remnant
- Dermoid cyst.

Chylolymphatic Cyst

- Commonest
- From misplaced lymphatic tissue
- No efferent connection with lymphatic system
- Thin walled, flat epithelium, contains lymph
- Unilocular, solitary
- Independent blood supply.

Enterogenous Cyst

- Arise
  - From sequestered diverticulum of the mesenteric border of the intestine
  - From duplication of intestine
- Thicker wall, lined by mucous membrane and muscle
- Common blood supply with intestine
- Removal of cyst requires resection of portion of gut.

Clinical Features

- Pain less abdominal lump
- Recurrent attacks of abdominal pain.
- Central abdominal mass mobile at right angle to attachment of mesentry
- Area of resonance around lump

Complications

- Torsion
- Rupture
- Hemorrhage
- Infection.

Investigations

- Ultrasonography
- CT abdomen

Treatment

- Chylolymphatic cyst
  - Enucleation of cyst
- Enterogenous cyst
  - Resection of cyst along with adherent portion of gut.

Mesenteric Ischemia

- Bowel ischemia is a complex disease caused by a drastic reduction in blood supply to the mesentery, that can be due to
  - Lack of arterial blood flow
  - Venous occlusion
  - Low cardiac output.

Incidence

- Overall incidence is 1% of all patients hospitalized for acute abdomen
- Described by Beniviene in 1509
- Cokkinis stated in 1921 that prognosis is hopeless, and the treatment almost useless, but advances in diagnostic imaging and vascular intervention, prognosis is not that dismol

Pathophysiology

- Acute ischemia can cause
  - Diffuse abdominal pain, and often without abdominal distention
  - Vasospasm, which causes *gut emptying* or profuse vomiting and diarrhea
  - Mucosal sloughing occurs and concomitant GI bleeding.

Causes of Mesenteric Ischemia

- Arterial occlusion (~50% of cases)
  - Emboli due to Atrial fibrillation , mural thrombi due to dyskinesia
  - Thrombotic occlusion due to pre-existing atherosclerotic vessel disease
  - Acute obstruction with underlying chronic mesenteric Ischemia
    ◊ Cardiac valvular lesions/vegetations
    ◊ Atheroemboli
    ◊ Dissecting aortic aneurysm
    ◊ Fibromuscular dyplasia
    ◊ Trauma
    ◊ Endotoxin induced shock
  - Non-occlusive mesenteric ischemia (~20–30% of cases)
    ◊ Systemic hypotension
- Cardiac failure
- Septic shock
- Mesenteric vasoconstriction (owing to sympathetic response)
- Venous occlusion (~5–15% of cases)
  - Primary vein thrombosis
  - Secondary vein thrombosis.

Clinical Features

- Pain is disproportionately exaggerated relative to physical findings

- Fever, diarrhoea, nausea and anorexia are commonly reported
- Malena/Frank blood in stool.

Diagnosis

- High index of suspicion
- History of Atrial fibrillation
- Older than 60 years of age
- Patients with postprandial abdominal pain and weight loss
- Aim to have early diagnosis to minimise gut infarction.

Laboratory

- Profound leukocytosis
- Metabolic acidosis
- Hemoconcentration on the complete blood count.
- Widened anion gap and increased lactic acid levels.

Radiology

- Plain films
  - Pneumatosis intestinalis along with gas in the portal vein
- CT scans Multi-slice spiral
- Angiography Gold standard for diagnosis
  - Both diagnostic and therapeutic option (Thrombolysis/Papaverine injection)
- MRI/MRA identify stenotic lesions in chronic ischemia.

Treatment

- Mainstay of treatment is surgical exploration
- Embolectomy
- Vascular reconstruction using a saphenous vein graft for aortomesenteric bypass
- Resecting compromised bowel.

76 | Spleen Injury

- Traumatic
- Iatrogenic

Traumatic

- Road traffic accident
- Blunt abdominal trauma
  - Fall from height
  - Direct blow to left upper quadrant
  - Sports injury
- Penetrating trauma
  - Stab wound
  - Gunshot injury

Iatrogenic

- During gastrectomy
- During left colon resection
- During pancreatic injury
- During left nephrectomy

Clinical Presentation

- Patient deteriorates and succumbs rapidly due to massive bleeding probably due to complete avulsion of spleen from its pedicle or associated injuries. This type of presentation is rare.
- Initial shock (due to blood loss) → Recovery due to tamponade effect → signs of late bleeding
- Delayed type of presentation: Following trauma there is a period of freedom from symptoms and this period can be extremely deceptive with patient appearing absolutely normal. Patient presents 4–5 days later after injury with sudden onset signs of internal haemorrhage and shock. Splenectomy is urgently indicated. Delay in bleeding can be due to greater omentum shutting off the portion of the general peritoneal cavity from the immediate vicinity of spleen or a blood clot temporarily seals the rent or a subcapsular haematoma forms which ruptures later on as it enlarges. Each of these factors at one time or another contributes in arresting serious bleeding temporarily.

Local Signs

- Left quadrant guarding/tenderness is present in more than 50% of cases
- Abdominal distension (meteorism) starts occurring 3–4 hours after accident due to paralytic ileus because of presence of blood in peritoneal cavity.
- Generalized tenderness/guarding
- Hyperesthesia over left shoulder (Kehr's sign) along with referred pain to left shoulder is often present. If patient is not complaining of any pain over shoulder, the patient is asked to lie flat on back in bed with foot end elevated by 0.5 meter. Wait for 10 minutes for the liquid blood in the peritoneal cavity to gravitate towards diaphragm and patient often complain of pain over shoulder which does not get worsened by movement of shoulder

- Shifting dullness in flanks
- Rectal examination – fullness in pelvis

Delayed Presentation

- Initial signs go unnoticed → delayed rupture of capsular hematoma
- Can be classified into three categories
  - Hemodynamically normal (normal blood pressure and heart rate)
  - Transient responders
    ◊ Present with low blood pressure and tachycardia → respond initially to I.V. infusion of colloids and crystalloids → again manifest abnormal vital signs indicating ongoing bleeding
  - Hemodynamically unstable patient who show no response to crystalloid infusion

Investigations

Focused Abdominal Sonography for Trauma (FAST)

- Detects free fluid in abdomen
- Operator dependent
- Portable, rapid, non-invasive

Diagnostic Peritoneal Lavage (DPL)

- Small infra-umbilical incision
- Dialysis catheter introduced into peritoneal cavity
- 1 litre of normal saline infused and then siphoned back
- Siphoned fluid is examined for RBC/ WBC/ Amylase
- DPL is considered positive if
  - Aspiration of 10 ml of gross blood
  - $>10^5$ RBC/cumm
  - >500 WBC/cumm
  - Evidence of gut contents
  - Amylase positive in fluid
- Indications
  - Useful in unstable patients
  - Extremely sensitive but low specificity
  - Does not differentiate between solid organ and hollow viscus injury

CT Scan

- Investigation of choice for stable patient
- Detects and defines solid organ injury
- Essential for non-operative management

CT Grading of Splenic Injury

Grade	Injury
I	Subcapsular hematoma <10% surface area (S.A.) Capsular tear with <1cm parenchymal depth of laceration
II	Subcapsular hematoma, 10–50% S.A. Intraparenchymal hematoma < 5 cm diameter Laceration 1–3cm parenchyma depth which does not involve trabecular vessel
III	Subcapsular hematoma, >50% S.A., Expanding, Ruptured Intraparenchymal hematoma, >5cm or expanding Laceration, >3cm parenchymal depth or involving trabecular vessels
IV	Laceration involving segmental or hilar vessels
V	Completely shattered spleen Hilar vascular injury

Non-Operative Management

- Patient should be monitored in critical care environment
- Operating facilities should be available in the event of sudden bleed/deterioration

Indications

- Hemodynamically stable patient
- Minimal or no abdominal findings
- Mode of injury is blunt and not penetrating
- There is no associated injury requiring surgery
- Total blood transfusion requirement does not exceed two units
- Injury should be grade I to III on CT scan.

More Successful in Children

- 70–90% of children with splenic injury can be treated non-operatively in contrast to only 40–50% of adults with splenic injury can be treated non-operatively
- Reasons for more success in children are:
  - Elastic cartilaginous rib cage provides protection to spleen
  - More elastin in the spleen in children producing contraction and some degree of hemostasis
  - Mechanism of injury more often due to
    ◊ Sports injury
    ◊ Falls
    ◊ Pedestrian collision
    ◊ Bicycle crash

Operative Management

Indications

- Hemodynamically unstable patient
  - Systolic BP <90 mmHg
  - Tachycardia >120/min
  - No immediate response to 1–2L of colloid infusion
- Grade IV or V injury on CT Scan
- Other associated injuries requiring laparotomy
- Blast/gun shot injury to left upper quadrant of abdomen
- Penetrating injuries
- Failure to respond non-operative management
  - Increasing fluid requirement
  - Blood transfusion requirement to maintain haemoglobin >10gm%
  - Increasing hemoperitoneum in serial imaging
  - Peritoneal signs or rebound tenderness

Operations

Splenorrhaphy

- Repair of splenic tear
  - Suture repair
  - Absorbable mesh repair
  - Resection of polar segment

- Superficial hemostatic agents, e.g. oxidized cellulose, absorbable gelatin sponge, topical thrombin

Splenectomy

- For shattered spleen
- For pedicle injuries.

Vaccination

- 2–3 weeks prior to elective splenectomy against *Pneumococci*, *H. influenzae* type B, and Meningococci for the primary immune response to be elective
- In trauma, patient is given the vaccines in post-operative period usually 10 after surgery except pneumococcal vaccine which is given immediately, as in immediate post operative period there is immunosuppssion

Patient education

- Carry splenectomy card
- Close surveillance and supply of stand by oral antibiotics of penicillin group with instructions to start them at the onset of febrile illness or rigors if there is no access to immediate medical evaluation
- Regular follow up visits to ensure compliance with antibiotics and vaccine prophylaxis
- Seek medical attention at the first sign of infection.

77 | Splenectomy

Functions of Spleen are:

A. Acts as site of quality control for red blood cells

B. Removes old damaged or fragmented erythrocytes from circulation.

C. Remodels the surface of maturing RBC and maintains normal relationship between membrane surface area and volume. After removal of spleen target cell with high ratio of membrane to intra- cellular hemoglobin appear in the circulation.

D. By process known as pitting intra-erythrocyte inclusions are removed from spleen. They are Howell Jolly bodies.

E. *Hematopoiesis:* From one and half to six and half months of intrauterine life it is site of production of myelocytes and platelets. From three and half to five months it also produces Red blood cells which can get reactivated in children if the bone marrow compensatory activity is exceeded.

F. It is the site for production of IgM, opsonins and Tuftsins.

G. Spleen is the site of filtration of encapsulated bacteria and foreign antigen through macrophages and reticuloendothelial system through phagocytosis.

H. It is the storage site for iron.

I. It is the site for sequestration of 30 % of circulating platlets.

Indications of Splenectomy

Definite Indications

- Spleen injury where spleen cannot be saved or salvaged
  - Hilar injuries
  - Shattered spleen
  - Blast injures to left upper quadrant
  - Multiple associated injuries
  - Unstable patient
  - Marked intra-abdominal contamination
- During en-bloc resection of adjacent organs
  - Proximal gastric cancer
  - Neoplasm of tail of pancreas
- Neoplasm of spleen
- Splenic abscess, if
  - Large
  - Multiple
  - Failed percutaneous drainage
- Hydatid cyst
- Rupture of splenic artery aneurysm
- Bleeding gastric varices from splenic vein thrombosis
- Spontaneous rupture of diseased spleen, e.g. Hodgkin's lymphoma, chronic malaria

Desirable Indications

- In following conditions on failure of medical treatment (with steroids and human IgG)
  - Hereditary spherocytosis
  - Idiopathic thrombocytopenic purpura
  - AIDS related thrombocytopenia

- Acquired haemolytic anemia
- Some cases of red cell enzyme defects, e.g. pyruvate kinase deficiency
- In sickle cell disease if there is
  - Hypersplenism
  - Massive splenic infarct
  - Major splenic sequestration
- Congestive splenomegaly associated with neutropenia
- To reduce blood transfusion requirement inhemoglobinopathies like thallesemia.

Debatable Indications

- Non-parasitic splenic cysts
- Lymphoma
  - Part of staging laparotomy (in pre CT era)
  - With specific cytopenia or pancytopenia
- Myeloproliferative disorders
- Thrombotic thrombocytopenic purpura.

Complications of Splenectomy

Incidence

- In 10% patients after open splenectomy.

Early Complications

- Bleeding
  - Slipped ligature of splenic artery
  - Oozing from raw surface of diaphragm or retroperitoneum after removal of large spleen
  - Dense vascular adhesions
- Subphrenic collection
- Left basal atelectasis/pleural effusion
- Gastric dilatation
- Hematemesis from gastric mucosal congestion
- Damage to the greater curvature of the stomach resulting in gastric fistula
- Trauma to the tail of pancreas
  - Pancreatic ascites
  - Pancreatic fistula
  - Subphrenic collection
- Damage to the splenic flexure of the colon
  - Fecal fistula
- Thrombocytosis with hypercoagulable state which may result in deep venous thrombosis.

Late Complications

- Overwhelming post splenectomy sepsis (OPSI)
- Migratory thrombophlebitis

- Deep venous thrombosis
- Recurrence of the disease due to hypertrophy of missed accessory spleen/spleniculi.

Overwhelming Post Splenectomy Infection (OPSI)

- Common in asplenic patients
- These patients have 40–50 fold increase in risk of infection due to
  Streptococcus pneumoniae, Hemophilus influenzae, Hemophilus pertussis, Neisseria meningitides, E. coli.

Greatest Risk in

- Infants and children <5 years of age
- In those adults where spleen is removed for thallesemia or reticulosis or lymphoma
- If splenectomy patients are treated with chemotherapy.

Lowest Risk in

- Young adults with splenectomy for trauma.

Contributing Factors for OPSI

- Impaired Filtration
- Diminished phagocytosis
- Decreased IgM levels
- Loss of opsonin/tuftsin
- Reduction in percentage of CD4+ T-cells.

Clinical Course

- Onset – insidious with non-specific viral like illness/malaise
- Course – Rapidly take fulminant form with
  - High grade fever
  - Nausea/vomiting
  - Dehydration
  - Hypotension
  - Death

Treatment

- Should be aggressive and without undue delay with broad spectrum antibiotics.

Prevention

- Prophylactic antibiotics to be given in children (till 10 years of age) and high risk adults
- Antibiotics used are – oral penicillin, erythromycin, amoxicillin or co-amoxyclav.

78 | Inflammatory Bowel Disease

- Chronic inflammatory diseases of unknown etiology
  - Ulcerative colitis (UC) - affects only the large intestine
  - Crohn's disease (CD) - most frequently attacks the distal third of the small intestine and the colon
- Diagnosed using clinical, endoscopic and histological criteria
- No single finding is absolutely diagnostic for one disease or the other
- Approx. 20% of patients have indeterminate colitis
- Wide spectrum of the treatment available
- Extra intestinal manifestations may be present
- Approx. 1 million people have Inflammatory Bowel Disease (IBD)
- Common in industrialized nations
- Lowest in developing regions
- Higher rate in urban areas vs. rural areas
- Incidence higher in Jews
- Incidence is slightly higher in females than males
- Vast majority diagnosed between ages 15–40 years

Pathophysiology

- Not known
- Defect in function of the intestinal immune system (breakdown in defense barrier)
- Exposure of mucosa to microorganisms results in inflammatory process causing ulceration, bleeding and loss of fluids and electrolytes
- Genetic predisposition (esp. when ileal segment is involved)

Etiology

Ulcerative Colitis

- 15 percent have first degree relative with IBD
- No organisms can be incriminated
- Relapse associated with bacterial dysenteries
- Smoking has a protective effect
- Prevalence - 160 per 10000 population
- Sex ratio-
  - Equal for first four decades
  - After 40 years it becomes less common in females
- Uncommon before 10 years
- Most patients between 20–40 years at diagnosis

Crohn's Disease

- DNA of *Mycobacterium paratuberculosis* is found in 60% cases in intestine of patients with Crohn's disease
- No immunological reaction is seen
- Focal ischemia is causative factor
- Smoking increases risk by three fold
- Family history in 10 percent
- Association with ankylosing spondylitis

Pathology

Crohn's Disease

- **Ileal disease:** 60 percent
- Limited to colon in 30 percent
- Anal lesions common
- Fibrous thickening of bowel with narrow lumen
- All layers of gut involved (trans mural inflammation)
- Internal fistulae formation very common
- Cobblestone appearance of mucosa
- Skip lesions often seen.

Ulcerative Colitis

- Affects the large intestine
- Starts in rectum and is continuous until some proximal part of the colon
- Involves the mucosa and sub-mucosa only
- Ulcerated, friable and granular appearance of mucosa
- Formation of crypt abscesses
- In chronic cases, colon becomes rigid and loses its haustral (pouch-like) markings
- Confined to rectum in 25% of cases; sigmoid colon in 30 percent
- Spread up to splenic flexure in 20 percent

Clinical Features

- Waxing and waning course in intensity and severity
- Symptoms correspond with degree of inflammation
- When patient is actively symptomatic, significant inflammation leads to flare-up of IBD
- When asymptomatic, inflammation absent (or less) resulting in remission

Ulcerative Colitis

- Watery or bloody diarrhoea
- **Rectal discharge:** mucus , blood stained or purulent
- Pain unusual
- Tenesmus or urgency

Disease severity

- **Mild:** Diarrhea less than 4 per day, no systemic signs of the disease
- **Moderate:** More than 4 motions per day, no systemic signs of the disease
- **Severe:** More than 4 motions per day with one or more systemic illness
  - Fever > 37.5°C
  - Pulse rate > 90/min
  - Serum albumin < 3gm%
  - Weight loss > 3kg

Crohn's Disease (CD)

- Known as "Granulomatous or Regional Enteritis", "Granulomatous Ileitis" or "Ileocolitis".
- Can affect any part of gut
- Can have non-continuous lesions (Skip lesions) with areas of severe inflammation with intervening normal mucosa
- Most frequently affects distal third of small intestine and the colon
- Affects all layers of the affected bowel
- Complicated by strictures, fistulae and abscesses
- Histologically, may show granulomas (aggregates of giant cells)
- Late in disease, mucosa develops a cobblestone appearance (deep ulcerations intervening with normal mucosa)
- Major patterns of involvement
  - Disease in ileum and cecum (40%)
  - Disease confined to small intestine (30%)
  - Disease confined to colon (25%)
  - Less commonly involves more proximal parts of GI tract (tongue, esophagus, stomach and duodenum)
- Increased incidence of gall stones and kidney stones (due to malabsorption of fats and bile salts)
- Additional mortality:
  - Multiple surgeries reduce the absorptive capacity of the small bowel
  - Multiple recurrences
  - Recurrent infections
  - Long-term use of steroids and cytotoxic drugs
  - Suicide

Extraintestinal Manifestations of IBD

- Iritis
- Episcleritis
- Arthritis
- Skin involvement, e.g. pyoderma nodosum
- Pericholangitis
- Sclerosing cholangitis

Ulcerative Colitis vs. Crohn's Disease

See Table 78.1

S. No.	Ulcerative colitis	Crohn's disease
	Table 78.1: Clinical and pathological differneces between warative colitis and crohn's disease	
1	Rectal bleeding common	Occasional rectal bleeding
2	Abdominal pain uncommon	Abdominal pain common
3	Rectal involvement almost 100%	Rectal involvement 50%
4	Fistula formation rare	Fistula formation common
5	Stricture and obstruction rare	Stricture and obstruction common
6	Perirectal, perianal abscesses uncommon	Perirectal, perianal abscesses common
7	Continuous involvement	Discontinuous involvement
8	Mucosa and submucosa involved	Transmural
9	Small bowel not involved	Small bowel often involved
10	Risk of malignancy greatly increased	Risk of malignancy less

Risk of Malignancy in IBD

- In Crohn's disease, increased risk of cancer of the affected areas.
- In ulcerative colitis, 8–10 years after initial diagnosis, there is a steady, significant increased risk of developing cancer.
- Prognostic factors increasing malignancy risk in UC:
  - Duration of disease 10 years or more
  - Pancolonic involvement
  - Continuous progressive disease
  - Severe initial onset
  - Associated liver disease

Differential Diagnosis

- Anorexia nervosa
- Appendicitis
- Celiac sprue
- *Clostridium difficile* colitis
- Giardiasis
- Lactose intolerance
- Chronic pelvic pain
- Diverticulitis
- Pseudomembranous colitis
- Salmonellosis
- IBS (irritable bowel syndrome)

IBS (Irritable Bowel Syndrome)

- Recurrent abdominal pain with constipation and/or diarrhea
- No detectable structural disease
- Cause unknown; associated with stress or anxiety and may follow severe infection
- No impact on mortality

Clinical History (UC)

- Bloody diarrhea common
- Abdominal pain, fever, cramping and weight loss in severe cases
- Greater extent of involvement, greater probability of diarrhea
- As degree of inflammation increases, more systemic symptoms develop (low-grade fever, sweats, dehydration, tachycardia, arthralgias)
- In chronic disease, there may be regenerative patches of mucosa called pseudopolyps rising above the diseased surface
- Formed stools indicate UC confined to rectum.

Findings on Imaging Studies and Endoscopies

- Irregular colon with "thumb printing" (air in colonic wall)
- *Toxic megacolon :* Long, continuous segment of air-filled colon greater than 6 cm in diameter (esp. in transverse colon)
- On barium enema, shortened colon in UC, with loss of haustrations and destruction of mucosal pattern ("lead pipe colon")
- Skip areas and rectal sparing in CD
- In CD, areas of segmental narrowing with loss of normal mucosa, fistula formation and string sign (narrow band of barium flowing through an inflamed or scarred area)
- Ileitis in UC (without the skip pattern)
- CT and U/S best for demonstrating mesenteric inflammation, intra-abdominal abscesses and fistulas
- Mucosal surface irregular and friable (esp. in UC)
- Colonoscopy recommended for making diagnosis and determining severity of disease.

Investigations in IBD

- CT and USG best for demonstrating mesenteric inflammation, intra-abdominal abscesses and fistulas

- Mucosal surface irregular and friable (esp. in UC)
- Colonoscopy recommended for making diagnosis and determining severity of disease.

Complications

- Toxic megacolon (can be caused by narcotics, cathartics, enemas, antidiarrheal medications) in UC-inflammation impedes ability to contract (peristalsis) and move gas; abdominal pain, distention
- Dilated colon – allows bacteria to leak into bloodstream, increases risk of perforation and peritonitis
- If no improvement, patient is usually treated with colectomy
- Strictures can lead to obstruction
- Fistulas and abscesses (more common in CD, but also 20% UC)
- *Fistula types:* enterovesical, enteroenteric, enteromesenteric, enterocutaneous, recto-vaginal and perianal
- Stenosis and obstruction
- In CD, obstructive hydronephrosis can be seen due to compression of right ureter
- Sepsis, malnutrition in Crohn's disease.

Extraintestinal Complications

- Arthritis
- Ankylosing spondylitis (HLA-B27)
- Episcleritis (3–4%)-parallels course of disease
- Iritis
- Erythema nodosum (often at disease onset)-esp. anterior tibia
- Pyoderma gangrenosum
- Aphthous ulcers.

Others

- Pericholangitis
- Chronic active hepatitis
- Primary sclerosing cholangitis
- Gall stones
- Hypercoagulable state.

Treatment

Aims of Treatment

- Inducing remission
- Maintaining remission
- Restoring and maintaining nutrition
- Maintaining patient's quality of life
- Surgical intervention (selection of optimal time for surgery).

Medical Treatment

- Anti-inflammatory agents (aminosalicylates, corticosteroids)
- Immunosuppressant
- Antibiotics
- TNF (Tumor necrosis factor) inhibitors
- Anti-diarrheal agents
- Antispasmodic agents
- Supportive therapy
- *** 75% of ulcerative colitis patients respond well to medical management*

Anti-Inflammatory Agents (Aminosalicylates)

Sulfasalazine (Azulfidine) - Combination of Sulfapyradine (Anti-bacterial) + 5-aminosalicylic acid (5-ASA)

- Greatest effect on IBD; mainstay of outpatient medical treatment for mild-moderately active UC and CD
- Possesses both anti-inflammatory and antibacterial properties
- Partially absorbed in jejunum but remainder passes to colon
- Mechanism of action
  - Inhibition of prostaglandin and leukotriene synthesis
  - Free radical scavenging
  - Impairment of white cell adhesion and function
  - Inhibition of cytokine synthesis

Mesalamine Group - Asacol, Pentasa, Rowasa

- Coating 5-ASA with acrylic resins- permits drug delivery to distal bowel and colon
- Effective for ileal and colonic involvement
- Rapid absorption
- Enemas and suppositories
- Fewer side effects than sulfasalazine
- Olsalazine - delayed absorption; useful in colonic disease

Corticosteroids

- Treatment of choice for acute attack of IBD (including IV treatment; enemas for acute proctitis)
- Generally used for moderate-severe IBD

- Not to be used for maintaining remission due to multiple and severe side effects
- **Prednisolone**
  - Synthetic glucocorticoid; powerful anti-inflammatory action
  - Usually tapered doses
  - IV use - methylprednisolone, dexamethasone
- **Budesonide** - newer type
  - Synthetic steroid coated with ethylmethylcellulose which delays its release until ileum and descending colon
- Side effects often outweigh benefits if used for prolonged period of time.

Immunosuppressants

- Reduce inflammation by suppressing immune system's response (which might damage digestive tissue) to invading virus or bacterium
- Azathioprine and mercaptopurine
  - Help reduce signs and symptoms of IBD and heal fistulas from CD
  - Inhibits mitosis
  - Increases risk of neoplasia
  - Serious hepatic, renal, and hematological side effects
- Methotrexate - used for patients who do not respond to other medications
- Cyclosporine.

Antibiotics

- IBD is associated with frequent bacterial infections especially with toxic megacolon, fistulas and fulminant disease
- Most effective antibiotics: metronidazole, ampicillin, cephalosporins, aminoglycosides, ciprofloxacin.

TNF (Tumor Necrosis Factor) Inhibitors

- TNF is a protein produced by the immune system; chemical messenger that can cause inflammation and tissue damage
- Etanercept; TNF receptor blocker; binds to alpha and beta TNF
- Used to treat rheumatoid arthritis (demote)
- Infliximab
  - Neutralizes cytokine TNF alpha
  - Increased risk infections (reactivation of TB or granulomatous disease)
  - Usually for moderate-severe disease
  - May be used for long-term therapy.

Antidiarrheal Agents

- Decrease peristalsis and therefore intestinal motility
- Improves diarrhea and prevents loss of fluid and electrolytes
- Loperamide, Atropine
- Cholestyramine- inhibits enterohepatic reuptake of bile salts.

Antispasmodic Agents

- Treat functional disturbances of GI motility
- Dicyclomine- anticholinergic; blocks action of acetylcholine at parasympathetic sites in secretory glands, smooth muscle and CNS.

Supportive Therapy

- In addition to adequate nutritional support also administer
  - Vitamin B12
  - Iron
  - Folic acid.

Surgical Treatment

- Surgical removal of large bowel (colectomy) will result in cure of ulcerative colitis
- Surgical removal of the affected bowel segment in CD *will not prevent the later appearance* of disease at an adjacent or distant site.

Ulcerative Colitis

- Main indications:
  - Failure of medical treatment
  - Complications (toxic megacolon, perforation)
  - Risk of malignancy
- Resection of colon and rectum (panproctocolectomy) is curative
- Fecal diversion via ileostomy or ileo-anal anastomosis in the form of ileal pouch
- Pouch may cause mechanical problems (40% develop inflammation resembling UC, 15% may need further surgery)
- 10% will have colectomy during 1st year
- 4% will have surgery during 2nd year
- 1 % annually in subsequent years
- Colectomy rate for patients with pancolitis is 32%
- Complications of surgery: Ileal Pouch-Anal Anastomosis (IPAA)
  - Pelvic sepsis
  - Leakage

– Incontinence
– Intestinal obstruction
– Anastomotic strictures
– Sexual dysfunction
– Pouchitis
– Female infertility.

Crohn's Disease

- For dealing with complications such as stricture formation, perforation and fistulae
- 30% need surgery within 1st year
- For the remainder, surgery rate is 5% per year
- Following resection, 30% will require further surgery within 5 years, and 50% within 10 years
- Least invasive procedures desirable.

Mild Ulcerative Colitis

- Distal or rectal involvement only
- 4 or fewer stools/day
- Treatment with retention enemas or oral anti-inflammatory medication
- *No systemic or extracolonic manifestations*
- ESR normal.

Moderate Ulcerative Colitis

- >4 stools per day
- No currently active pancolitis
- Mild systemic symptoms
- No serious complications
- No worse than mild anemia
- ESR mildly raised

- Treatment may require intermittent use of oral steroids or other cytotoxic drugs.

Severe Ulcerative Colitis

- ≥ 6 stools per day
- Active pancolitis with frequent diarrhea, abdominal pain
- Severe and typical systemic findings
- Bloody diarrhea, fever, tachycardia, anemia
- Weight loss > 10% of body weight
- Lab results reveal moderate - severe anemia and/or hypoalbuminemia
- ESR>30mm/hour
- Recent (within 5 years) toxic megacolon or multiple surgeries
- Treatment requires high doses of steroids or multiple cytotoxic medications.

Crohn's Disease - Favorable Factors

- Normal CBC
- Ileal involvement only
- Stable weight
- Non-steroidal medications only
- Colonoscopies every 12–24 months
- Older age

Crohn's Disease - Unfavorable Factors

- Low blood counts on CBC
- Multiple sites in GI tract
- Low and/or fluctuating weight
- Steroid use
- Surgical intervention (multiple)
- Poor follow-up/compliance

79 Acute Appendicitis and Right Iliac Fossa Mass

- Most common cause of acute abdomen
- Appendicectomy is the most common emergency operation performed through out the world
- The diagnosis is essentially clinical

ANATOMY

- Appendix is a blind muscular tube communicating with the cecum.
- It has four layers — it denotes underdeveloped distal end of cecum
- It arises from postero-medial aspect of cecum, about 2.5 cm below and lateral to the ileocecal junction
- Base is located at a point where taenia coli of the colon meet, a fairly constant finding that helps in identification of the appendix
- Tip of the appendix is variable
  - Retrocecal   65–74%
  - Pelvic   21–31%
  - Subcecal   1.5–2.5%
  - Pre-ileal   1%
  - Right paracolic   0.5–2%
  - Post-ileal   0.5%
- Length of appendix varies from 1 to 25 cm (average 5–7 cm) and lumen diameter ranges from 1–3 mm
- Appendicular artery is a
  - Branch of ileocolic artery
  - Runs in mesoappendix
  - Falls short at tip
  - Is an end artery
- Accessory appendicular artery is present in 1/3rd of cases
  - Branch of posterior cecal artery

Acute Appendicitis

- Uncommon before 2 years of age
- Peak incidence in the first decade and early twenties
- After middle age the risk reduces
- M:F ratio is 3:2 uptill 25 years

Types

Obstructive

- Obstruction of lumen due to
  - Fecolith
  - Swelling of lymphoid tissue in the wall
  - Kinking
  - Adhesions
  - Fibrosis, parasites and tumors
- Obstruction → closed loop → appendix gets distended with mucus → bacteria multiply → pressure atrophy of mucosa → bacteria gain entry to appendicular wall → infection spreads to serosa → outside appendix, infection spreads to appendicular artery → thrombosis → gangrene → peritonitis.

Non-Obstructed

- Bacterial invasion of lymphoid tissue in the appendicular wall

- *Streptococci* common
- Course is generally gradual
- Gangrene is rare
- Acute infection can resolve

Clinical Features

- Pain
  - At first the pain is colicky, periumbilical, due to distension of appendix (visceral) associated with nausea and vomiting (vomiting is reflex in nature due to protective pylorospasm)
  - Pain then shifts to right iliac fossa when irritation to parietal peritoneum starts
  - Classical shift is seen in 50% patients
  - Atypical pain can be seen in elderly and in case of pelvic appendicitis (which may present with suprapubic discomfort and tenesmus)
- Temperature – mildly raised (99 to 100°F)
- Constipation
- Diarrhea may be seen in pediatric age group, pre-ileal appendicitis and pelvic appendicitis.

Clinical Signs

- Anxious look, pulse and temperature mildly raised
- Dry tongue
- On inspection, limitation of movement of right lower abdomen with respiration
- Tenderness and rebound tenderness in right iliac fossa
- Rigidity
- Hyperasthesia in Sherren's triangle
- Rovsing's sign positive—pressure in left iliac fossa elicits pain in the right iliac fossa
- Psoas sign in retrocecal appendicitis
- Obturator sign if inflamed appendix lies on obturator internus
- In case of pelvic appendicitis
  - Irritation of urinary bladder may cause frequency
  - Irritation of rectum may cause diarrhea or tenesmus
  - No abdominal signs may be seen
  - Tenderness on per-rectal or per-vaginal examination
- In case of post-ileal appendicitis
  - Pain may not shift
  - Diarrhea is present
  - Intractable vomiting may be present

Scoring System for Appendicitis — Alvarado (MANTREL) Score

- Symptoms
  - Migratory right iliac fossa pain   1
  - Anorexia   1
  - Nausea/vomiting   1
- Signs
  - Tenderness in right iliac fossa   2
  - Rebound tenderness   1
  - Elevated temperature   1
- Laboratory investigations
  - Leucocytosis   2
  - Shift to left   1
- **Total**   **10**

Score 7 or more strongly predicts appendicitis.

Score of 5–6 is equivocal, abdominal ultrasound or CECT scan may be needed to confirm the diagnosis.

Radiological Investigations

- Indicated if Alvarado score is 5–6 or less
- Non-specific signs or symptoms

Plain X-ray Abdomen (Supine and Erect)

- Presence of pneumoperitoneum indicates other hollow viscus perforation
- Non-specific signs of appendicitis
  - Fecolith
  - Localized ileus
  - Loss of peritoneal fat stripes
  - Gas in appendix

Ultrasound

- Graded compression on ultrasound
- Sensitivity >85%, specificity >90%
- Sign of appendicitis
  - Non-compressible appendix of 7 mm or more in antero posterior diameter
  - Presence of appendicolith
  - Interruption of continuity of echogenic sub-mucosa
  - Periappendiceal fluid or mass
- To rule out other pathologies like tubal/ovarian disease or ureteric calculi

CT Scan

- 5 mm cuts obtained
- Distended or thickened appendix giving a 'Halo' or 'Target' appearance

- Periappendiceal inflammation
  - Abscess
  - Fluid collection
  - Edema — appears as clouding of mesenteric fat

Nuclear Scan

- Experimental
- Using radiolabelled WBC (Tc99m WBC) or radiolabelled IgG (Tc99m IgG)
- Injected IV — localization at the site of appendicular inflammation

Differential Diagnosis

In Children

- Gastroenteritis
- Mesenteric lymphadenitis
- Meckel's diverticulitis
- Intussusception

In Adult Male

- Ureteric colic
- Regional ileitis (Crohn's disease)
- Rectus sheath hematoma
- Amebic typhlitis
- Carcinoma cecum
- Perforated peptic ulcer

In Adult Female

- Salpingitis
- Ectopic pregnancy
- Torsion or rupture of ovarian cyst

Fate of Acute Appendicitis

- Surgical removal
- Appendicular lump
- Appendicular abscess
- Peritonitis
- Gangrene, perforation, fecal peritonitis
- Mucocele of appendix
- Fibrosis
- Resolution — least common

Treatment

- Appendicectomy after pre-operative preparation
  - IV fluids
  - Antibiotics
- Appendicectomy can be
  - Conventional (open method)
  - Laparoscopic

- History of appendicectomy
  - Claudius amyand (1736) — removed appendix from hernia sac
  - Lawson tait (1880) — appendicectomy for acute appendicitis

Etiology and Management of Right Iliac Fossa Mass (RIF)

Etiolgy

Mass in RIF can arise from following structures:

Structures Normally Present in RIF

- Cecum
- Appendix
- Right ovary and tube (females)
- Lymph nodes
- Iliac vessels
- Psoas muscle with sheath
- Iliac bone

Structures which can be Present in RIF

- Undescended testis
- Unascended kidney
- Fundus of gallbladder
- Liver in massive enlargement

Cause of RIF Mass

- Infective
- Neoplastic
- Inflammatory
- Vascular
- Miscellaneous

Infective Causes

- Appendicular lump
- Appendicular abscess
- Ileocecal tuberculosis (hyperplastic type)
- Ameboma of cecum
- Actinomycosis
- Pyogenic psoas abscess
- Tubercular psoas abscess
- Infective iliac lymphadenitis
- Pyosalpinx
- Tubo-ovarian mass due to PID

Neoplastic Causes

- Carcinoma cecum/ascending colon
- Secondary in iliac lymph nodes
- Lymphoma of iliac lymph node
- Bony tumors of iliac bone

- Tumor in an undescended testis
- Ovarian cyst or ovarian tumor in females
- Fibroid uterus in females

Inflammatory Causes

- Crohn's disease
- Sarcoidosis

Vascular Causes

- Iliac artery aneurysm
- Hematoma following ruptured inferior epigastric artery

Miscellaneous Causes

- Spigelian hernia
- Kidney transplant
- Pelvic kidney enlargement due to varied etiology like hydronehrosis
- Ileo-colic intussusception

Clinical Features

History

- There can be history of mass without any symptoms
- Patient can present with recent onset three "A" — anorexia, anemia, asthenia in carcinoma cecum especially in middle aged or old persons
- Altered bowel habits in hyperplastic ileocecal tuberculosis
- Altered blood in stool in amoeboma or carcinoma cecum
- Colicky abdominal pain due to recurrent attacks of subacute intestinal obstruction
- Constitutional symptoms, e.g. loss of weight or loss of appetite especially in malignancy
- Urinary symptoms in pelvic kidney pathology
- Restricted mobility of hip joint in psoas abscess
- History of absence of testis
- Lower limb swelling due to iliac vein compression due to lymph nodes

Examination

- Malnutrition or cachexia
- Pallor
- Lymphadenopathy
- Pedal edema
- Flexion deformity of hip joint

Local Examination

Inspection

- Shape and extent of swelling
- Visible peristalsis or pulsations
- Cough impulse at hernia sites

Palpation

- Ascertain if the swelling is parietal or intra-abdominal
- Tenderness
- Confirm findings of inspection
- Mobility of lump
- Consistency, surface and margins of lump
- Genitalia examination to rule out undescended testis
- Groove sign— in psoas abscess there is no groove palpable between swelling and iliac crest in contrast to appendicular lump
- Per rectal examination
- Per vaginal examination

Percussion

- Shifting dullness or fluid thrill

Auscultation

- Increased bowel sounds

Investigations

Aims

- To establish anatomical diagnosis
- To establish the pathological diagnosis
- To assess the extent of disease
- To assess fitness for surgery

Ultrasonography

- First investigation of choice as it is non-invasive/cost effective
- Indicate organ of origin
- Can decide diagnosis, e.g. appendicular lump
- Detect free fluid
- Lymph nodes >1.0 cm can be detected

Barium Studies

Barium studies are being performed less commonly as they are being replaced by contrast enhanced CT (CECT). CECT gives much more information than barium studies. Barium studies are being only done if CT facility is not available or there is contra-indication to perform CT.

- Barium study can be double contrast barium enema or barium meal follow through. It can give useful information in:
  - Tuberculosis
  - Terminal ileitis
  - Malignancy of cecum

Colonoscopy

Advantages of colonoscopy include ability to visualise whole of colon and terminal ileum. One can take biopsy from suspected lesions. In one third of cases, due to acute bent in transverse colon one may not be able to reach up to the cecum. It is very useful in

- In carcinoma cecum
- Terminal ileitis

Dynamic Spiral CT/Virtual Colonoscopy

- 3D reconstruction of whole colon is possible
- Small mucosal lesions can be detected
- Unnecessary diagnostic colonoscopy can be avoided
- Staging of malignancy can be carried out
- Kidney pathology can be detected

Image Guided FNAC of Mass

- Tuberculosis
- Psoas abscess
- Lymph node enlargement.

Treatment

Appendicular Lump

- Conservative management
- Ochsner-Sherren regimen
  1. Nil by mouth
  2. Antibotics
  3. IV fluids
  4. Analgesia
  5. Regular monitoring of Temp./Pulse/symptoms

- Outcome – 3 "S"
  - Subside
  - Suppurate
  - Spread

Appendicular Abscess

- Drain abscess

Hyperplastic Ileocecal Koch's

- No features of obstruction with pain
  - Liquid diet
  - Anti-tubercular therapy
- Recurrent or acute obstruction
  - Surgery (limited resection)
  - With ATT

Carcinoma Cecum

- Confirm diagnosis
- Stage the disease
- Rule out synchronous lesion
- Right hemicolectomy
- Chemotherapy if indicated

Ameboma

- Emetine or dihydroemetine
- If it does not regress then surgery

Psoas Abscess

Pyogenic

- Drain abscess
- Antibiotic therapy

Tubercular

- Antitubercular therapy
- If big drain by catheter
- Bed rest if spine involved

Unascended Kidney

- If normal and there is no pathology, it can be observed
- If hydronephrotic treat the cause

INCIDENCE

- One of the commonest malignancy being second only to lung cancer as a cause of cancer death
- If diagnosed early and treated adequately, large gut cancer has a good prognosis. Almost 1/3rd patients can be cured
- Generally occurs in individuals >50 years of age
- *Male:* Female ratio is 3:1

Pathogenesis

- Most of the large gut cancer arises from adenomatous polyps
- Adenomatous polyps are present in the colon of >30% of population
- <1% of these become malignant. Change is more common in
  - Sessile (flat based) polyps
  - Villous adenomas — 3 times more common than in tubular adenoma
  - If size >2.5 cm, risk of malignancy is 10%; if 1.5–2.5 cm, risk is 2–10%; if <1.5 cm, the risk is <2%.
- Adenomatous polyps require >5 years to become malignant

Etiology and Risk Factors

- Diet
  - More common in persons consuming animal fat
  - Less common in persons consuming high fiber diet

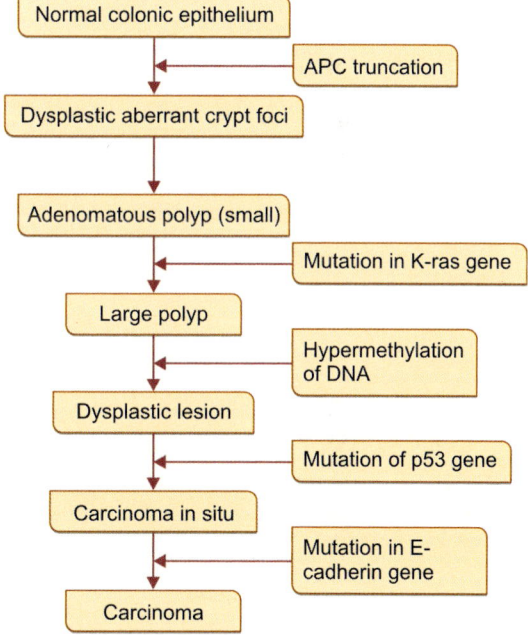

Fig. 80.1: Flowchart showing various genetic mutations in the development of carcinoma colon

- Hereditary syndrome
  - More common in patients suffering from Familial adenomatous polyposis
  - Characterized by the appearance of thousands of adenomatous polyps throughout the large gut
  - Associated with deletion in long arm of chromosomes

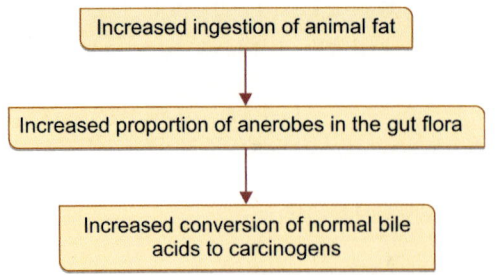

Fig. 80.2: Flowchart showing role of excessive animal fat in development of carcinoma colon

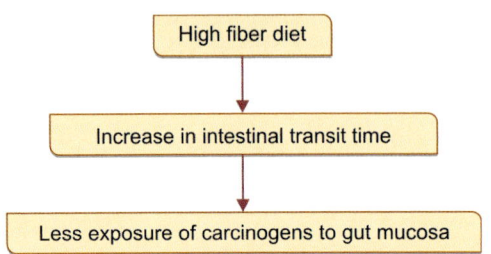

Fig. 80.3: Flowchart showing role of high fiber dist in preventaions of carcinoma colon

- – If not treated surgically, cancer develops in almost all patients before 40 years of age
- Inflammatory bowel disease
  - – Long standing ulcerative colitis of >25 years carries a risk of 8 to 30%
  - – Risk is 1% per year after initial 10 years with the disease
- *Streptococcus bovis* bacteremia
  - – Patients suffereing from endocarditis or septicemia have high risk of occult colorectal tumors
- Ureterosigmoidostomy
  - – 5–10% risk after 15–30 years of procedure
- Tobacco use

Morphology
- Location
  - – Rectum and rectosigmoid junction — 50%
  - – Sigmoid colon — 25%
  - – Rest 25% are equally distributed between cecum, ascending colon, transverse colon and descending colon
- 2–5% patients have more than one colorectal cancer, i.e. synchronous tumor
- 3–5% patients develop another colorectal tumor subsequent by after one colorectal cancer has been resected, i.e. metachronous tumor

Types
Gross Tumor
- Annular stricture — common in left colon
- Tubular stricture — common in rectosigmoid junction
- Ulcerative lesion — common on right side
- Proliferative lesion — common on right side

Histological Type
- Adenocarcinoma

Clinical Features
Local
- Change in bowel habits
  - – Increasing constipation
  - – Sense of incomplete evacuation
  - – Constipation alternating with diarrhea
  - – Early morning spurious diarrhea
- Rectal bleeding
  - – From growth in distal colon dark blood
  - – From secondary piles developing due to proximal growth
- Abdominal pain — dull aching or colicky
- Acute intestinal obstruction — due to left side 'annular' growth
- Palpable mass
- Acute appendicitis — in cecal malignancy
- Intussusception — in right sided malignancy
- Perforation or fistula — gastrocolic or vesicocolic.

General Effects
- 3 'A's — anemia, anorexia, asthenia occurs due to tumor toxins, e.g. TNF-α, IL-6.

Secondary Deposits
- Jaundice
- Ascites
- Hepatomegaly
- Nodules at umbilicus — sister Joseph nodules
- Left axillary lymph nodes — irish lymph nodes

Spread of Tumor
Local Spread
- By continuity through muscle coat — mainly circumferential, longitudinal spread limited
- By contiguity to invade adjacent viscera

Lymphatic Spread (EPIC)

- Epicolic lymph nodes
- Paracolic lymph nodes
- Intermediate lymph nodes
- Central lymph nodes

Blood Borne Spread

- Liver
- Lung
- Bone

Transperitoneal Spread

- Implantation in omentum, ovaries (Krukenberg Tumor), rectouterine or rectovesical pouch (Blummer's Shelf).

Staging

Duke's Staging with Modification by Kirklin, Astler and Coller, Turnbull (Modified Dukes Staging)

- A   Intramucosal tumor limited up to muscularis mucosae without any spread in to mucularis propria
- B_1 Spread into muscularis propria but not beyond
- B_2 Spread through the wall into peritoneal tissue
- C_1 B_1 + Lymph node involvement
- C_2 B_2 + Lymph node involvement
- D   Tumor with distant metastasis

Investigations

Hematological

- Complete blood count.

Biochemical

- CEA estimation
- Liver function test

Radiological

- Double contrast barium enema to localize the growth
  - Shouldering
  - Apple core deformity
  - Filling defect
- Chest X-ray for secondaries

Endoscopy

- Flexible sigmoidoscopy/colonoscopy to take a biopsy from growth.

CT Scan/ MRI

- To stage the disease.

Treatment

- Surgery after pre-operative gut preparation
- Chemotherapy
  - 5-Fluorouracil/Cisplatin/Oxaloplatin. Chemotherapy can be adjuvant or neo-adjuvant chemotherapy
- Radiotherapy has role only in carcinoma rectum.

81 Rectum–Anatomy and Proctitis

- 18–20 cm long which begins from rectosigmoid junction at sacral promontory and ends at anorectal junction where puborectalis muscle encircles it to form anorectal angle
- It follows curve of sacrum and has three lateral curvatures
  - Upper and lower curvatures are convex to the right
  - Middle curvature is convex to the left
  - On mucosal sides they correspond to semicircular folds (called Houston's valves)
- Part of the rectum between middle and lower valve is widest — called Ampulla
- Relation with the peritoneum
  - Upper 1/3 rd of the rectum has peritoneal covering all around
  - Middle 1/3 rd has peritoneal covering anteriorly and laterally
  - Lower third is extraperitoneal
- Lower rectum is separated from other organs by fascial condensation
  - Anterior — Denonvillier's Fascia
  - Posterior — Waldeyer's Fascia.

Mesorectum

- Present in posterior and lateral aspect of extraperitoneal portion of the rectum
- Derived from hindgut
- Contents
  - Superior rectal artery/branches
  - Superior rectal vein/branches
  - Lymphatics and lymph nodes
  - Autonomic nerves
  - Loose areolar tissue
- Surrounded by fascia propria which is extension of pelvic fascia
- Mesorectum is excised along with rectum in surgery for carcinoma rectum — called "Total Mesorectal Excision (TME)".

Blood Supply

- Arterial Supply
  - Superior rectal artery — branch of inferior mesenteric artery
  - Middle rectal artery — branch of anterior division of internal iliac artery
  - Inferior rectal artery — terminal branch of internal pudendal artery
- Veins correspond to arteries

Lymphatics

- Mainly drain upward (upper 2/3rd) to inferior mesenteric nodes and para-aortic nodes
- Laterally (inferior 1/3rd) to internal iliac nodes

Proctitis

- It is the inflammation of mucosa and submucosa.

Types

- It may be acute or chronic.
- It may be infective or non-infective.

Acute Infective

- *Clostridium difficle*
- Bacillary
- Amebic
- Gonococcal
- HIV
- Primary syphilis

Chronic Infective

- Amebic granuloma

- Tubercular
- Bilharziasis

Non-Infective

- Non-specific
- Ulcerative colitis
- Crohn's disease
- Due to herbal enema
- Radiation proctitis

82   Rectal Prolapse

- Falling down of hindgut
- First described by papyrus
- In rectal prolopse, rectum comes out of anal opening

Types

- Complete — full thickness prolapse
- Partial — only mucosa gets prolapsed
  - Circumferential
  - Only portion of mucosa

Factors Preventing Prolapse

- Curvature of sacrum (underdeveloped sacral curve predisposes to prolapse)
- Tilt of pelvis
- Serpentine course of rectum
- Levator ani muscles — fixes rectum
- Puborectalis sling — tilt and elevate lower end of rectum

Etiology

- Congenital
- Poor bowel habits, e.g. constipation
- Neurological disease
  - Cauda equina syndrome
  - Spinal cord injury
  - Congenital anomaly, i.e. spina bifida
- Female gender
- Nulliparity
- Redundant rectosigmoid
- Deep pouch of doughlas
- Patulous anus
- Defect in pelvic floor
- After operation — hemorrhoidectomy, fistulectomy
- Free mesentery of entire rectum
- Lack of fixation of rectum to sacrum
- Torn perineum
- Straining at micturition

Clinical Features

- Something coming out of anal canal on straining, coughing or lifting weight
- Constipation present in 50% of cases
- Fecal incontinence
  - More common in long-standing complete prolapse
  - Due to stretching of pudendal and perineal nerves
  - Dilatation of anal canal and relaxation of anal sphincters
- Mucus discharge
- Bleeding rarely occurs in massive or irreducible prolapse

Differential Diagnosis

- Prolapsed hemorrhoid
- Large polypoidal lesion protruding through anus
- Long intussusception

Investigations

- Barium enema
- Colonoscopy
- Anorectal physiology
  - Low resting anal pressure
  - Low squeeze pressure
  - Poor anorectal sensation on electric stimulation

Treatment

- Surgical correction is the treatment of choice
- Non-operative treatment is indicated if
  - Surgery is contraindicated
  - Patient refuses surgery

Non-Operative Methods

- Adhesive strapping of buttocks
- Manual anal support during defecation
- Correction of constipation
- Perineal exercises
- Electrical stimulation
- Submucosal injection of phenol in almond oil
- Infrared coagulation

Surgical Treatment

- Partial prolapse
  - If partial circumference — simple excision of prolapsed part
  - If complete mucosal prolapse
    ◊ Circumferential excision
    ◊ Use of circular stapler (used for stapled hemorrhoidectomy)
- Acute irreducible rectal prolapse
  - Reduction under anesthesia (to relax anal sphincter)
  - Taping the buttocks together
  - Trendelenburg's position
  - Placement of sugar/salt topically to reduce edema
  - Injection of hyaluronidase
  - If prolapsed rectum is not viable then resection of the part
- Complete rectal prolapse
  - Perineal approach
  - Abdominal approach
    ◊ Open
    ◊ Laparoscopic

Perineal Operations

- Have higher recurrence rates than abdominal operations

Indications

- Pediatric age group
- Frail/very elderly patients
- Injury or disease of spinal cord

Thiersch Repair

- Anal canal is tightened by passing a silver wire/nylon/silicone rubber in perineal space.

Delorme's Procedure

- Prolapsed part of rectum is fully denuded of its mucosa
- Underlying rectal musculature plicated
- Defect of mucosa repaired

Altmeir's Procedure

- Rectosigmoidectomy through transanal route

Abdominal Operations

- Suspension or fixation of the rectum to sacrum or pubis
- Rectum is fully mobilized
  - Lateral peritoneal reflections are incised
  - Dissection done till levators
  - Lateral rectal ligaments divided
- Rectum is fixed to the sacrum by
  - Teflon mesh (Ripstein, 1972)
  - Simple sutures
  - Ivalon sponge (polyvinyl alcohol) (Well's procedure, 1959)

Resection Procedure

- Redundant sigmoid and rectum are resected.
- Descending colon fully mobilized till splenic flexure.
- Anastomosis is constructed 12 cm above anal verge.

Resection Rectopexy (Frykman and Goldberg, 1969)

- It involves anterior resection and fixation of rectum to presacral fascia.

83 | Management of Piles

- Pile — a Latin word meaning a ball
- Hemorrhoids (Greek word meaning Hema = blood, Rhoes = flowing).

Etiology

- Down ward sliding of anal cushions.

Anal Cushions

- Three in number
- Located at left lateral, right anterior medial and right posterolateral (3, 7, 11 o'clock positions)
- They lie in sub mucosal plane
- Comprises of arterioles, venules, arteriolvenular communication, smooth muscles and elastic connective tissue

Function of Anal Cushions

- Close the anal canal during rest
- Aids in the continence of anal canal

Cause of Sliding of Anal Cushions

- Disintegration and atrophy of
  - Anchoring and supportive connective tissue
  - Terminal fibers of longitudinal muscles

Classification

- Internal hemorrhoids
- External hemorrhoids
- Mixed hemorrhoids

Grades of Hemorrhoids

Four Grades

- First degree — remains inside the anal canal
- Second degree — Prolapse during defecation but reduce spontaneously
- Third Degree — need to be reduced manually
- Fourth degree — permanently prolapsed (Fig. 83.1)

Clinical Features

- Bleeding
- Prolapse
- Mucous discharge
- Pruritis
- Pain
- Anemia.

Complications

- Ulceration
- Fibrosis

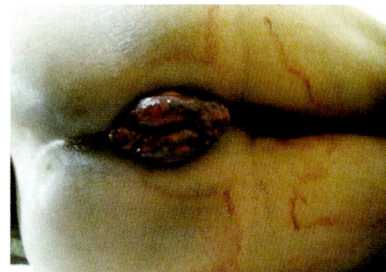

Fig. 83.1: Grade 4 piles

- Strangulation
- Thrombosis
- Gangrene
- Infection and suppuration
- Pylephlebitis and pyemia

Evaluation

- Inspection: To look for external piles
- Proctoscopy to visualise the pulse
- Colonoscopy as indicated
- Common in >40 yrs of age
- Family history of colorectal cancer
- Recent change in bowel habits

Treatment

- General measures
  - High fibre diet
  - Stool softener
  - Increased fluid intake
  - Avoidance of straining

Injection Sclerotherapy

- Described by Mitchell
- Useful in first degree and early second degree piles
- Injection into sub mucosa at the apex above dentate line
- 1–3 ml injected
- Substances used
  - 5% phenol in almond oil
  - Quinine urea
  - Sodium tetradecyl sulphate (STS)

Rubber Band Ligation

- Described by Barren
- Indicated in first and second degree piles
- Rubber band applied 1–2 cm above dentate line
- Mucosa is grasped above dentate line, pulled in to the rubber band applier
- Ligator is fired
- Ring goes over the mass and strangulates it
- Ischemic necrosis of pile mass occurs

Complications of rubber band ligation

- Pain
- Urinary retention
- Infection
- Secondary hemorrhage

Infrared Photocoagulation

- For piles that do not prolapse
- Applied at apex to coagulate the underlying venous plexuses
- Described by Leicester

Cryosurgery

- Liquid nitrogen at –196 degree
- Causes coagulation
- Diffuse mucous discharge and pain

Surgical Treatment

Indications: Third degree piles, Fibrosed piles, Interno-external piles

Types of Hemorrhoidectomy

- Closed hemorrhoidectomy (Park and Ferguson)
- Open hemorrhoidectomy (Milligan and Morgan)
- Whitehead hemorrhoidectomy
- Stapler hemorrhoidectomy

Complications

- Post-operative pain
- Urinary retention (10–15%)
- Reactionary bleeding
- Fecal impaction
- Secondary bleeding
- Infection
- Incontinence
- Anal stenosis
- Anal fissure

Lower GI Bleeding (Differential Diagnosis)

Causes

- Piles
- Anal fissure
- Diverticular disease
- Angiodysplasia
- Neoplasm
- Colitis
  - Infective
  - Idiopathic
  - Ischemic
  - Radiation-induced
- Solitary rectal ulcer syndrome
- NSAID ulcer or colitis
- Lymphonodular hyperplasia
- Aorto-colic fistula (rare)
- Vasculitis

Investigations of Lower GI Bleeding

- Digital examination
- Proctoscopy
- Sigmoidoscopy in <40 years or younger patients with history of bleed
- Colonoscopy
- 99mc technetium scan
- Angiography

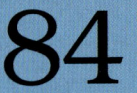

84 Anal Fissure

Anal canal starts at the upper border of pubo-rectalis muscle (internal sphincter muscle) and ends at the anal verge. The average length of anal canal is 3–4 cm. The dentate line corresponds to mid-point of anal canal.

Definition

Anal fissure is an elongated ulcer in the epithelium of anal canal along its long axis distal to the dentate line.

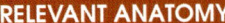

Table 84.1: Location of anal fissure	
Males	*Females*
Mid line posterior 90%	Mid line posterior 60%
Mid line anterior 10%	Mid line anterior 40%

Anatomical Factors

- Sharp bend between posterior wall of rectum and anal canal
- Posterior anal mucosa is relatively unsupported by muscle
- Hard fecal matter presses on the posterior anal tissue, which stretches overlying epithelium leading to ischemia and ulceration.

Precipitating Factors

- Constipation
- *Difficult childbirth:* Trauma by fetal head on anterior ano-rectal wall
- Incorrectly performed operation for piles

- Inflammatory bowel disease, e.g. Crohn's or ulcerative colitis
- Sexually transmitted diseases.

Pathology

Acute Anal Fissure

- Characterized by spasm of anal sphincter muscle
- No inflammatory edema or induration of edges occurs.

Chronic Anal Fissure

- Induration of edges
- Fissure is guarded by a tag of edematous skin at the lower end, known as sentinel pile
- Scar tissue and fibrosis occurs at the base of the fissure or internal sphincter fibers
- Hypertrophic anal papilla may occur at upper end of the fissure
- There may be a small subcutaneous fistula or abscess formation underlying the sentinel pile
- There may be a specific cause, e.g. Crohn's tuberculosis or carcinoma anal canal.

Clinical Features

- Common in females
- Uncommon in aged due to muscular atony
- Can lead to acquired mega-colon if it occurs in children.

Symptoms

- Pain on defecation which is severe in nature and lasts up to 1–2 hours after passing stools

- Bleeding which is characterized by streaking of stools in contrast to piles when bleeding is marked and separate from stools
- Mucus discharge
- Constipation is present in almost all cases.

Signs

- Sentinel skin tag is present
- Lower end of fissure is seen by gently separating the buttocks
- Intense anal spasm is present so digital examination of rectum should be avoided

If essential, apply 5% lignocaine jelly and wait for 5 minutes before proceeding for per rectal examination.

Differential Diagnosis

- Carcinoma of the anal canal in early stages
- Tubercular ulcer
- If ulcers multiple then rule out
  - Skin diseases
  - Crohn's disease
  - Sexually transmitted diseases
  - Homosexual practices

Treatment

- Aimed at complete relaxation of anal internal sphincter

- Conservative management in the form of laxatives so that stools are soft and bulky. High fiber diet is advised. Fiber supplement in the form of bran and isphagula is given.
- Local application of lignocaine jelly
- Chemical sphincterotomy using glyceryl trinitrate or diltiazem ointment. It acts by relaxing anal internal sphincter by donating nitric oxide and by improving blood flow
- Botulinum toxin injection causes temporary muscle paralysis and relief

Operative

Indications

- Chronic fissure
- Failure of medical treatment
- Recurrent fissure

Surgical Methods

- Anal dilatation (not done these days)
- Lateral anal sphincterotomy (30% internal sphincter fibers cut)
- Dorsal fissurectomy and sphincterotomy.
- Anal advancement flap: Indicated in woman and those with normal or low resting anal pressures. After excision of the fissure, the resultant defect is covered with an inverted rectangular shaped flap of perianal skin.

85 Ano-rectal Abscess

It can be defined as abscess occurring around the anal canal and rectum.

Classification

These are classified according to the spaces they occupy:
- Submucosal (5%)
- Perianal (60%)
- Intersphincteric (4%)
- Ischiorectal (30%)
- Perirectal (1%)

Etiology

In 70–80% cases, patients have no obvious cause and sepsis arises in the anal glands only.

In 20% cases there is a predisposing factor like:
- Inflammatory bowel disease
- Ano-rectal cancer
- Anal fissure
- Complicated hemorrhoids
- Local trauma
- Extension of cutaneous boil
- Blood borne infection
- Diabetes and AIDS.

Bacteriology

- *E. coli* (60%)
- *Staph. aureus* (23%)
- Bacteroids, proteus and streptococcus in others

Associated anal fistula is a more likely possibility if pus culture grows *E. coli* or bacteroids.

Submucous Abscess

- Occurs above the dentate line
- Common after injection sclerotherapy for hemorrhoids.

Pelvi-rectal Abscess

- Occurs between upper surface of levator ani and pelvic peritoneum
- May occur secondary to appendicitis, diverticulitis or Crohn's disease
- May burst into the rectum or penetrate downwards, through levator ani and present as ischiorectal abscess.

Presentation

- Patient of perianal abscess present with history of well localised pain along with a tender palpable lump around the anal margin.
- In ischiorectal abscess, symptoms are poorly localised, as there is large fat filled space in the ischiorectal fossa with much less tissue tension.
- Examination of buttock reveals, diffusely swollen buttock with generalized induration.

Management

Treatment is mainly surgical with incision and drainage of abscess.

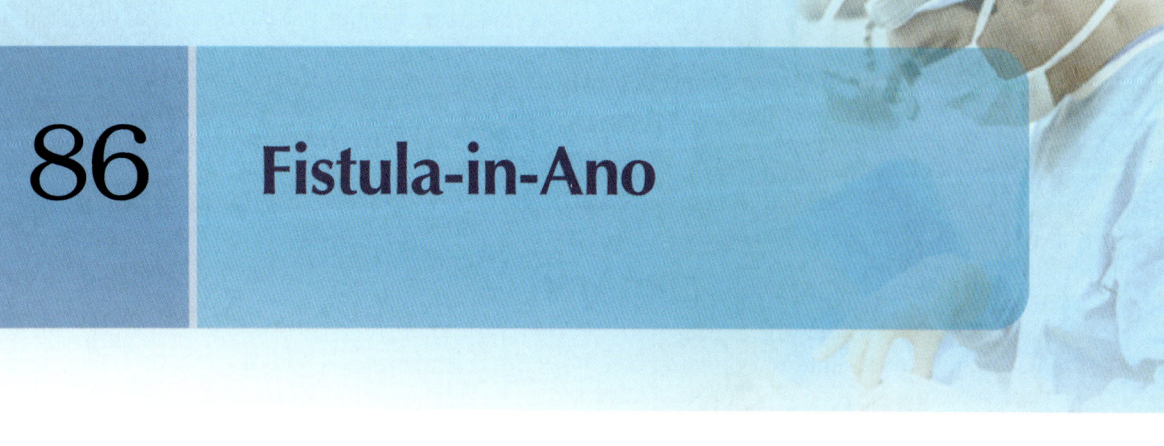

86 Fistula-in-Ano

- Abnormal communication between the perineal skin and either the anal canal or rectum is called Fistula-in-Ano.
- It is lined by unhealthy granulation tissue and fibrous tissue.

ETIOLOGY

Usually Results From

- Anorectal abscess which ruptures spontaneously or is inadequately drained
- Tuberculosis
- Ulcerative colitis
- Crohn's disease
- Carcinoma of colon
- Actinomycosis
- Lymphogranuloma venerum.

Types

Low Level

- Internal opening is below the anorectal ring
- Can be laid open without fear of anal incontinence.

High Level

- The internal opening is above the anorectal ring
- There is fear of damage to anorectal ring and hence external sphincter if the tract is laid open leading to anal incontinence
- It should be managed by a staged procedure.

Classification

Standard Classification

- Subcutaneous
- Submucus
- Low anal
- High anal
- Pelvirectal.

Park's Classification (Fig. 86.1)

- Intersphincteric
  - Tract runs between internal sphincter and external sphincter

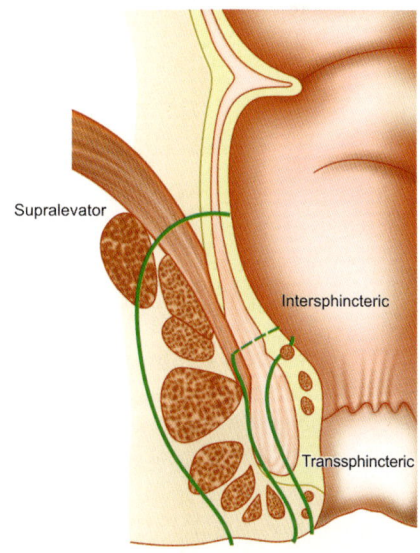

Fig. 86.1: Park's classification of anal fistula

- Trans-sphincteric
  - Sphincteric portion of tract passes through internal sphincter
  - May be high or low
- Supra-sphincteric
  - Tract passes above the external and internal sphincter.

Clinical Features

- Seropurulent discharge that dates back to years
- Pain is not a feature if the opening is large enough for the pus to escape
- External opening within 3–4 cm of anal canal
- Induration of skin around the fistula
- Digital examination – internal opening can be felt as a nodule on the wall of anal canal. Invariably there is one internal opening
- Proctoscopy will reveal internal opening. Hypertrophied papilla is suggestive of internal opening.

Goodsall's Rule

- Fistulae with external opening in relation to anterior half of rectum or anus tends to be direct type, fistula is radially ending into the anal canal
- If the external opening is in relation to posterior half of anal canal opening, the fistula is a curved one, opening internally in the midline posteriorly.

Investigations

- Probing and fistulography have no role
- Endoluminal ultrasound or MRI can be done to map the complex fistulae or in cases of recurrent fistulae. Endoluminal ultrasound is done with instillation of hydrogen peroxide in the fistula tract. MRI can demonstrate secondary extension.
- CT scan has limited indication if extrasphincteric fistula is suspected.

Treatment

Surgery is Mandatory

Low fistula

- Fistulotomy
  - Fistula tract is laid open
  - Whole granulation tissue is removed.

High fistula

- Lower portion of the fistula is laid open and a *seton* (ligature of silk or nylon) is inserted along a fistula tract and tied loosely
- Seton acts to
  - Provide ongoing drainage
  - Stimulate fibrosis of sphincteric muscle, so that subsequent cutting will not result in retraction of muscle
  - Provide means of assessing the depth and extent of sphincteric muscle involvement
- Seton is tightened gradually to cut through the sphincter.

87 Malignant Lesion of the Anus and Anal Canal

- Squamous cell carcinoma
- Basiloid carcinoma
- Mucoepidermoid carcinoma
- Basal cell carcinoma
- Malignant melanoma
- Anal intraepithelial neoplasia

Incidence

- 2% of all colorectal cancer
- Usually in 6th and 7th decade of life
- 70% anal tumors arise from the anal canal (The anal canal is 4 cm in length extending from anal margin till anorectal ring).
- 30% anal tumors arise from anal verge (The anal verge starts from anal margin and includes 4 cm of the perianal skin all around).

Clinical Features

Symptoms

- Rectal bleeding
- Mucus discharge
- Tenesmus
- Sensation of lump in the anus
- Change in bowel habit
- Inguinal lymph node enlargement due to metastasis

Signs

- Ulcerating hard, tender, bleeding mass in anal canal or at anal verge (Fig. 87.1).

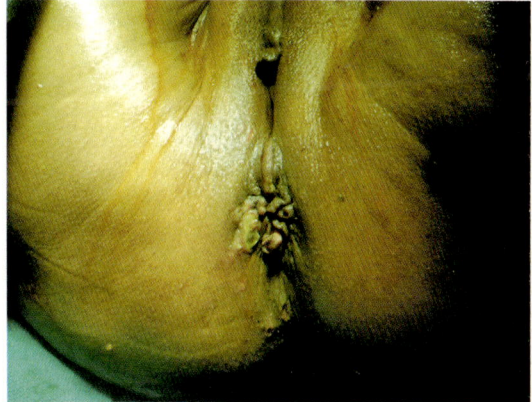

Fig. 87.1: Anal carcinoma

- Lesions can fungate and appear on the anal skin
- Can present as fistula or fissure

AJCC Staging for Anal Carcinoma

T Staging

T staging depends upon size of primary tumor in its greatest dimension

Tx – Primary tumor cannot be assessed

T0 – No evidence of any primary tumor

Tis – Carcinoma *in situ* (Bowen's disease, high grade squamous intraepithelial lesions, anal intrathelial neoplasm)

T1 – Tumor less than 2 cm

T2 – Tumor larger than 2 cm but less than 5 cm

T3 – Tumor larger than 5 cm

T4 – Tumor of any size invading adjacent organs, e.g. vagina, urethra, bladder.

N staging

Nx – Regional lymph nodes cannot be assessed
N0 – No regional lymph node metastasis
N1 – Metastasis in perirectal lymph nodes
N2 – Metastasis in unilateral internal iliac and/or inguinal lymph nodes
N3 – Metastasis in perirectal and inguinal lymph nodes and/or bilateral internal iliac and/or inguinal lymph nodes

Treatment

Anal Verge Tumor

- Wide excision of tumor with a margin of 2.5 cm all around
- Block dissection of groin lymph nodes if the lymph nodes are involved

Anal Canal Tumor

- Chemoradiation forms the mainstay of the treatment (first described by Nigro and associates)

External beam radiation to primary tumor and pelvic and inguinal lymph nodes is started on day one and continued till 15 days in the fractions of 200 cGy/day with total dose of 3000 cGy.

Systemic chemotherapy in the form of 5FU is started as continuous infusion in the dose of 1000 mg per sq meter for 24 hours and is given for four days starting from day one. The 5FU is again repeated on 28th day for 4 days. Mitomycin C is given as bolus dose of 15 mg per sq meter on day one.

- 2/3rd of all patients respond to chemo-radiation alone.

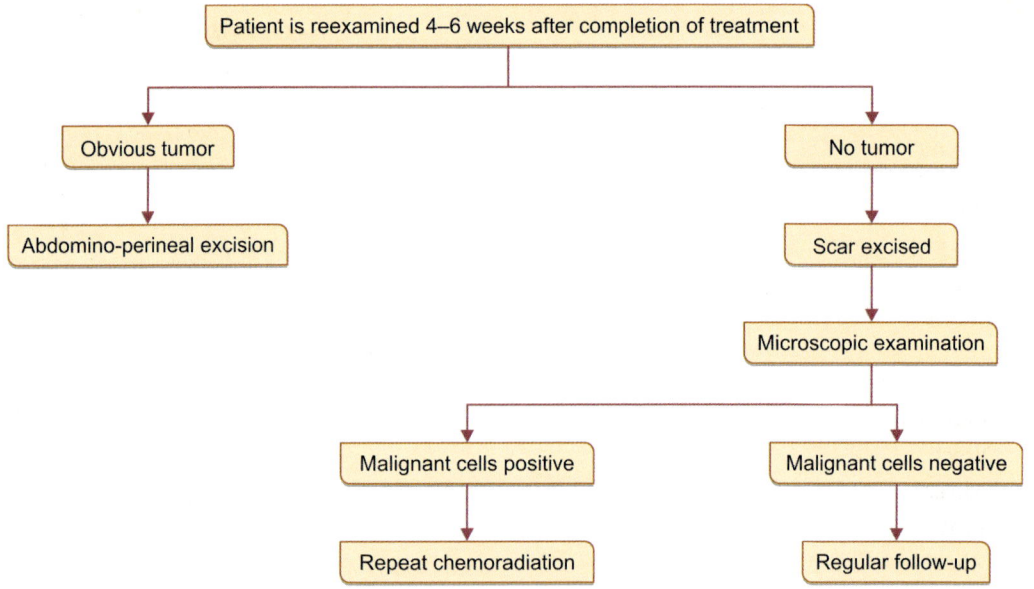

Fig. 87.1: Flowchart showing followup of anal carcinoma patients after completion of chemoradiation

88 | Hernia–An Overview

It can be defined as protrusion of viscus or part of viscus through an opening or weakneses in the wall of the cavity containing it.

- Hernias by themselves usually are harmless, but nearly all have a potential risk of having their blood supply cut off (becoming strangulated).
- If the blood supply is cut off at the hernial opening in the abdominal wall, it becomes a medical and surgical emergency.

Types of Hernias

- Inguinal hernia
  - Direct
  - Indirect
- Femoral hernia
- Umbilical hernia
- Incisional hernia
- Spigelian hernia
- Obturator hernia
- Epigastric hernia

Inguinal Hernia

- Makes upto 75% of all abdominal wall hernias and occurs up to 25 times more often in men than women.
- Two types of inguinal hernias: Indirect inguinal hernia and direct inguinal hernia.

Indirect Inguinal Hernia

- Symptomatic patent processus vaginalis.
- This processus normally closes before birth but remains a possible site for a hernia.
- Sometimes the hernial sac may protrude into the scrotum.
- This type of hernia may occur at any age but becomes more common as people age.

Direct Inguinal Hernia

- This occurs medial to the site for the indirect hernia, through posterior wall of inguinal canal, in a place where the abdominal wall is naturally weak.
- It rarely will protrude into the scrotum.
- The direct hernia almost always occurs in the middle-aged and elderly because their abdominal walls weaken as they age.

Femoral Hernia

- The femoral canal is the way through which the femoral artery, vein, and nerve leave the abdominal cavity to enter the thigh.
- Although normally a tight space, sometimes it becomes large enough to allow abdominal contents (usually intestine) into the canal.
- This hernia causes a bulge below the inguinal crease in the thigh.
- Rare and usually occurring in women, these hernias are particularly at risk of becoming irreducible and strangulated.

Umbilical Hernia

- These common hernias (10–30%) are often noted at birth as a protrusion at the umbilicus.
- This is caused when an opening in the abdominal wall, which normally closes before birth, does not close completely.
- Even if the area is closed at birth, these hernias can appear later in life because this spot remains a weaker place in the abdominal wall.
- They most often appear later in elderly people and middle-aged women who have had children.

Incisional Hernia

- Abdominal surgery causes a flaw in the abdominal wall that must heal on its own.
- This flaw can create an area of weakness where a hernia may develop.
- This occurs after 2–10% of all abdominal surgeries, although some people are at higher risk.
- After surgical repair, these hernias have a high rate of recurring (20–45%).

Spigelian Hernia

- This rare hernia occurs along the edge of the rectus abdominis muscle, which is several inches to the side of the middle of the abdomen.

Obturator Hernia

- This extremely rare abdominal hernia happens mostly in women.
- This hernia protrudes from the pelvic cavity through obturator foramen.
- This will not show any bulge but can present as bowel obstruction and cause nausea and vomiting.

Epigastric Hernia

- Occurring between the umbilicus and the xiphisternum, these hernias are composed usually of fatty tissue and rarely contain intestine.
- Formed in an area of relative weakness of the abdominal wall, these hernias are often painless and difficult to be pushed back into the abdomen when first discovered.

CAUSES OF HERNIAS

- Any condition that increases the pressure of the abdominal cavity may contribute to the formation or worsening of a hernia.

- Obesity
- Heavy lifting
- Coughing
- Straining during a bowel movement or urination
- Chronic lung disease
- Fluid in the abdominal cavity
- Hereditary

Signs and Symptoms

- The signs and symptoms of a hernia can range from noticing a painless lump to a painful, tender, swollen protrusion of tissue that you are unable to push back into the abdomen— possibly a strangulated hernia.

Asymptomatic Reducible Hernia

- New lump in the groin or other abdominal wall area
- May ache but is not tender when touched.
- Sometimes pain precedes the discovery of the lump.
- Lump increases in size when standing or when abdominal pressure is increased (such as coughing)
- May be reduced (pushed back into the abdomen) unless very large

Irreducible Hernia

- Usually painful enlargement of a previous hernia that cannot be returned into the abdominal cavity
- Some may be long term without pain
- Can lead to strangulation
- Signs and symptoms of bowel obstruction may occur, such as nausea and vomiting

Strangulated Hernia

- Irreducible hernia where the entrapped intestine has its blood supply cut off
- Pain always present followed quickly by tenderness and sometimes symptoms of bowel obstruction (nausea and vomiting)
- The patient may appear ill with or without fever
- Surgical emergency
- All strangulated hernias are irreducible (but all irreducible hernias are not strangulated)

Diagnosis

- Clinical examination is adequate to make a diagnosis.

- There is no role of ultrasound or herniography, although described in literature.

Treatment

- Treatment of a hernia depends on whether it is reducible or irreducible and possibly strangulated.
- Reducible
  - Elective surgery

- Irreducible
  - All acutely irreducible hernias need emergency treatment because of the risk of strangulation.
  - An attempt to push the hernia back can be made (*taxis*).
- Strangulation
  - Emergency surgery is required.

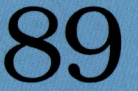

89 | Ventral Hernia

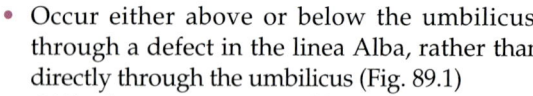

- Occur either above or below the umbilicus, through a defect in the linea Alba, rather than directly through the umbilicus (Fig. 89.1)
- 90% of cases are acquired hernia in adults
- More common in women than men
- High morbidity and mortality because of high tendency of incarceration and strangulation
- Due to narrow neck of the hernia, strangulation is very common
- Early repair after diagnosis is advised.

Contents

- Greater omentum (commonest)
- Small intestine
- Transverse colon
- Urinary bladder.

Predisposing Factors

- Extreme obesity
- History of multiple pregnancies with prolonged labor

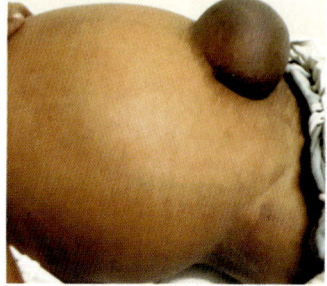

Fig. 89.1: Umbilical hernia

- Ascites
- Large abdominal tumors

Various Operations for Umbilical Hernia in Adult

- *Mayo's repair:* Tissue repair if the defect is up to 4 cm. Double breasting of upper and lower flap is done.
- *Simple suture repair:* The fascial defect is closed primarily by interrupted non absorbable sutures. Defects up to 2 cm are suitable
- *Mesh repair:* If defect is more than 4 cm in diameter and in cases of recurrent hernia.
- *Laparoscopic repair:* Role still evolving.

Mayo's Repair

- For defects up to 4 cm in diameter
- Infraumbilical incision
- Double breasting of rectus sheath using non-absorbable suture.

Mesh Repair

- This procedure is indicated if the hernial defect is more than 4 cm in diameter and in cases of recurrent hernia.
- A polypropylene mesh is placed in an inlay or sublay fashion and anchored circumferentially with interrupted sutures to the surrounding healthy fascia.

Incisional Hernia

- Incisional hernia is defined as visible or palpable bulge at the site of previous surgical

intervention which is more apparent during erect position or on coughing
- The incidence of 3–20%.

Clinical Presentation

- More than half occur within the first two years after primary operation
- A diffuse bulge directly under or adjacent to a previous incision
- Increased protrusion with valsalva manoeuvre or standing
- Cosmetic concerns
- Interference with work or activity is a common complaint
- Pain is unusual unless there are incarcerated or strangulated structures
- As they enlarge, they become symptomatic
- CT or ultrasound
  - In obese patients
  - Patients with significant rectus diastasis
  - Patients with laxity due to spinal injury
  - Patients who have had multiple prior abdominal surgeries.

Risk Factors

- Age above 65 or 70
- Malnutrition
- Sepsis
- Anemia
- Uremia
- Ascites/liver failure
- Diabetes
- Pulmonary disease
- Smoking
- Abdominal distension
- Obesity
- Coughing/retching
- Urinary retention
- Post-operative Ileus
- Peritoneal dialysis
- Wound infection
- Corticosteroids
- Chemotherapy
- Immunosuppression.

Etiology

- Mechanical factors – Intra-abdominal pressure overwhelming a weakness in the abdominal wall.
- Pathologic changes in collagen that adversely affect wound healing.

- Type I collagen is dominant in a mature scar
- Type III collagen dominates in the early stages of wound healing
- Factors such as smoking, malnutrition, immuno-compromise, wound infection and underlying diseases are now understood to interfere with normal collagen metabolism.

Prevention of Incisional Hernias

- The strength of a wound lies in the musculo-aponeurotic layer.

Incision

- Abdominal incisions are based on anatomical principles
  - They must allow adequate access to the abdomen
  - They should be capable of being extended if required
  - Ideally muscle fibers should be split rather than cut
  - Nerves should not be divided.

Midline Incision

- The most common and most versatile approach.
- The following structures are divided:
  - Skin
  - Linea alba
  - Transversalis fascia
  - Extraperitoneal fat
  - Peritoneum
- The incision can be extended by cutting through or around the umbilicus
- Above the umbilicus, the Falciform ligament should be avoided
- The bladder can be accessed via an extra-peritoneal approach through the space of Retzius
- The wound can be closed using a mass closure technique
- The most popular sutures are either non-absorbable or absorbable monofilaments
- At least 1 cm bits should be taken 1 cm apart
- Requires the use of one or more sutures four times the wound length
- Bites incorporating all layers of the abdominal wall except skin and fat — no need to close the peritoneum.

Suture Characteristics

- Non-absorbable suture
  - Has better tensile strength

– Can persist and become a focus of infection or a draining sinus tract
- Monofilaments and inert materials are less likely to be associated with wound infection
- Braided materials knot more securely than monofilament and are less likely to stretch.

Suture Techniques

- "One centimeter back and one centimeter apart."
- Bite – it should be placed at least 2 cm from the wound edge
- Spacing – sutures stitches are placed about 2 cm apart
- Continuous *vs* interrupted sutures – continuous suturing may better distribute the tension but if one bite pulls loose it compromises the whole closure
- Tension sutures – full thickness sutures that help prevent dehiscence in cases of difficult abdominal closure.

Prevention of Trocar Site Hernias

- The incidence of trocar site hernia has been shown to be 0.65–2.80%
- Midline, periumbilical port sites greater than 5 cm and made with bladed introducers often result in incisional hernia if not closed.

Why Incisional Hernias should be Repaired?

- Incisional hernias can cause following serious complications:
  – Incarceration of gut in 6–15% of cases
  – Strangulation in 2% of cases. Strangulated gut rapidly becomes ischemic, necrotic and perforates if hernia is not reduced rapidly
  – Many patients who are suffering from large incisional hernia are forced to change their life style or give up their gainful employment leading to major social and economic implications.

Classification of Incisional Hernia

Incisional hernias may be classified as:
- Small if the defect is less than 5 cm in diameter
- Medium if the defect is between 5–10 cm
- Large or giant if the defect is more than 10 cm.

Indications for Surgical Intervention

- Symptomatic hernias
- Enlarging hernias

- Hernia with a small fascial defect and a large sac with incarcerated contents.
- Cosmetic concerns.

The Risk Factors for Recurrence

- Obesity
- Comorbidities related to obesity
- Patients on steroids
- Large fascial defects
- Postoperative wound infection
- Postoperative hematoma formation
- Postoperative abdominal distension
- Chronic pulmonary disease
- Advanced age
- Size of hernia – If the hernia defect is large, there are more chances of recurrence
- Type of repair – Suture repair carries more chances of recurrence
- Recurrence is more common after repair of recurrent incisional hernia
- Incisional hernia following surgery for abdominal aortic aneurysm.

Types of Incisional Hernia Repair

Types of incisional hernia repaired can be grouped in one of the following types:
- Open suture repair
- Open mesh repair
- Laparoscopic mesh repair.

Anatomical Repair or Simple Fascial Closure

- This repair is suitable when the defect is less than 3 cm and the patient has adequate muscle tone
- Lateral margins of defects are approximated to each other using continuous or interrupted no 1 monofilament suture or a loop suture.

Principles of repair
- Tension free repair
- Incision — Chosen to provide good exposure of the defect
- Do not expose bowel to reactive mesh
- Clear adequate margins of the defect
- Skin hygiene
- Antibiotic prophylaxis
- Choice of anesthesia (general anesthesia preferred)
- Avoid counter-incisions.

Cardiff Repair

- This technique is suitable for small and medium sized defects

- Sac is excised and peritoneum is closed by chromic catgut or polyglactin suture
- Abdominal wall closure is performed by interrupted non absorbable suture using "Cardiff far and near suture".

Mayo Technique

- Anterior rectus sheaths are double breasted using interrupted monofilament sutures.
- Overlapping is performed in two layers employing two layers of sutures.

Keel's Operation

- Appearance of repair is like inverted beam of the old ship or boat in bottom
- Sac is gradually inverted inside peritoneal cavity by pleating by application of continuous or interrupted sutures one over another till the margins of defects get approximated to each other.

Nuttall's Repair

- This operation is done for lower midline incisional hernia.
- Attachments of rectus muscles are detached
- Two rectus muscles are crossed over each other and are reattached to opposite pubic bones to create a firm abdominal wall support by crossed rectus muscles.

Shoelace Darn Technique

- This technique restores the normal anatomy of abdominal wall by reconstruction of new strong linea alba
- Suture creates a new linea alba and pushes the sac inside peritoneal cavity.

Complications

- Wound infection
- Local hematoma formation
- Stitch sinus formation
- Flap necrosis
- Respiratory complications.

Open Mesh Repair

- Onlay mesh
- Inlay mesh
- Extra-peritoneal or subfascial (Rive stoppa's repair).

Complications of Incisional Hernia Repair

- Enterotomy
- Wound infection
- Mesh infection
- Persistent seroma
- Prolonged pain
- Ileus
- Bleeding/Hematoma
- Recurrence
- Respiratory distress
- Abdominal compartment syndrome or IVC compression.

Wound and Mesh Infection

- Many wounds are inflamed but not necessarily infected
- Infected wounds need to be opened
- Avoid exposing the underlying mesh if possible
- Infections that involve polypropylene meshes can be managed with surgical drainage, excision of exposed, segments and antibiotics
- Meshes (ePTFE) require removal in most cases because they lack tissue ingrowth that could combat the infection.

Seroma

- The development of seroma is virtually guaranteed after lap incisional hernia repair and probably after repair with mesh in general. They typically resolve spontaneously without intervention and are not considered a complication unless they are clinically apparent more than 8 weeks postoperatively.

Prolonged Pain

- In Rive-Stoppa's or other open mesh implantation it occurs in more than 10% of patients
- Trans-abdominal suture site pain after laparoscopic ventral hernia repair occurs in 1–3% of patients.

Possible Advantages of Laparoscopic Repair

- Minimization of soft-tissue dissection
- To visualize much of the abdominal wall leads to fewer missed hernias
- In obese patients
- Recurrent hernias— Avoids dissection through the previous operative site.

90 | Groin Hernia

A protrusion of a viscous or a part of a viscous through an opening or weakness in the wall of the cavity containing it.

Common Presentations

- A lump
  - Comes and goes
  - Appears on straining/coughing
- A pain
  - Dragging pain/pain on exertion
- Incidental finding on examination/imaging
- Presenting as a complication
  - Incarceration/intestinal obstruction

Inguinal Hernia

- Commonest external hernia in both sexes
- Male preponderance
- Infant/adult
- Direct/indirect/combined
- Weakness/increased pressure
- Causes pain/discomfort
- Carries risk of complications
- Treated surgically

History

- Objectives
  - Establish differential diagnoses
  - Identify risk factors and significant co-morbid pathologies

- Increased intra-abdominal pressure due to
  ◊ Ascites
  ◊ Chronic airways disease
  ◊ Chronic constipation
  ◊ Bladder outlet obstruction
  ◊ History of lifting heavy weights
  ◊ History of previous lower abdominal surgery
- History of
  - Onset
  - Duration
  - Symptoms
  - Other hernia(e)
  - Irreducibility
  - Gastrointestinal system
  - Respiratory system
  - Surgery/anesthesia

Examination

- Surface markings
  - Anterior superior iliac spine
  - Pubic tubercle
  - Midpoint of inguinal ligament
- Objectives
  - Confirm diagnoses
  - Out rule differentials
  - Establish type
  - Determine contents
  - Reducibility
  - Identify co-morbid pathologies

Table 90.1

Direct inguinal hernia	Indirect inguinal hernia
Posterior wall	Deep ring
Less common	70%
Older	Congenital
Smaller	Scrotal
Hasselbach's triangle	Deep ring
Medial	Lateral
Lower risk of complications	Strangulation more often

- Examination
  - In standing and lying down position
  - Cough impulse
  - Reducibility
  - Contents
  - Bowel sounds
  - Scrotal contents

Differential Diagnosis

- Direct/indirect/combined
- Femoral hernia
- Hydrocele
- Lipoma
- Lymph node
- Testicular tumor
- Saphenous varix

Inguinal Anatomy

- The inguinal canal represents the oblique passage through the anterior abdominal wall for the vas deferens (round ligament)
- It is 3.75 cm long and lies directly above the medial half of the inguinal ligament
- Three nerves
  - Ilioinguinal nerve
  - Sympathetic fibers
  - Genitofemoral nerve
- Three layers of fascia
  - Internal spermatic fascia (transversalis fascia)
  - Cremastric fascia (conjoint tendon)
  - External spermatic fascia (external oblique muscle)
- Three arteries
  - Testicular artery (branch of aorta)
  - Artery to the vas (branch of external iliac artery)
  - Cremasteric artery (branch of inferior epigastric artery)
- Three other structures
  - The vas deferens
  - The pampiniform plexus of veins
  - Lymphatic (to aortic nodes)

- Factors preventing formation of inguinal hernia
  - Obliquity of inguinal canal
  - Plugging action of cremasteric reflux
  - Shutter like mechanism of conjoint muscle or tendon
  - Sliding mechanism of transversus fascial ring

Hernia Complications

- Incarceration
- Strangulation
- Intestinal obstruction

Classification based on Operative Findings

Gilbert Classification of Groin Hernia (Per operative classification)

Type 1 – indirect normal internal ring
Type 2 – indirect dilated internal ring<4 cm
Type 3 – indirect internal ring >4 m encroaching direct space and displacing inferior epigastric vessels
Type 4 – direct generalized bulge of posterior wall
Type 5 – direct localized bulge of posterior wall less than 2 cm

Rutkow and Robbin's Added

Type 6 – Both direct and indirect
Type 7 – Recurrent hernia.
For type I hernia → treatment is simple herniotomy
For type II hernia → treatment is herniotomy and narrowing of internal ring (Lytl's repair).
For type III to type VII hernia → treatment is mesh hernioplasty.

Special Types of Inguinal Hernia

- Maydl's hernia — W loop of intestine
- Richter's hernia — partial inclusion of intestinal wall
- Sliding hernia — bladder, Sigmoid colon/ appendix.

Management

Investigations

- None required for routine uncomplicated case
- Plain X-ray for suspected bowel obstruction
- Ultrasound in case of diagnostic uncertainty
- Herniogram rarely used
- Routine pre-operative investigations

Surgery

- Mainstay
- To relieve symptoms
- To prevent complications

Truss

- Patient unfit for surgery
- Inguinal hernia which is reducible

Operations for Groin Hernia

Operations

- Open hernia repair
- Laparoscopic hernia repair
  - Total extra-peritoneal (TEP)
  - Trans-abdominal pre-peritoneal (TAPP)

Anesthesia

- General
- Spinal
- Local

Laparoscopic Repair

Unilateral Hernia

- No advantage except slightly less pain and 2 days earlier return to work
- Drawbacks
  - High recurrence rate
  - Difficult to learn
  - Cannot be performed under local anesthesia
  - All cases not fit for laparoscopy
  - Small but definite risk of serious vascular/gut injuries
- Indications for laparoscopic hernia repair
  - Bilateral hernia
  - Recurrent hernia

Hernia Repair — Operations

- *Herniotomy:* Isolation of sac, reduction of contents, transfixation at neck or pushing back in peritoneal cavity.
- *Herniorrhaphy:* Herniotomy + repair of posterior wall of inguinal canal by locally available tissues.
- *Hernioplasty:* Herniotomy + strengthening posterior wall of inguinal canal by exogenous material.

Herniotomy

- Basic operation
- Steps
  - Dissecting out sac from cord structures
  - Opening the hernial sac
  - Reducing sac contents
  - Either transfix the sac at neck and remove remaining portion
  - Or push the sac inside peritoneal cavity without transfixing
- Sufficient for
  - Infants
  - Adolescents
  - Young adults
  - Type 1 and 2 hernia, as there is no weakness of posterior wall

Herniorrhaphy

- Strengthening of posterior wall of inguinal canal by locally available tissue
- Known as tissue repair
- Types
  - Marcy repair
  - Bassini's repair
  - Shouldice repair
  - Mcvay's repair
- Drawback
  - Repair under tension
  - High recurrence rate

Hernioplasty

- Tension free mesh repair (Lichenstein's) repair
- Gold standard
- Low recurrence rate
- Posterior wall strengthened by placing 8 × 15 cm of prolene mesh placed over fascia transversalis
- Steps are described in chapter of common surgical operations.

Femoral Hernia

- Herniation through femoral canal
- Appears below and lateral to pubic tubercle
- Relatively uncommon
- Common in females
- Contains omentum or small intestine
- High risk of strangulation
- Repaired surgically

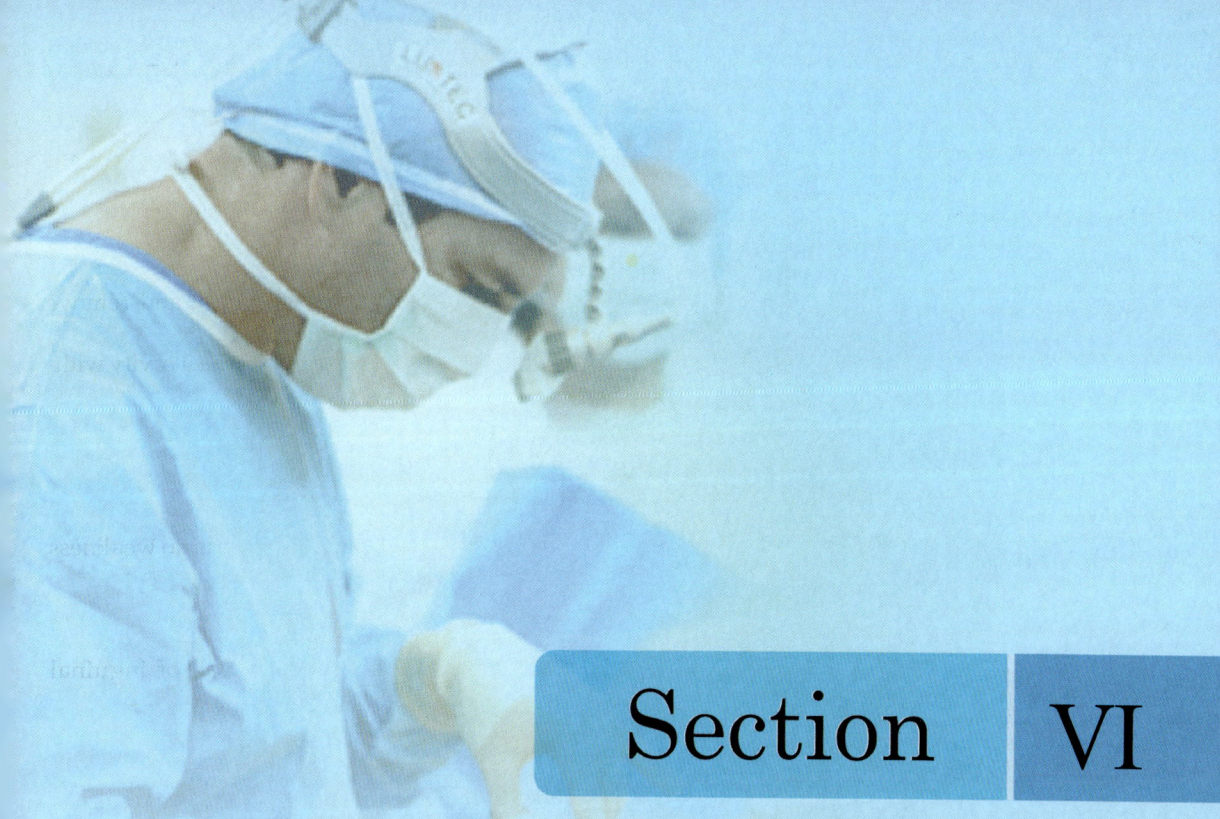

Section VI

91. Common Surgical Operations

91 Common Surgical Operations

Following Operations will be Described
- Cholecystectomy
- Appendectomy
- Inguinal hernia repair
- Modified radical mastectomy
- Thyroidectomy

Pre-Operative Work Up
- Informed consent
- Mark the site to be operated
- Investigations for the fitness of patient for anesthesia
- Specific investigations pertaining to that surgery

Informed Consent
- Specific for procedure
- Should be in patient's language
- Taken by surgeon competent to perform procedure
- Other treatment options must be discussed
- Benefits of surgery must be outlined
- Possible complications must be enumerated

Cholecystectomy
Indications
- Symptomatic cholelithiasis
- Calculus cholecystitis acute or chronic
- Cholesterosis or porcelain gall bladder
- Gall bladder polyps
- Part of other surgical procedures
- Trauma to gall bladder
- Torsion of gall bladder
- Carcinoma gall bladder

Types
Based on Access
- Laparoscopic — gold standard
- Open

Based on Extent
- *Simple:* Gall stone disease
- *Radical:* For carcinoma gallbladder
- *Partial:* Difficult case, frozen Calot's triangle

Open Cholecystectomy
- *Position:* Supine with sand bag under right lower chest
- *Anesthesia:* General with good muscle relaxation
- Pre requisites
  - Good exposure
  - Good light
  - Good relaxation

Incisions
- Kocher's subcostal incision
- Midline vertical
- Right paramedian vertical

Steps
- Hand between liver and diaphragm
- Three packs and retraction of stomach and colon

- Exposure of Calot's triangle (Fig. 91.1)
- Cystic duct isolation and CBD palpation

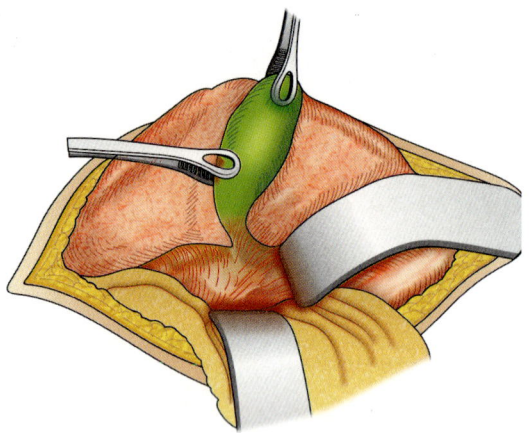

Fig. 91.1: Exposure of Calot's triangle

- Cystic duct and artery ligation (Fig. 91.2)

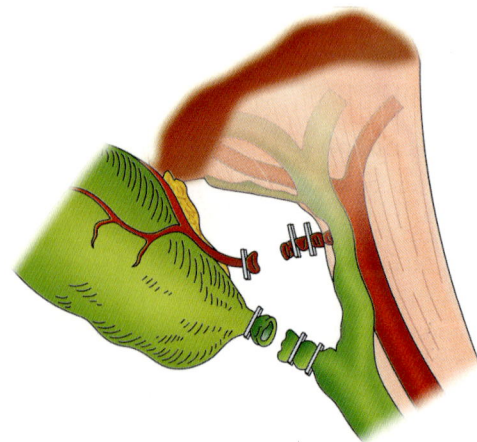

Fig. 91.2: Cystic duct and artery ligation

- Removal of gallbladder from fossa (Fig. 91.3)
- Hemostasis in gall bladder fossa

Laparoscopic Cholecystectomy

Gold standard

Contraindications for Lap Cholecystectomy

- Unwilling patient
- Untrained surgeon
- Carcinoma gall bladder
- Cirrhosis of liver with portal hypertension
- Gangrene of gallbladder
- Mirizzi syndrome

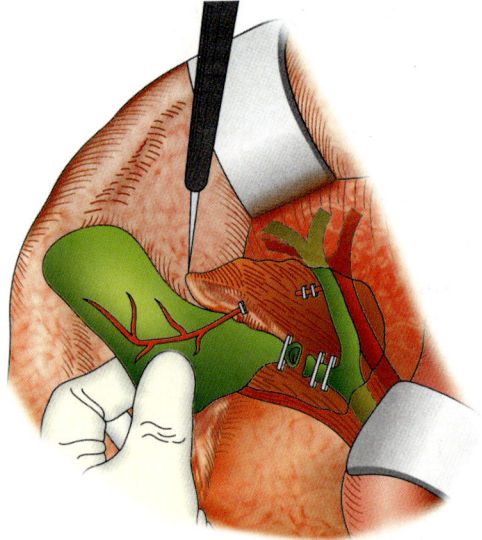

Fig. 91.3: Removal of gallbladder from liver bed

- Third trimester of pregnancy
- Patients with difficult access to peritoneum, i.e. multiple operations in upper abdomen
- Pulmonary disease with raised pCO_2

Port Placement

- Infraumbilical port (10 mm)
- Epigastric port (10 mm)
- Right subcostal port (5 mm)
- Right lumbar port (5 mm)

Steps

- Dissection in Calot's triangle — posterior dissection first to avoid injury to common bile duct
- Isolation of cystic artery and duct
- Clip and divide cystic artery and duct
- Extraction of gallbladder
- Delivery of gallbladder — epigastric or umbilical port; may need extraction of stones/enlarging incision

Appendectomy
Indications

- Acute appendicitis
- Recurrent appendicitis
- Interval appendectomy
- As a part of Ladd's procedure for intestinal malrotation

- After reduction of appendicular intussusception, if appendix appears congested or gangenous
- Appendicular diverticulae
- Appendicular carcinoid if <2 cm and cecal base not involved
- If appendix is lead point for intussusception

Procedure

- *Position of patient:* Supine
- *Anesthesia:* Spinal or general
- Incisions
  - Grid iron (Fig. 91.4)
  - Transverse (Lanz' incision)
  - Lower midline

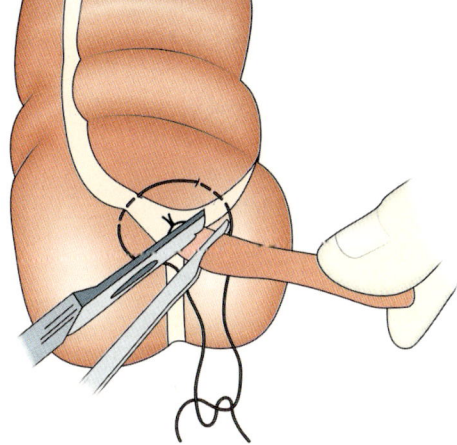

Fig. 91.5: Removal of the appendix

Appendicular Stump

- Inversion by purse string sutures not required
- Drawbacks of inversion
  - Stump appendicitis
  - Lead point of intussusception
  - Mimic cecal tumor on future imaging

Laparoscopic Appendectomy

Advantages

- Thorough exploration of peritoneal cavity
- Definitive treatment for non-appendiceal lesions
- Reduced hospital stay
- No need for extension of incision for abnormal location of appendix
- No post-operative discomfort and narcotic requirement
- Early resumption of routine work
- Thorough peritoneal toilet in case of appendicular perforation

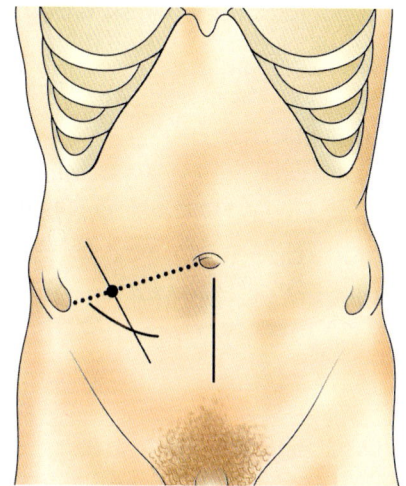

Fig. 91.4: Grid iron incision for appendicectomy

Steps

- External oblique incised
- Internal oblique and transverses muscles split along the direction of muscle fibers
- Peritoneum incised
- Deliver the appendix
- Secure the appendicular vessel
- Crush the appendicular base
  - Helps in secure ligation of base
  - Inverts mucosa
  - Blocks lymphatic and prevents migration of bacteria when appendix being divided
- Ligate the appendicular base and remove appendix (Fig. 91.5)
- Closure of peritoneum
- Internal oblique approximated
- Closure of external oblique

Position of Patient

- Supine with a sand bag below the pelvis
- Surgeon on the left, assistant caudal to left of the surgeon
- Scrub nurse on the right side
- Video monitors on right of the patient

Port Placement

- Infraumbilical port (10 mm)
- Hypogastric port (5 mm)
- Right lumbar port (5 mm)

Steps

- Exploration of abdomen for confirming the diagnosis
- Identification of appendix
- Ligation of appendicular artery
- Meso-appendix divided
- Base of appendix defined
- Base of appendix ligated
- Retrieval of appendix

Mastectomy

- Simple mastectomy
- Total mastectomy
- Modified radical mastectomy
- Radical mastectomy
- Wide local excision
- Skin sparing mastectomy

Simple Mastectomy

- Removal of breast up to its palpable limits
- 2nd to 6th rib craniocaudally
- Midline anteriorly to mid axillary line

Total Mastectomy

- Removal of breast up to anatomical limits, i.e. clavicle to costal margin in mid-clavicular line
- Mid line to posterior axillary line in horizontal plane

Modified Radical Mastectomy (MRM)

- *Definition:* Enbloc excision of breast, nipple areola complex, skin overlying tumor and 2 cm around with axillary dissection.

Types of MRM

- **Patey's Type:** Pectoralis minor removed
- **Autchincloss:** Pectoralis minor retracted
- **Scanlon:** Pectoralis minor divided at the tip of coracoid process and reflected down

Axillary dissection

- Level 1 and 2 lymph nodes removed
- Minimum of 8–10 lymph nodes removed for adequate dissection
- All lymph nodes and fibro-fatty tissue below axillary vein removed
- Following must be preserved
  - Axillary artery and vein
  - Nerve and artery to lattisimus dorsi
  - Nerve to serratus anterior

- Intercosto-brachial nerve and lateral pectoral nerve may be divided

Steps

- Position of patient — supine with sand below shoulder; paint and drape to allow free movement of upper limb for axillary dissection
- Raising skin flaps – plane between subcutaneous fat and fat of breast tissue
- Breast and pectoral fascia lifted
- Lateral border of pectoralis major defined
- Pectoralis major retracted and pectoralis minor seen
- Axillary vein identified
- Fibro fatty tissue dissected down
- Axillary dissection completed
- Wound closed after putting suction drains.

Inguinal Hernia Operations

- Herniotomy
- Herniorrhaphy
- Hernioplasty.

Herniotomy

- Basic operation
- Dissecting out sac from cord structures
- Opening the hernial sac
- Reducing sac contents
- Either transfix the sac at neck and remove remaining portion or push the sac inside the peritoneal cavity without transfixing
- Sufficient for
  - Infants
  - Adolescents
  - Young adults
  - Type 1 and 2 hernia
  - In these cases there is no weakness of the posterior wall.

Other indications of hernitomy are:
1. Congential hydrocele
2. Herniotomy is a part of orchidopexy for undescended testis as patent processes vaginalis is present in 80% of cases.

Herniorrhaphy

- Strengthening of posterior wall of inguinal canal by locally available tissue
- Known as tissue repair
- Commonly performed herniorrhaphy
  - Bassini's repair
  - Shouldice repair

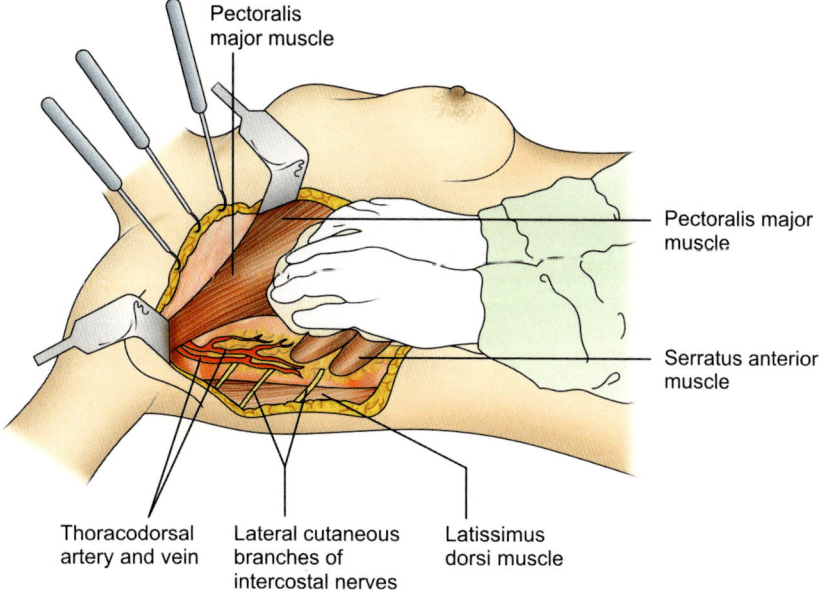

Pectoralis
major muscle

Pectoralis major
muscle

Serratus anterior
muscle

Thoracodorsal
artery and vein

Lateral cutaneous
branches of
intercostal nerves

Latissimus
dorsi muscle

Fig. 91.6: Raising the upper flap

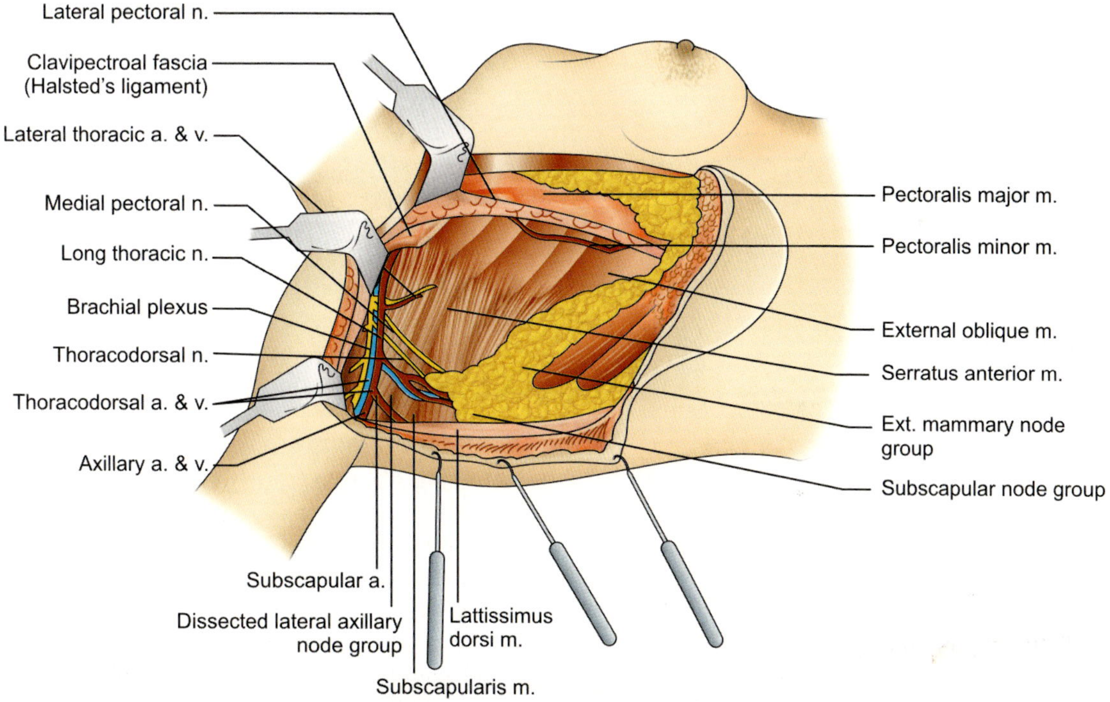

Lateral pectoral n.

Clavipectroal fascia
(Halsted's ligament)

Lateral thoracic a. & v.

Medial pectoral n.

Long thoracic n.

Brachial plexus

Thoracodorsal n.

Thoracodorsal a. & v.

Axillary a. & v.

Pectoralis major m.

Pectoralis minor m.

External oblique m.

Serratus anterior m.

Ext. mammary node
group

Subscapular node group

Subscapular a.

Dissected lateral axillary
node group

Lattissimus
dorsi m.

Subscapularis m.

Fig. 91.7: Axillary dissection completed

- Drawbacks
  - Repair under tension
  - High recurrence rate

Hernioplasty

- Tension free mesh repair (Lichtenstein) repair
- Gold standard
- Low recurrence rate
- Posterior wall strengthened by placing 8 × 15 cm of prolene mesh over fascia transversalis.

Steps

- Incision over medial 2/3rd of inguinal ligament 1/2 inch above it
- External oblique aponeurosis incised in the line of skin incision
- Cremastric fascia incised
- Sac isolated from cord
- Sac dissected till internal ring and ligated
- Posterior inguinal canal wall strengthened and inguinal canal closed
- Incision closed in layers

Mesh Hernioplasty

- Mesh placed over the posterior wall under the spermatic cord
- Mesh fixed to pubic tubercle, inguinal ligament and conjoint tendon

Bassini's Repair

- Posterior wall reinforced by approximating conjoint tendon to inguinal ligament using non-absorbable suture.

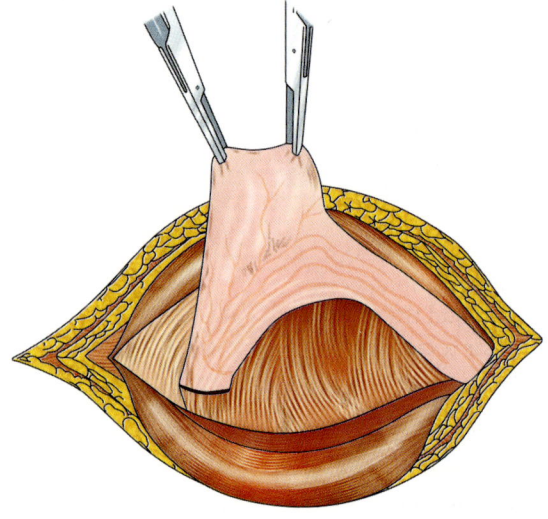

Fig. 91.9: Isolation of sac

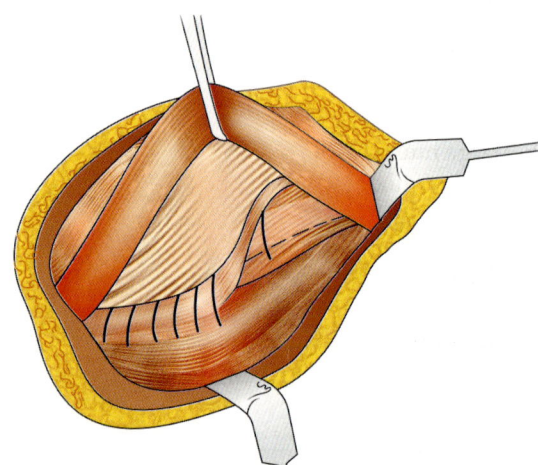

Fig. 91.10: Closure of floor and incision in layers

Approximation should be without tension and interrupted sutures should be used.

Laparoscopic Repair

- Unilateral hernia
  - No advantage except slightly less pain and earlier return to work
- Drawbacks
  - Difficult to learn
  - Cannot be performed under local anesthesia
  - All cases not fit for laparoscopic repair
  - Small but definite risk of serious vascular or gut injuries

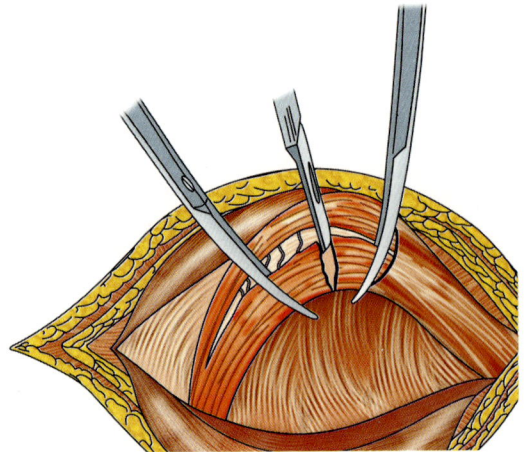

Fig. 91.8: Isolation of cord and incision of cremastric fascia

Indications for Lap Hernia Repair

- Bilateral hernia
- Recurrent hernia

Approaches for Lap Hernia Repair

- Total extraperitoneal (TEP)
- Transabdominal pre peritoneal (TAPP)

Thyroidectomy

- Hemithyroidectomy
- Subtotal thyroidectomy
- Near total thyroidectomy
- Isthmusectomy

Indications

Hemi-thyroidectomy

- Solitary nodule with follicular pathology
- Multi-nodular goiter confined to one lobe
- Dominant cold nodule in a multi-nodular goiter (MNG)
- Young women with lower risk group if papillary or follicular cancer is less than 1 cm

Subtotal Thyroidectomy

- Large multi-nodular goiter
- Graves' disease

Near Total Thyroidectomy

- Thyroid cancer
- MNG
- Thyrotoxicosis

Steps

- Position of patient — extended neck and stablised
- Skin incision marked - skin crease (Kocher's incision)
- Upper skin flaps raised up upper border of thyroid cartilage
- Lower skin flap raised up to sternal notch
- Deep cervical fascia incised vertically in the mid line
- Strap muscles retracted laterally
- Ligation of superior thyroid vessels
- Recurrent laryngeal nerve identified
- Inferior thyroid artery branches ligated on surface of thyroid
- Isthmus divided
- Division of lobe
- Hemostasis secured
- Closure with or without drain

Complications

Intra-operative

- Bleeding
- Injury to recurrent laryngeal nerve
- Injury to external laryngeal nerve
- Devascularization of parathyroid gland

Post-operative

- Bleeding with hematoma formation
- Hypothyroidism
- Hypoparathyroidism

Index